Coronasphere

This book presents a broad overview of the challenges posed by COVID-19 in India and its neighbouring countries. It studies the differing responses to COVID-19 infections across South Asia, the variegated impact of the pandemic on its societies, communities and economies, and emerging challenges, which require an interdisciplinary understanding and analysis.

With a range of case studies from India, Bangladesh, Myanmar, Pakistan, Nepal, Bhutan, and Sri Lanka, this book:

- Analyses the socio-economic impact of the pandemic, including the structural challenges faced by farmers in the agricultural production and migrant workers in the informal sectors.
- Examines the shifting trends in migration and displacement during the pandemic.
- Explores the precarity faced by LGBTQ+, transgender, Dalit, tribal, senior citizens, and other marginalised communities during the pandemic.
- Discusses the gendered impact of the pandemic on women and girls, combining with multiple and intersecting inequalities like race, ethnicity, socio-economic status, age, geographical location, and sexual orientation.
- Sheds light on the position of health infrastructure and healthcare services across different countries, and the transitions experienced in their education sectors as well, in response to COVID-19.

A holistic read on the pandemic, this book will be of interest to scholars and researchers of sociology, medical anthropology, sociology of health, pandemic and health studies, political studies, social anthropology, public policy, and South Asian studies.

Chandan Kumar Sharma is Professor of Sociology at Tezpur University. He did his B.A. from Cotton College, Guwahati, and M.A., M.Phil. and Ph.D. from Delhi School of Economics, Delhi. His research areas include development, environment, urbanisation, migration, and identity politics with special reference to northeast India and he has published his works in various journals and edited volumes. He was a Charles Wallace Visiting Fellow to Queen's University, Belfast, in 2008. He has also been a visiting fellow to several Indian Universities including Delhi School of Economics and Jawaharlal Nehru University (JNU). He is the founder editor of *Explorations*, the e-journal of the Indian Sociological Society. His latest publications include *Fixed Borders, Fluid Boundaries: Identity, Resources and Mobility in Northeast India* (Routledge, 2020) (co-edited).

Reshmi Banerjee is Political Scientist based in London, the United Kingdom, and is currently a visiting research fellow at the King's India Institute (KII), King's College, London. She is also a visiting research fellow at the Institute of Social Sciences, New Delhi, India. She was previously an academic visitor at the Asian Studies Centre (Programme on Modern Burmese Studies) in St Antony's College, University of Oxford, a research associate at the School of Oriental and African Studies (SOAS), University of London, a post-doctoral fellow at the department of international relations, University of Indonesia (UI), and a researcher in the Indonesian Institute of Sciences (LIPI), Jakarta. She has been a visiting professor in Jamia Millia Islamia and a fellow in the Rajiv Gandhi Institute for Contemporary Studies and has taught in Delhi University and in the University of Indonesia. She completed her M.A., M.Phil. and Ph.D. from the Centre for Political Studies (CPS), Jawaharlal Nehru University (JNU), New Delhi.

With a specialisation in food security, agricultural policies, and cross-border studies on the Indo-Myanmar region, she is the author of *Land Conflicts across Frontiers: Contested Spaces in Myanmar and North East India* (2018), and has co-edited three books: *Fixed Borders, Fluid Boundaries – Identity, Resources and Mobility in Northeast India* (Routledge, 2020), *Gender, Poverty and Livelihood in the Eastern Himalayas* (Routledge, 2017) and *Climate Change in the Eastern Himalaya: Impact on Livelihoods, Growth and Poverty* (2015). She also has a master's degree in museum cultures from Birkbeck, University of London and has worked as a volunteer with the London Museum of Water and Steam. Currently, she volunteers in the Royal College of Music (RCM) Museum in London. In 2022, she published *12 Months* (a short memoir) and *Potpourri: Yearning and Learning* (a collection of essays on travel).

Coronasphere

Narratives on COVID-19 From India and Its Neighbours

Edited by Chandan Kumar Sharma and Reshmi Banerjee

Routledge
Taylor & Francis Group
LONDON AND NEW YORK

pro-feminist thinker and has written about "men and feminism" in the EPW special volume on Men and Feminism in India in 2015. He also serves on the international advisory committee of Community Development Journal Published from OUP, the United Kingdom and Ireland. His forthcoming edited volume from Routledge entitles "Sexuality, Abjection and Queer Existence in Contemporary India".

Rajdeep Singha is Assistant Professor at the Centre for Labour Studies and Social Protection at the Tata Institute of Social Sciences (TISS), Guwahati Campus, Assam, India. Prior to joining TISS, he was teaching at the Department of Economics of St. Joseph's College of Arts and Science, Bengaluru, and Research Associate at the Indian Institute of Management Bangalore (IIMB). He obtained a Ph.D. in Economics from the Institute for Social and Economic Change (ISEC), Bengaluru. He is the co-editor of *Employment and Labour Market in Northeast India: Interrogating Structural Changes* (Routledge, 2018), and *Work, Institutions and Sustainable Livelihood: Issues and Challenges of Transformation* (Palgrave Macmillan, 2017). He has published several articles in peer-reviewed journals and chapters in edited books. His areas of research and teaching interest include development economics, poverty, agrarian studies, industrial economics, and labour economics. He was engaged in various research projects on issues related to poverty, employment, inequality, and labour supported by the United Nations Development Programmes (UNDP), International Centre for Integrated Mountain Development (ICIMOD), International Water Management Institute (IWMI), Oxfam Germany (ODE), Assam Rural Infrastructure and Agricultural Services Society (ARIAS Society) under Government of Assam, ONGC, New Delhi North Eastern Electric Power Corporation Limited (NEEPCO), and Action Aid.

Ramila Bisht is Professor at the Centre of Social Medicine and Community Health, Jawaharlal Nehru University (JNU), New Delhi. She holds an M.A. in Psychology and M.Phil. and Ph.D. in social sciences in health from JNU. Her research interests centre round health policy and reforms in India, comparative health systems and policies, urbanisation, environment and health, and the gendered social and cultural determinants of women's health. Working largely in India, most of her research has been in highland economies and in the states of Maharashtra and Delhi. She was awarded the *British Society of Population Studies LEDC Visitor award, 2010*. She was an embedded fellow in 2010 in the ESRC Rising Powers Network Award entitled "India's challenge in a globalising healthcare economy: social science directions".

Reshmi Banerjee is Political Scientist based in London, the United Kingdom, and is currently a visiting research fellow at the King's India Institute (KII), King's College, London. She is also a visiting research fellow at the Institute of Social Sciences, New Delhi, India. She was previously an academic visitor at the Asian Studies Centre (Programme on Modern Burmese Studies) in St Antony's College, University of Oxford, a research associate at the School of Oriental and African Studies (SOAS), University of London, a post-doctoral fellow at the department of international relations, University of Indonesia (UI), and a researcher in the Indonesian Institute of Sciences (LIPI), Jakarta. She has been a visiting professor in Jamia Millia Islamia and a fellow in the Rajiv Gandhi Institute for Contemporary Studies and has taught in Delhi University and in the University of Indonesia. She completed her M.A., M.Phil., and Ph.D. from the Centre for Political Studies (CPS), Jawaharlal Nehru University (JNU), New Delhi.

With a specialisation in food security, agricultural policies, and cross-border studies on the Indo-Myanmar region, she is the author of *Land Conflicts across Frontiers: Contested Spaces in Myanmar and North East India* (Notion Press, 2018), and has co-edited three books: *Fixed Borders, Fluid Boundaries – Identity, Resources and Mobility in Northeast India* (Routledge, 2020), *Gender, Poverty and Livelihood in the Eastern Himalayas* (Routledge, 2017) and *Climate Change in the Eastern Himalaya: Impact on Livelihoods, Growth and Poverty* (Academic Publishers, 2015). She also has a master's degree in museum cultures from Birkbeck, University of London, and has worked as a volunteer with the London Museum of Water and Steam. Currently, she volunteers in the Royal College of Music (RCM) Museum in London. In 2022, she published *12 Months* (a short memoir) and *Potpourri: Yearning and Learning* (a collection of essays on travel).

Ritu Priya has been Faculty Member from the medical stream at the Centre of Social Medicine and Community Health, Jawaharlal Nehru University (JNU), New Delhi, since 1990. Her work links epidemiology, popular culture, political economy and health systems research for decentralised planning, policy formulation and analysis, and technology assessment. It has been specifically focused on the politics of knowledge between healing systems and between experts and laypeople; health perceptions of Dalits and other marginalised groups; urban health; nutrition and communicable diseases especially TB and HIV. She has co-edited a volume titled "Dialogue on AIDS: Perspectives for the Indian Context". In 2008 and 2009, she was on deputation as Advisor (Public Health Planning) with the National Health Systems Resource Centre under the National Rural Health Mission, Government of India. She is Coordinator of the Trans-disciplinary Research Cluster on Sustainability Studies and founder member of the Trans-disciplinary Research Cluster on Plural Health Care: Knowledge, Technology, Practice and Policy at JNU.

Rukmini Sen is Professor in Sociology at the School of Liberal Studies of Ambedkar University Delhi (AUD). She is currently Director of the Centre for Publishing at AUD. She has previously worked at The WB National University of Juridical Sciences, Kolkata, and Centre for Women's Development Studies, New Delhi. She teaches courses on Law and Society, Relationships and Affinities, Gender and Society, Social Research, and Women's Movements. She is member of the Core Group on Women, National Human Rights Commission since 2019. Previously, she has been a member of the Expert Committee in the National Commission for Women. She has been in the Executive Committee of Indian Association for Women's Studies.

Shaheen Anam is the Executive Director of Manusher Jonno Foundation (MJF), a nongovernmental organisation working for Human Rights and Good Governance in Bangladesh. She has a master's degree in Psychology and Social work from Dhaka University and Hunter College School of Social Work, New York. Her work revolves around supporting movements and coalitions to ensure human rights of marginalised groups, protect women and children from violence and policy advocacy on behalf of vulnerable groups. She is known nationally and regionally as a human rights and women rights activist.

Shailaja Menon teaches Modern Indian History at the School of Liberal Studies, Ambedkar University, Delhi. Her area of research includes modern Indian history, urbanisation, gender, and cultural studies. She has published in various national and international journals and conducted projects.

Shaveta Menon is assistant professor (Public Health) at Eternal University, Himachal Pradesh. A dentist by graduation and a master's degree in Public Health (gold medallist), she holds her M.Phil. and Ph.D. from the Centre of Social Medicine and Community Health, Jawaharlal Nehru University (JNU), New Delhi. She carries an experience in community research with strong focus on policy-related issues and the associated implications on health of the population. Having worked in the areas ranging from oral health to tobacco use in Punjab, her area of interest is Health Policy and Systems Research. Her research focus is to bring the inter-disciplinary approach of public health to the forefront moving beyond the biomedical realm and language of public health.

Sonam Kinga works at the Royal Research and Advisory Council. He teaches Bhutan's Political History at the Royal Institute of Governance and Strategic Studies in Bhutan. He was earlier a visiting professor at the Graduate School of Asian and African Area Studies in Kyoto University, a visiting research fellow at the Institute of Developing Economies (IDE) in Tokyo, and a founding member and researcher at The Centre for Bhutan Studies.

He served for two terms (2008–2013) as member of Parliament having contested elections during Bhutan's historic transition to democracy. In his second term, he served as the Chairperson of the National Council, the second chamber of Parliament.

She has been co-investigator, in the research project: Feminist Taleem: Teaching Feminisms, Transforming Lives: Questions of Identity, Pedagogy and Violence in India and the UK (2017–20). This project is funded by UGC-UKERI in collaboration with the University of Edinburgh, Scotland. She has curated "City through Feminist Lens", a walking tour across the city of Delhi, as part of this project. She has also been a co-investigator for a project titled "A History of Gender Training in Delhi" (November 2016–February 2017) under the Dyason Fellowship award, University of Melbourne.

Some of her recent publications are Doing Feminism in the Academy (2020, co-editor), Zubaan Publications, New Delhi, Trust in Transactions (2019, co-editor), Orient Blackswan, New Delhi, "Indian Feminisms, Law Reform and Law Commission of India: Special issue in Honour of Lotika Sarkar" (2018, special issue; co-editor), for the Journal of Indian Law and Society, published by WB National University of Juridical Sciences, Kolkata, Stay Home Stay Safe: Interrogating Violence in the Domestic Sphere in EPW Engage Vol 55, Issue No 25, June 2020 www.epw.in/engage/article/stay-home-stay-safe-interrogating-violence, Life after COVID-19: A Society of Empaths or More Socially Distant, 30 March 2020 www.newsclick.in/author/Rukmini%20Sen/articlelist

Vallala Sravya is pursuing a master's degree in Sociology. She co-founded Queer Collective at University of Hyderabad in 2019. She has also been a student volunteer for the Gender Equality Awareness Committee, School of Social Sciences since 2020. Her research interests lie in questions of gender and sexuality, state mechanisms, and society and law. She is currently in the final year of her master's degree and working on the same-sex marriage debate in India.

Virginius Xaxa is currently Visiting Professor at the Institute for Human Development (IHD), Delhi. He was Chairman of the High-Level Committee on Socio-Economic, Health and Educational Status of Tribal Communities of India, Government of India (2014). He is the author of *Economic Dualism and Structure of Class: A Study in Plantation and Peasant Settings in North Bengal* (Cosmo, 1997) and *State, Society, and Tribes: Issues in Post-Colonial India* (Pearson, 2008).

Introduction

Chandan Kumar Sharma and Reshmi Banerjee

The Arrival of the Pandemonium

The arrival of the COVID-19 virus and the resultant pandemic are the most critical health calamity of the century since the Second World War, which has destroyed both lives and livelihoods. It is a human, economic, and social crisis. Although the virus has not discriminated and has easily crossed frontiers, its lethal impact has been disproportionately felt by the poorer and the marginalised sections of every country and region in the world. Measures to tackle the deadly virus have ranged from closing borders and setting up quarantine centres to physical distancing, from restricting large gatherings to partial or complete lockdowns. Various cultural, religious, sport, and political mass events were either cancelled or curbed including the Tokyo Olympics.

Working hours were massively reduced due to the pandemic with pre-existing structural inequalities (based on gender, age, and race) getting aggravated within our social production and labour market. Workers in the informal sector were hit the hardest. The globalised world's unequal development and economic models have been given visibility by the pandemic, thus providing a pressing need to amend these highly discriminating socio-economic structures with equality and environmental sustainability (Ryder et al., 2020). Many families have been pushed into poverty. Migrants, refugees and IDPs, women, Indigenous communities, older people, that is the vulnerable sections existing already on the periphery of society including in policies have faced severe challenges. Violence against women, including domestic violence, has also increased during this crisis period. Sexual exploitation and child marriages might go up in poor countries arising out of desperate economic conditions.

Since the lockdown, unpaid work for women at home has increased with patriarchy and social norms placing undue load on young girls. UN Women survey results from Asia and the Pacific show that women are losing their livelihoods faster than men with many employed in the informal sector. Gender is combining with multiple and intersecting inequalities like race,

DOI: 10.4324/9781003282815-1

ethnicity, socio-economic status, age, geographical location, and sexual orientation to complicate matters even further (UN Women, 2020).

Every country has had its own story to narrate. In the United States, New York was the initial epicentre. However later, Texas, Florida, Arizona, and California emerged as areas with high cases of virus infections. Data has shown that members of the Black, Latino, and ethnic minority communities have been disproportionately affected like the Latinos account for around 39% of California's population but accounted for 56% of the total cases (as of 30 June 2020) (BBC, 2020).

There are, however, smaller countries with much fewer resources, which have performed reasonably well in tackling the crisis situation. Vietnam has done well in containment with strict quarantine rules, proactive prevention, and people-centric measures. Early awareness of the pandemic helped the country (Alam, 2020). Anna Jones has remarked that the country is respectful of infectious diseases and knows them well from past experiences like SARS in 2003 to avian influenza in 2010. The country practiced very effective localised containment with the one-party machinery and its local party cadres being used to spread awareness. However, Phil Robertson of Human Rights Watch argues that there were definitely human rights violations in the process of maintaining this rigid control over society (Jones, 2020).

South Asian countries struggled to control the rate of infections although Bhutan did well in tackling the virus with the King, the officials, and members of civil society each playing their part in this moment of national crisis. In Pakistan, Coronavirus has exposed its digital weakness and inequalities with millions of students not having Internet, which in turn has affected their online studies. Internet facilities are especially poor in Balochistan, Khyber Pakhtunkhwa, and Gilgit-Baltistan (Zahra-Malik, 2020).

Bangladesh saw thousands of people assembling in a special prayer session for protection against the virus in Lakshimpur without having the local government's permission. Amidst the crisis, voting also took place in three constituencies. Lockdown witnessed many people leaving Dhaka and the bigger cities by travelling in overcrowded public transport, thus posing huge risks of disease transmission. Cox's Bazar, where many Rohingyas live, witnessed a special lockdown (Anwar et al., 2020). Amena Mohsin has observed that the Bangladesh government was averse to using the word lockdown. Instead it termed it as "*Sadharan Chutti*" (general holiday). She also states that the number of "new poor" may rise in the country with the Chittagong Hill Tracts area badly affected (75% of CHT do not have access to Internet) (Mohsin, 2020).

In Nepal, people are still recovering from the massive earthquake which occurred five years back. As a result, many still live in structures which are vulnerable as formal reconstruction rate has been only around 65%. Thus many do not even possess a home to feel safe in. The international migrants contributing 30% to Nepal's GDP have also been affected badly. Remittances were an important source of income for many families, the absence of which could put them in a precarious condition in the future (Shneiderman et al., 2020).

Crippling Contagion: India's Journey

India's 1.4 billion people went into one of the world's strictest lockdown on 24 March 2020 for 21 days. Around 140 million vulnerable workers found their earnings collapse as they were suddenly thrust into a crisis. Strained public resources along with increased central and state deficits have been accompanied by diversion of resources from the welfare schemes of mid-day meals in schools and vaccinations to tackle the pandemic. Schools and businesses shut down with tech and industrial hubs struggling to keep their momentum going (Kazmin, 2020).

Each state within India has had a different trajectory of COVID-19 infections and resultant differing responses at times. Several sectors of the country and different communities were impacted by the pandemic which this volume addresses in its chapters. The struggle to choose between saving people's lives and reviving a declining economy has been a tough one. Unemployment has reached an all-time high with the migrant population most adversely affected. Thousands have walked home with some dropping dead on the way out of exhaustion, whereas others have been sprayed with disinfectants on arrival in their home states. With no food and cash, they have been pushed to the brink of starvation and extreme human indignity.

Anindita Adhikari who contributes to reporting by the Stranded Workers Action Network (SWAN) has pointed out that there are two types of stranded: the visible (seen in shelters) and the invisible (sleeping on footpaths or living under flyovers or stuck in slums). SWAN found that 89% of the stranded workers had not been paid wages and most had only just Rs. 200 ($3) left in their pockets. Small businesses were also often unable to pay their workers as their own condition was in a precarious state (Adhikari as quoted in Pandey, 2020).

Manish K. Jha and Ajeet Kumar Pankaj have argued that flight and plight characterised the status of the migrant workers: either they were seen as subjects of pity or they were considered as carriers of disease and fear. The crisis seemed to have turned the human body into a biological body disconnected with socio-political life. Further, Jha and Pankaj felt that the village scene was set to change with purity-pollution concepts and patron-client relationships set to return with cases of violence also set to increase (already villages had seen stigmatisation of the return migrants) (Jha and Pankaj, 2020).

The ILO has projected that 400 million people in India could fall into poverty. Most informal workers are with micro-, small-, and medium-sized enterprises (MSMEs) with the small and micro enterprises comprising 99.2% of all MSMEs. The country could see rising economic and social tensions if the economy is unable to bounce back soon. The cash transfers to poor households, MNREGA, and an urban employment scheme could all go a long way in addressing the immediate concerns (Kugler and Sinha, 2020). The government announced a $266 billion support package (said to be worth around 10% of India's GDP) (Roy Choudhury, 2020).

Online classes have exposed the digital divide and existing socio-economic faultlines with poor students having limited or no access to Internet. About 86% of them are unable to explore online learning (according to reports), which in turn is thus enhancing the rich-poor divide as well as the rural-urban divide in India. Many students who got jobs through campus interviews may not be able to join these jobs eventually with many private educational institutions facing eventual closures (Biswas, 2020). Social distancing has made the elderly population not only lonely and isolated but many also suffer from restricted mobility and lack of financial security.

Proper functioning of courts has been hampered even though virtual courts came up to handle urgent cases. Mental health crisis could be India's next major worry as depression, anxiety, and suicides are rising. Social isolation, loss of jobs, domestic abuse, and violence are all leading people to take drastic decisions. The Indian Psychiatry Society's recent survey found that there was an increase of 20% in the number of mental illness cases since the lockdown. Children can be affected adversely as they are not only seeing increased family violence but also going through extended period of isolation. Alcohol-related problems will also rise (Sharma, 2020).

Media has suffered from various challenges ranging from difficulties faced in gathering information to the inability to meet people. Many have relied only on government information. The economic impact on media channels has also affected their functioning like Tasungtetla Longkumer; the manager of the English daily *Nagaland Page* stated that people stopped taking newspapers as they feared that the virus would spread through newspapers. Even the hawkers stopped taking them (Dodum, 2020).

Indian doctors have faced social boycott and attacks with the Indian Medical Association condemning these attacks. Many were evicted from their rental homes as people feared that doctors would pass on the infections to them. The medical community thus had to fight two battles: within and outside the hospitals (Sarkar, 2020). There are groups in our society who have always been forced to remain invisible like the LGBTQ community who have during the lockdown turned to social media and online communication for support (Aljazeera, 2020). People working on the streets like street vendors and those living on the streets like street children have faced various kinds of hardships. India is also home to asylum seekers and refugees. Vatsal Raj has argued that the refugees not only lack government documentation and social security but they are also not part of any national pandemic response plans (Raj, 2020). The UNHCR has temporarily suspended all refugee status determination (RSD) activities, thus affecting the cases of not only the asylum seekers but also those who are yet to register with the UNHCR (Shankar and Raghavan, 2020).

The pandemic has made us realise the need for robust grass root institutions to access people and their problems. Several NGOs have been helping during the pandemic like Minds Foundation, Neptune Foundation, The Banyan, and Diya Foundation among others who have been spreading awareness, providing necessary care and essential commodities, helping people with mental health issues and stress-related problems (Balaji, 2020). The service provided by the NGOs has been recognised by the Supreme Court (The Hindu, 2020) as well as by the NITI Aayog. The Supreme Court praised individuals who came forward and helped migrants. The NITI Aayog also requested help from over 92,000 NGOs to assist the government. Amir Siddiqui's "*Project Umeed*" in New Delhi, BG Foundation's "*Umeed Ki Kiran*" in Gurugram, and children from Delhi schools starting an initiative called "*Masks for India*" are some of the initiatives springing from civil society (Marwaha, 2020). Kolkata's *Gana Tadaroki Udyog* started by activists regularly has posted news of Bengali migrant workers stranded in other states and requested for support (Sarmin, 2020). The NGOs also worked with the private sector to collectively address the challenges faced by the common people.

The pandemic also raised the issue of cooperative federalism. All states from Kerala to Odisha and from Punjab and West Bengal to Assam not only followed the broad guidelines of the centre but also created their own local/ state centric protocols. Amartya Lahiri has argued that "federal structure encourages policy experimentation by constituent states", thus leading to faster learning since we learn from multiple sources rather than one (Lahiri, 2020). Health also belongs to the state list, so the role of the states will continue to be critical.

Ranabir Samaddar has argued for a new "biopolitics from below" – a new kind of public power with trust being an essential element to it. Role of neighbourhood committees, local clubs, and associations would be important to build this solidarity, which would involve caring for each other (Samaddar, 2020a). Sandro Mezzadra also called for a "care of the common". He said, "Coronavirus is a threat to something essential, to the common" (Mezzadra as quoted in Samaddar, 2020b). The pandemic has raised some larger questions of justice, humanitarian law, rights, belonging, and citizenship. There is need to revisit the role of the welfare state in a crisis situation. It has made us also realise that our knowledge is limited reminding us of what Socrates had said: "the only true wisdom is in knowing you know nothing". One therefore needs to constantly learn for a better progressive tomorrow even while we struggle in our turbulent today.

Aim of the Book

The main purpose of this endeavour is to study the impact of COVID-19 in India and in the South Asian region in all its totality. The pandemic has changed forever the way our socio-economic and political systems operate, and therefore it is important to know the ways and means in which this change is impacting and transforming us. It is also important to study the responses that we need to have for the future. The book titled *Coronasphere: Narratives on COVID-19 From India and Its Neighbours* has attempted to capture the stories of challenges and adaptations which can truly inform the readers of the resilience and skills needed for tackling an unprecedented human calamity. The goal has been to not only examine India but also study the experiences of its regional neighbours to have cross-border learning.

The book is divided into four sections. The first section (A) titled *Impact on Economy* has three chapters covering the impact of the pandemic on our economy. The second section (B) titled *Unforeseen Transformation* has four chapters on the impact of the pandemic on sectors like health, education, and NGOs. The third section (C) titled *On the Periphery* has five chapters discussing the adverse impact of the lockdown on specific groups like women, Dalits, tribes, elderly persons, and homosexuals/transgender. Finally, the last section (D) titled *Regional Narratives* has six chapters providing a glimpse to the ways and means in which our regional neighbours have been coping with the deadly virus.

We hope that this volume will not only make some useful contribution in understanding the myriad and complex ways in which COVID-19 has placed its footprints in our lives but also provide us strength and hope for the future with the belief that together "we shall overcome".

Note: The chapters in the book cover the pandemic from its beginning in early 2020 till September 2021. Since then, the virus has mutated several times with varied impact and repercussions. It is an evolving situation, which both the editors and the contributors are cognisant of. Also, we are aware of the impact of the pandemic on citizenship, media, and judiciary besides several other sectors. However, the book could not capture all the phases and issues because of constraints of word limit, although some of these issues have been addressed in different chapters.

References

Alam, Sorwar (2020), "Vietnam: A success story in fight against COVID-19", *AA*, 5 June, www.aa.com.tr/en/asia-pacific/vietnam-a-success-story-in-fight-against-covid-19/1866670, accessed 24 July 2020.

Anwar, Saeed, Nasrullah, Mohammad and Jakir Hosen, Mohammad (2020), "COVID-19 and Bangladesh: Challenges and how to address them", *Frontiers in Public Health*, 30 April, https://frontiersin.org/articles/10.3389/fpubh.2020.00154/full, accessed 25 July 2020.

Balaji, Roshni (2020), "These NGOs are helping people deal with mental health issues amid the coronavirus pandemic", *Social Story*, 26 April, https://yourstory.com/socialstory/2020/04/ngos-helping-people-mental-health-coronavirus, accessed 29 July 2020.

Biswas, Atanu (2020), "COVID-19 and the blow to the education sector", *The New Indian Express*, 1 May, https://newindianexpress.com/opinions/2020/may/01/

covid-19-and-the-blow-to-the-education-sector-2137682.html, accessed 27 July 2020.

Coronavirus lockdown 'lonely' and 'dangerous' for LGBTQ Indians (2020), *Aljazeera*, 22 June, https://aljazeera.com/news/2020/06/coronavirus-lockdown-lonely-dangerous-lgbtq-indians-200622084040019.html, accessed 31 July 2020.

Coronavirus: What's behind alarming new US outbreaks? (2020), *BBC*, 30 June, https://bbc.co.uk/news/world-us-canada-53228134, accessed 24 July 2020.

Dodum, Ranju (2020), "Journalism in the time of Covid-19", *The Citizen*, 21 April, https://thecitizen.in/index.php/en/NewsDetail/index/9/18629/Journalism-in-the-Time-of-Covid-19, accessed 28 July 2020.

Explainer: How COVID-19 impacts women and girls (2020), *UN Women*, https://interactive.unwomen.org/multimedia/explainer/covid19/en/index.html, accessed 23 July 2020.

Jha, Manish K. and Pankaj, Ajeet Kumar (2020), "Insecurity and fear travel as labour travels in the time of pandemic", in R. Samaddar (ed), *Borders of an Epidemic – Covid 19 and Migrant Workers*, Calcutta: Calcutta Research Group.

Jones, Anna (2020), "Coronavirus: How 'overreaction' made Vietnam a virus success", *BBC*, 15 May, https://bbc.co.uk/news/world-asia-52628283, accessed 24 July 2020.

Kazmin, Amy (2020), "Modi stumbles: India's deepening coronavirus crisis", *Financial Times*, 27 July, https://ft.com/content/53d946cf-d4c2-4cc4-9411-1d5bb3566e83, accessed 27 July 2020.

Kugler, Maurice and Sinha, Shakti (2020), "The impact of COVID-19 and the policy response in India", *Brookings*, 13 July, https://brookings.edu/blog/future-development/2020/07/13/the-impact-of-covid-19-and-the-policy-response-in-india/, accessed 28 July 2020.

Lahiri, Amartya (2020), "Indian states can absorb diverse Covid response models, but Modi govt using one size for all", *The Print*, 6 May, https://theprint.in/opinion/indian-states-can-absorb-diverse-covid-response-models-but-modi-govt-using-one-size-for-all/415244/, accessed 1 August 2020.

Marwaha, Sana (2020), "Power of the people: NGOs and Samaritans bolster India's fight against COVID-19", *TimesNowNews.Com*, 25 May, https://timesnownews.com/india/article/power-of-the-people-ngos-and-samaritans-bolster-india-s-covid-19-fightback/596336, accessed 29 July 2020.

Mohsin, Amena (2020), "Covid 19 in South Asia: Regional perspectives on vulnerabilities and dispossessions", *Webinar, Calcutta Research Group*, 24 August.

NGOs deserve all appreciation for helping migrants during COVID-19 pandemic: SC (2020), *The Hindu*, 9 June, https://thehindu.com/news/national/ngos-deserves-all-appreciation-for-helping-migrants-during-covid-19-pandemic-sc/article31786947, accessed 29 July 2020.

Pandey, Geeta (2020), "Coronavirus in India: Desperate migrant workers trapped in lockdown", *BBC*, 22 April, https://bbc.co.uk/news/world-asia-india-52360757, accessed 28 July 2020.

Raj, Vatsal (2020), "Covid-19 and refugees in India: A tale of exclusion and counter-exclusion", *Border Criminologies*, 23 July, https://law.ox.ac.uk/research-subject-groups/centre-criminology/centreborder-criminologies/blog/2020/07/covid-19-and-0, accessed 30 July 2020.

Roy Choudhury, Saheli (2020), "India's economy was hit by the coronavirus lockdown. These charts show how", *CNBC*, 22 June, https://cnbc.com/2020/06/22/

economic-impact-of-indias-coronavirus-lockdown-in-four-charts.html, accessed 28 July 2020.

Ryder, Guy, Barcena, Alicia and Valovaya, Tatiana (2020), "Building back better: Equality at the Centre", *ILO*, 16 July, www.ilo.org/global/about-the-ilo/newsroom/news/WCMS_750862/lang – en/index.htm, accessed 23 July 2020.

Samaddar, Ranabir (2020a), "Introduction", in Ranabir Samaddar (ed), *Borders of an Epidemic – Covid 19 and Migrant Workers*, Calcutta: Calcutta Research Group.

Samaddar, Ranabir (2020b), *Borders of an Epidemic – Covid 19 and Migrant Workers*, Calcutta: Calcutta Research Group.

Sarkar, Sonia (2020), "Indian doctors face censorship, attacks as they fight coronavirus", *Aljazeera*, 13 April, https://aljazeera.com/news/2020/04/indian-doctors-face-censorship-attacks-fight-coronavirus-200410063124519.html, accessed 29 July 2020.

Sarmin, Utsa (2020), "Hunger, humiliation, and death: Perils of migrant workers in the time of COVID-19", in Ranabir Samaddar (ed), *Borders of an Epidemic – Covid 19 and Migrant Workers*, Calcutta: Calcutta Research Group.

Shankar, Roshni and Raghavan, Prabhat (2020), "The invisible crisis: Refugees and COVID-19 in India", *Andrew and Renata Kaldor Centre for International Refugee Law*, 19 May, https://kaldorcentre.unsw.edu.au/publication/invisible-crisis-refugees-and-covid-19-india, accessed 30 July 2020.

Sharma, Aditya (2020), "Coronavirus triggers mental health crisis in India", *DW*, 1 July, https://dw.com/en/coronavirus-triggers-mental-health-crisis-in-india/a-54011738, accessed 28 July 2020.

Shneiderman, Sara, Baniya, Jeevan and Billon, Philippe Le (2020), "Learning from disasters: Nepal copes with coronavirus pandemic 5 years after earthquake", *The Conversation*, 23 April, https://theconversation.com/planning-from-disasters-nepal-copes-with-coronavirus-pandemic-5-years-after-earthquake-134009, accessed 25 July 2020.

UN Women (2020), "Surveys show that COVID-19 has gendered effects in Asia and the Pacific", 29 April, https://data.unwomen.org/resources/surveys-show-covid-19-has-gendered-effects-asia-and-pacific, accessed 23 July 2020.

Zahra-Malik, Mehreen (2020), "The coronavirus effect on Pakistan's digital divide", *BBC*, 14 July, www.bbc.com/worklife/article/20200713-the-coronavirus-effect-on-pakistans-digital-divide, accessed 24 July 2020.

Part I

Impact on Economy

1 COVID-19 and the Challenges of Doubling Farmers' Income in India

Chitrasen Bhue

Introduction

Growth of the agrarian sector in India has got considerable attention by both policy-makers and researchers since the last two decades. There are at least two important reasons for this keen attention. One, farm sector has dominance in providing employment to a large section of the rural population. Secondly, agriculture is in crisis and it is evident by the increasing number of farmers' suicides. The crisis-ridden agriculture with such a huge dependency on it implies the slower rate of poverty reduction, which is an obstacle to development in India. Eswaran et al. (2009) have shown that 67% of total poor households belong to agricultural sector and depend on agriculture for their livelihood. Poverty reduction is closely associated with agricultural growth in India. Thus, agricultural growth is the prerequisite for the overall growth and development. But the agrarian sector in India is characterised by low productivity, and there are structural constraints to the low productivity in land, labour, and credit market. Production structure of the Indian agriculture is changing, and the emerging pattern of land, labour, and credit arrangement is becoming growth retarding in nature. With the present land, labour, and credit arrangement, the long run growth of the sector is challenging. Again, realising a higher income not only depends on high productivity of the sector but also depends on an efficient marketing system. The agricultural marketing system is inefficient in terms of infrastructure, information, and institution. Given the present marketing and production structure, doubling farmer's income is far away from reality.

The outbreak of COVID-19 in March 2020 has adversely affected all sectors including agriculture. It has worsened the already existing challenges of the farm sector. Although it is early to make a prediction, but there are certain direct impacts of COVID-19 on the agrarian sector. There are headlines, and studies which have focused on the impact of COVID-19 on the food supply chain, which is a direct impact on agriculture. But none of the studies are commenting on what could be the implication of COVID-19 on the growth retarding production structure of agriculture. This chapter

DOI: 10.4324/9781003282815-3

would be an initial reflection of the impact of COVID-19 on the production structure in Indian agriculture.

State of Indian Agriculture Before COVID-19

Decelerating Agrarian Growth Before COVID-19

COVID-19 has affected agriculture adversely disturbing its supply chain. But the situation of agriculture in India was not fascinating in the pre-COVID period as well. The share of gross value added (GVA) of agriculture is very low and it is declining at a very faster rate. The share of GVA of agriculture was nearly 50%, which has reduced to 12% in 2019–20 (see Figure 1.1). The decade before the green revolution was introduced in India; the growth rate of Net Domestic Product of agriculture was more than 3% (decade ending 1950–60). There was a continuous sluggish growth rate after that which reached to less than 2% in the decade ending 1966–67 (author's calculation from National Account Statistics, MOSPI, Government of India).

The introduction of green revolution made a major breakthrough in the growth of the agrarian sector. With the application of new technology, the growth rate started increasing from the decade ending 1967–68. The next following periods witnessed a turnaround in the growth rate of agricultural Net Domestic Product (NDP) and crossed the rate of 3% during the decade ending 1977–78. The growth rate continued to move in the range of 2% to 3% for the next three decades. It reached a level of more than 3% in the end of 1980s. Then a deceleration in the growth was witnessed in the first half of the reform period (mid-1990s) (author's calculation from National Account Statistics, MOSPI, Government of India; Chand, 1999; Singh, 2000).

The compound annual growth rate decelerated from more than 3% in the initial years of 1990s to nearly 2% in the subsequent years. It was followed by a recovery from the decade ending 2004–05 after which it started increasing. The growth rate became more than 3% in the decade ending

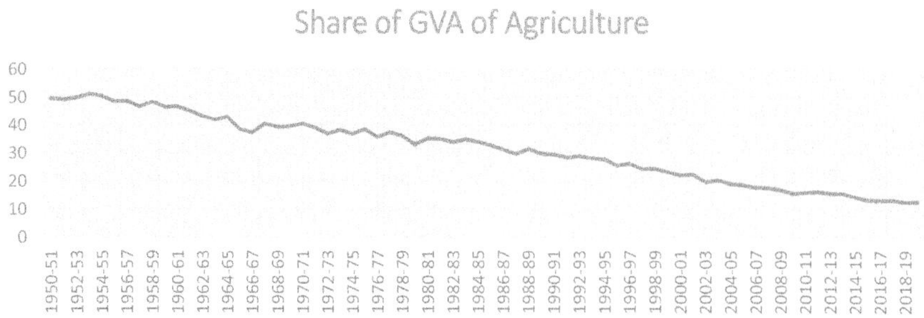

Figure 1.1 Share of Agricultural GDP

Source: National Account Statistics, MOSPI, Government of India

2012–13 (author's calculation from National Account Statistics, MOSPI, Government of India; Chand, 1999; Singh, 2000; Binswanger, 2013). In a nutshell, it can be concluded that the growth rate in the agrarian sector has witnessed different phases of growth. A similar phase-wise study at the all-India level can be found in the work of Chand and Parappurathu (2012). A huge regional disparity can also be seen in the agricultural performance among the states. The high agrarian growth in India was experienced in Punjab, Haryana, and Uttar Pradesh after the initiation of the green revolution but in the post-green revolution phase, the growth rate in Punjab and Haryana was decelerating.

Agricultural Growth During COVID-19

The quarterly estimates of agricultural gross domestic product (GDP) help us in understanding the situation of agriculture in terms of growth immediately before and after COVID-19. Figure 1.2 presents the quarterly estimates. It shows that in the beginning of COVID-19 in March 2020, which is covered in the last quarter (Jan–Mar) of 2019–20, the agricultural growth was 6.8%, which was reduced to 3.3% in the first quarter of 2020–21 when lockdown was imposed. In the subsequent quarter (Oct–Dec) in 2020–21, the growth rate again decreased to 3% with a marginal increase in the next quarter. The quarterly comparison of agricultural growth between 2019–20 and 2020–21 reveals that while the growth rate was consistent in 2019–20, there was a fluctuation in the growth rate during the COVID period.

In a nutshell it can be said that the performance of Indian agriculture was characterised by low growth with regional disparity. There could be multiple reasons for the present situation of agriculture but this chapter outlines

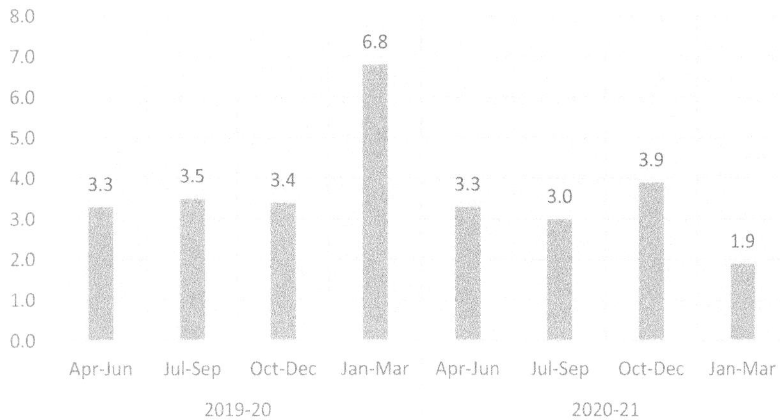

Figure 1.2 Quarterly Estimates of Agricultural GDP During COVID-19

Source: National Account Statistics, MOSPI, Government of India

some of the structural reasons in the land and labour market in the production site and structural issues of agricultural marketing. The outbreak of COVID-19 has influenced the agricultural performance, and the influence could be not only on the supply chain and agricultural marketing, but also on the already existing structural issues of agrarian sector. This has had a long-term impact on the income of farmers. The next section discusses the structural issues in landholding structure in agriculture followed by issues in labour market and agricultural marketing.

Issues of Landholding Structure in Indian Agriculture

Land is one of the important inputs in farm operation. The relationship between land and agricultural productivity in India has been analysed in line with the landholding size (farm-size productivity debate), land relation (tenancy and other contractual forms), and use of farm land. The studies highlight (a) relationship between farm size and agricultural productivity – is the small or large farm efficient? (b) relationship between the ownership of land and agricultural productivity and (c) is there a diversification of farm land for non-farm use which impacts agricultural productivity? Another important fact in Indian agriculture is the land market and labour market, which are highly interlinked to each other.

Marginalisation of Landholding in India

The average size of landholding in Indian agriculture is declining. The average size of operational holding was 1.41 ha in 1995–96, which has declined to 1.08 in 2015–16 (see Table.1.1). The distribution of size of landholding in Table 2 shows that along with the decline in average size of landholding, the

Table 1.1 Average Size of Operational Holding (in ha.)

Agricultural Census Year	*Average Size of Operational Holding in ha.*				
	1995–96	*2000–01*	*2005–06*	*2010–11*	*2015–16*
Assam	1.17	1.15	1.11	1.1	1.09
Arunachal Pradesh	3.31	3.69	3.33	3.51	3.35
Manipur	1.22	1.15	1.14	1.14	1.14
Meghalaya	1.33	1.3	1.18	1.37	1.29
Mizoram	1.29	1.24	1.22	1.14	1.25
Nagaland	4.82	7.28	6.93	6.02	4.87
Sikkim	1.65	1.57	1.48	1.42	1.27
Tripura	0.6	0.56	0.5	0.49	0.49
All India	1.41	1.33	1.23	1.15	1.08

Source: Various Agricultural Census Reports of India

number of marginal and small holding in India is also increasing. The size of marginal landholding has increased from 46.7% to 48.12% from 2010–11 to 2015–16. The marginal and small landholding together accounted for 68% of the total operational landholding, which accounted for nearly 24% of the total operated area in 2015–16. The average size of the operational landholding for small and marginal landholdings is lower than the other size of landholdings with the average size for these two categories declining over the years (various Agricultural Census Reports of India) (see Table 1.2).

There are at least two implications of the aforementioned structure of landholdings. Firstly, the marginal landholding (below 0.5 ha.) can be considered as effectively landless labour in agriculture (Basole and Basu, 2011). There are two options for the effectively landless category of households. Given the opportunities outside the farm sector, they can move to non-farm operation, which causes occupational diversification. The occupational diversification can happen with inter-state or intra-state migration. They can stay in the farm sector and enter into the agrarian production system as a cultivator taking land on lease for their survival. The limited capacity of small and marginal households to invest in agricultural operation could lead to low agricultural productivity. What is the evidence in Indian agriculture?

Tenancy and the Emergence of Non-Cultivating Peasant Households

With the increase in marginal and small landholding, one could expect an increase in tenancy if the small and marginal landholding category entered into the agricultural operation as a cultivator. If the landless turns themselves to a cultivator (pure tenant), they become the potential demander of land, and demand for land increases in the economy resulting in an increase in tenancy. The number of pure tenant households has increased from 7.15% in 2003 to 11.51% in 2013 (Bhue and Vijay, 2017). The increase in the share of pure tenant households also creates another structure in the agrarian economy. The increase in the number of pure tenants' households increases the demand for land. It becomes lucrative for the households who own land but do not self-cultivate to give the land in tenancy and earn rent. This rent-seeking behaviour has been seen in the agrarian economy, which takes a part of agricultural produce from the investment channels. Bhattacharyya (2011) mentions that the worst performance in terms of agricultural investment and productivity is in the areas where the landlords have property rights as compared to the areas where the cultivators have property rights. One possible reason for the declining investment in the regions where larger share of land is under tenancy could be the higher rental rate, which goes out of the flow of investment.

Athreya et al. (1990: 106), in a field survey in Tamil Nadu, found that the rental rate was around 40% of the gross value production. Similarly, Vijay and Sreenivasulu (2017), in a field survey in the three villages of

Table 1.2 Size of Landholding in India: 2010–11 to 2015–16

		2010–11			*2015–16*		
Category of Land Holding	*Land Holding Size (ha.)*	*Percentage of Operational Holding*	*Percentage of Area Operated*	*Average Size of Operational Land Holding*	*Percentage of Operational Holding*	*Percentage of Area Operated*	*Average Size of Operational Land Holding*
Marginal	Below 0.5	46.7	9.68	0.24	48.12	10.44	0.23
	0.5–1.0	20.03	12.81	0.73	20.34	13.59	0.72
Small	1.0–2.0	17.91	22.08	1.42	17.6	22.91	1.4
Semi-medium	2.0–3.0	6.97	14.51	2.4	6.71	14.81	2.38
	3.0–4.0	3.07	9.11	3.42	2.84	9.03	3.42
Medium	4.0–5.0	1.76	6.74	4.43	1.62	6.63	4.42
	5.0–7.5	1.81	9.48	6.03	1.62	8.96	6.01
	7.5–10.0	0.67	4.97	8.5	0.58	4.57	8.55
Large	10.0–20.0	0.58	6.57	13.13	0.47	5.74	13.08
	20.0 & above	0.13	4.02	36.94	0.1	3.32	36.18

Godavari Delta Zone, found that 41% of the output was paid as rent by the tenant households and among them, the marginal farmers pay the highest rent of 48% of the output. If a major share of production goes as rent, the investment capacity of the cultivator shrinks as the cultivator has to pay for other inputs used in the production process in addition to the survival of his/her family. Again, Vijay (2012) and Bhue and Vijay (2016) have found the increasing importance of household who owns land but does not self-cultivate. An increase in these households implies a separation between the owner and the operator of the land, which constrains the incentive to invest. Secondly, there is a high chance of shifting the land from farming to non-farming activities by the Non-Cultivating Households (NCH). Bhue and Vijay (2016) have studied the land use pattern of cultivator and non-cultivator households in rural India. They found that the non-cultivating households have shifted their land from agricultural operation to residential purpose. In 2002–03, the share of crop irrigated and un-irrigated area was around 70% with residential area of 12% out of the total area owned by the non-cultivating households. In 2013, the share of residential area became 71% with a significant decline in crop area to 25%.

This existing structure of landholding is growth retarding in nature, which is one of the reasons for the low agricultural productivity in India. In order to achieve the objective of doubling famers' income, the state has to play an important role in altering the existing structure of land relation. The imposition of lockdown due to the outbreak of COVID-19 might strengthen the existing structure of land relation. Tenancy might increase when the migrant labour return and engage themselves in agricultural sector as many of them are small and marginal farmers.

Structural Issues in Labour Market in Agriculture: Reflecting on COVID-19

Well-functioning labour market is necessary for the productivity growth in Indian agriculture. With the marginalisation and increasing tenancy, the land-man ratio in Indian agriculture is increasing, which could be one of the reasons for low productivity. The dependency in Indian agriculture is still high with the decrease in share to total GDP of the country. The labour force participation in agriculture is declining at a slower rate as compared to the decline in share of agriculture in total GDP (Binswanger, 2013). Figure 1.1 shows that during January–December 1983, the share of male labour usually employed based on their principal status was 77% in the Primary Sector, which includes agriculture and allied activities. It has reduced to 59% in 2012. But the decline in the share of agricultural GDP is faster than the decline in the share of labour force. Figure 1.1 shows that in 2019–20, the share of GVA of agriculture was only 12% (National Accounts Statistics, MOSPI, Government of India).

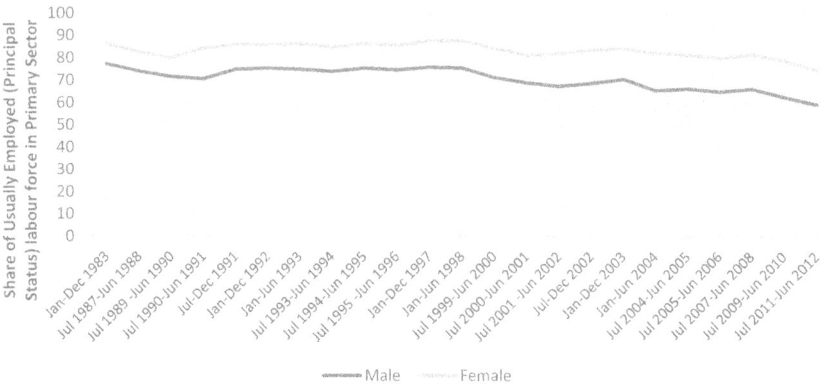

Figure 1.3 Labour Force Participation in Agriculture

Source: Different rounds of NSSO

This has an implication for poverty reduction until and unless either the growth rate in value generation in agriculture is very high or opportunities are created outside of agriculture to absorb the excess labour. The policy in the last few decades has focused on how to transform the excess labour from the agricultural sector to the non-agricultural sector. This in one way could provide higher wages in the non-agricultural sector. The decrease in pressure on land might increase the agricultural productivity. It solves the purpose of reduction in poverty and increase in agricultural productivity. The discourse of structural transformation in India highlights some of the characteristics of labour market. Is there a diversification from farm to the non-farm sector? Who are diversifying from the farm to the non-farm sector?

There are at least three observations of diversification from the farm to the non-farm sector in the discourse of structural transformation. There is an emergence of rural non-farm sector, which provides an alternative source of income. Post-1980s, there was a significant growth of non-farm GDP, which contributed to the growth of non-farm employment (Binswanger, 2013; Jha, 2006,). Growth in non-farm sector acts as a dent to rural poverty by reducing it (Himanshu et al., 2011). Another view explains the rigidity of rural labour market. Although there is an expansion of the non-farm sector, the diversification of labour from farm to the non-farm sector is constrained by various factors. The non-farm sector demands skill labour. Chadha (1993), Samal (1997), and Eswaran et al. (2009) found that lack of education was one of the important factors for the labour to diversify their occupation from farm to the non-farm sector. Again, the diversification is limited to the young age group dominated by the male population. It has also been discussed in the discourse that the non-farm sector is also vulnerable in providing job security and other social security to the labour (Unni, 1998;

Binswanger, 2013). In the non-farm employment, the share of constriction is the highest and its ability to provide employment is questionable.

The third issue of rural labour market that has been discussed in the discourse is the question of who are diversifying from the farm sector. The production structure of Indian agriculture has been changing over time. The non-farm sector in India is not generating sufficient employment to absorb the rural labour engaged in agriculture. Having surplus labour in agriculture is leading to low productivity in this sector, which in turn is leading to low agricultural wage rate, which is insufficient for the labour to survive. Given less opportunity and low wage, the agricultural labour is entering into the agrarian production structure, taking land in lease (Bhue and Vijay, 2017). The landless agricultural labour households are not diversifying to non-farm sector and becoming pure tenant households. The share of pure tenant in the agrarian economy has increased from 7.15% in 2003 to 11.51% in 2013 (Bhue and Vijay, 2017).

These three structural issues of the labour market in the rural areas have a strong implication for doubling farmers' income. Firstly, the low agricultural productivity will persist because of the low rate of diversification and high land-man ratio. Secondly, the increasing share of pure tenant household in the agrarian production system pushes these households to both production and marketing risk. The landless agricultural labour households have limited capacity to invest in agriculture as they can't access the formal credit market. In the long run, the investment in agriculture will decrease, which might reduce agricultural productivity.

Returned Migrant During COVID-19 and Its Possible Impact on Rural Agrarian Labour Market

The recent COVID-19 will worsen the already inefficient labour market in the rural areas. The rural-urban migration has been low (Binswanger, other reference). Given the low rate of rural-urban migration, the imposition of lockdown in March 2020 forced a large section of the labour to return to rural areas for at least the warmth and empathy of the family. The data on reverse migration during COVID-19 is rarely reported by the state and other agencies. A report published in *The Hindu*, Special Correspondent on 15 June 2020 in correspondent with Railway Board Chairman V. K. Yadav, revealed that till 1 May, 60 lakh migrant workers had returned to their respective states in 4,450 Shramik Special Trains (The Hindu, 2020). Another evidence based on the written reply[1] by Santhosh Kumar Gangwar, Minister of State (IC) for Labour and Employment on 14 September 2020 in the Parliament shows that ten million migrant labourers returned to their home states. The written reply also gives the state-wise number of migrant labourers returning to the home states. However, actual reverse migration is far more than this number. Majority of the return migrants were engaged in the informal sectors in the cities and urban agglomeration.

Given the distress-driven Indian agriculture, it can't be a sustainable source of employment for all the rural population. The alternative sources of employment (other than agriculture) can be non-farm employment incorporating migrant workers to urban and semi-urban places. Dandekar and Ghai (2020) argue, "Large scale migration induced by greater and greener pastures of economic growth is a myth, as most of migrant is for subsistence and survival and falls under the category of distress migration". Majority of the reverse migrants who left their destination and ended up in rural areas are unskilled and semi-skilled workers. Given the limited capacity of non-farm sector to absorb the surplus labour, their last resort would be agriculture. It has been argued that other employment generation policy like MGNREGA has been able to provide employment to the returned migrant workers during the lockdown. But Rawal et al. (2020) show that for nearly a month after the lockdown, there was no employment opportunity and the reopening of employment in this scheme is very slow. Majority of the migrant labourers in India are landless small or marginal farmers (Dev, 2012). The return of the migrants into the agricultural operation will increase the land-man ratio, disguised unemployment and reduce the collective bargaining. It will lead to decline in the agricultural productivity and agricultural income. The second phase of lockdown in 2021 will adversely affect the agricultural operation of upcoming Rabi Crops. The impact will only be visible in the next couple of months. This has strong implications for the poverty reduction in India.

Issues of Agricultural Marketing in India: Reflecting COVID-19

Appropriate income of the farmers requires not only an efficient production system but also an efficient marketing system. Indian farmers face both production and marketing risks (Gulati et al., 2020). Marketing risk involves price risk. Farmers in India do not get appropriate prices for their product due to an inefficient marketing system. The efficient marketing system needs efficiency in Marketing Infrastructure, Marketing Information, and Marketing Institution. Inadequate marketing infrastructure, asymmetrical information, and inefficient marketing institutions create hindrances in the process of getting an appropriate price of the product to the farmers. Indian agriculture is operating with inadequate marketing infrastructure. The total number of cold storage and warehouses available was 8,038 and 2,145, respectively, in 2019. The total number of Principally Regulated markets under Agricultural Produce Marketing Committee (APMC) was 2,447 and the number of sub-market yards regulated by the respective APMC was 4,843 (Ministry of Finance, Government of India, 2017). The Ministry of Agriculture and Farmers' Welfare (2017) recommends a Farmer-centric National Agricultural Marketing System for realising an adequate price of the farm produce. The report highlights that the number of regulated

Table 1.3 Marketing Infrastructure in India

Number of Cold Storages in 2019	8,038
Number of Warehouses in 2019	2,145
Principal Regulated Markets Under APMC in 2016–17	2,447
Sub-market Yards Regulated by Respective APMC in 2016–17	4,843

Sources:

1 Central Warehousing Corporation
2 Lok Sabha Unstarred Question No. 501 (dated 25.06.2019)
3 Economic Survey 2016–17

markets is inadequate and suggests the need of restructuring marketing architecture consisting of 22,000 Primary Retail Agriculture Market and 10,000 Primary Wholesale Agricultural Market. It also suggests that these markets should be networked with online platform to facilitate a pan-India market access to increase farmers' income.

In India, the Minimum Support Price (MSP) acts as a benchmark price upon which the market price is decided. The Government of India has approved MSP and procuring agencies for 24 crops (for the crop year 2020–21). Bhue and Kikon (2020) have shown that only 17% of the farmers are aware about MSP out of which only 7% sell at MSP to the procuring agencies. They have also cited pre-pledging of crops as a structural issue in agrarian production system. Given the inefficient agricultural marketing structure, doubling farmers' income is far from reality.

Given the inefficient marketing structure, COVID-19 has directly affected the supply chain. The imposition of lockdown has disturbed the existing marketing channels for the farmers with small and marginal farmers affected highly by the disturbance. The direct impact is visible by the low market arrival and low price of different commodities during the lockdown.

Direct Impact of COVID-19 on Market Arrival and Prices of Commodities

The imposition of lockdown on 25 March 2020 affected the movement of essential commodities from the farmers to the market. The data given by the Agmarknet shows how market arrival of certain essential commodities had fallen due to the lockdown from March to May 2020. Table 1.4 shows the market arrivals of essential commodities like paddy, wheat, potato, and onion for the months of March, April, and May for 2019 and 2020. It helps to compare the market arrivals of different commodities during the lockdown with the same period in 2019.

It shows that the market arrivals of wheat, potato, and onion absolutely declined during the period of lockdown. The market arrivals of wheat in April 2020 were 6,952,400 tonnes lesser as compared to the same month in 2019. Similar was the case for potato and onions. The reduction in market

Table 1.4 Market Arrival (in Tonnes) of Essential Commodities in Different Phase of Lockdown

	Crop	*March*	*April*	*May*
2019	Paddy	834,089	686,501	1,039,493
	Wheat	1,347,457	10,677,784	7,373,685
	Potato	1,234,569	935,156	869,371
	Onion	1,211,485	1,285,273	1,164,664
		Lockdown: Phase 1 to Phase 4 (25th March to 31st May)		
2020	Paddy	726,480	712,770	1,317,523
	Wheat	1,035,111	3,725,385	7,372,731
	Potato	729,219	475,538	518,405
	Onion	900,619	459,810	777,688
Chane in Market Arrival from 2019 to 2020	Paddy	–107,609	26,269	278,031
	Wheat	–312,346	-6,952,400	-954
	Potato	–505,350	-459,618	–350,966
	Onion	–310,866	-825,463	–386,976

Source: AGMARKNET, Directorate of Marketing & Inspection (DMI), Ministry of Agriculture and Farmers Welfare, Government of India

arrivals implies that farmers have not been able to sell their commodities on time which can cause the price to shrink. Secondly, the non-arrival of these commodities in the market could raise the price and affect the consumers. Paddy and wheat are completely non-perishable and there is MSP for these two crops.

Despite MSP, due to the closing down of Mandis (Bhasole and Shelly, 2020; Raju, 2020) in different states due to COVID-19, there were media reports of selling of the commodities at less than the MSP. Rawal et al. (2020) have shown that wheat was sold at less than MSP in different Mandis of Rajasthan, Uttar Pradesh, Madhya Pradesh, Chhattisgarh, and Gujarat during the lockdown. Similar trend was observed for the price of onions in Maharashtra, Karnataka, Uttar Pradesh, and Telangana in the same study. Onions were sold at a price of Rs.2,000 per quintal before the lockdown but sold at Rs. 500–1,000 in different Mandis during the lockdown (Rawal et al., 2020). The situation of perishable commodities would be much more vulnerable than the non-perishables. Many of the non-perishable commodities are not covered under MSP. For those commodities, getting a fair price during normal times is tough for a farmer due to the inefficient marketing structure. Considering COVID-19 lockdown, the situation must have been more vulnerable.

Conclusion

COVID-19 has adversely affected the farm sector economy in India. Farmers and agricultural labourers in the rural areas are the worst affected. The impact has been felt throughout the disruption in the movement of farm produce due to the imposition of lockdown from March to May 2020. As a result of that, a large section of farmers in different parts of the country sold their commodities at a lower price, which could increase their indebtedness. The debt burden of returned migrants who have not managed to find work will also increase which will affect the trends of poverty and inequalities in rural India. One of the reasons for the adverse effect could be the lack of preparedness and sudden imposition of lockdown by the government, although it was anticipated much before when China was affected by COVID-19. This will adversely affect the objective of doubling farmers' income by 2022.

Doubling farmers' income is a larger goal and to achieve that goal, it is necessary to address the structural constraints of Indian agriculture. In the production structure, the land and labour market arrangement are growth retarding in nature. Tenancy (pure tenancy) is increasing with the rise of rent-seeking class who own the land but do not self-cultivate. As a result of that, the long-term investment in agriculture will be adversely affected as these households have no incentive to invest. The opportunities outside the agriculture are limited forcing the landless to enter into the production structure. India experienced a second wave of COVID-19 in 2021 with the return migration continuing. Agriculture being the lender of last resort for majority of the migrant workers, the labour market will be over-burdened with surplus labour resulting in lower agricultural productivity and low wage.

COVID-19 has unfolded the structural challenges that Indian agriculture faces in marketing and production since last few decades. The inadequate policy response to the marketing and production was revealed during the pandemic. While on the one hand, the disturbance in the food supply chain alarms the need of self-reliance in food production, it also reflects the inadequate marketing infrastructure to procure the produce. The APMC has to be strengthened by increasing the market and sub-market yards with more numbers of cold storage and warehouses. The supply of critical inputs should be available to the local agricultural cooperative to smoothen the process of agricultural operation. Closure of mandis had a severe impact on the procurement of many crops and had affected the farmer's income. As India witnessed a second wave in 2021, Government has to find out a way in the future to make the mandis more functional and develop alternative mechanism of procurement in the rural villages.

Along with reforms in marketing constraints, reform is also needed in Land, Labour, and Credit market structure of Indian agriculture. Employment opportunities outside the farm sector can reduce the labour force dependency, which will increase the wage and agricultural productivity. The Mahatma Gandhi National Rural Employment Guarantee Scheme (MGNREGS) has to be revamped to provide employment guarantees. Cooperative farming, Farmers' Producers Organization, and other forms of cooperative of small and marginal farmers have to be encouraged with incentive by the government. The government should expand the institutional lending to small and marginal farmers.

Note

1 http://164.100.24.220/loksabhaquestions/annex/174/AU138.pdf

References

Athreya, V. B., Djurfeldt, G. and Lindberg, S. (1990), *Barrier Broken Production Relation and Agrarian Change in Tamil Nadu*, New Delhi: SAGE Publication Pvt. Ltd, p. 106.

Basole, A. and Basu, D. (2011), "Relations of production and modes of surplus extraction in India: Part I – Agriculture", *Economic and Political Weekly*, 46(14), 41–58.

Bhasole and Shelly (2020), "Covid-19 impact: Fearful vegetable mandis threaten to shut shop", *The Economic Times*, 24 March, https://economictimes.indiatimes.com/news/politics-and-nation/fearful-vegetable-mandis-threaten-to-shut-shop/articleshow/74783100.cms?from=mdr, accessed 6 April 2021.

Bhattacharyya, S. (2011), "Five centuries of economic growth in India: The institution perspective", *MPRA, Paper No.67901*, https://mpra.ub.uni-muenchen.de/67901/MPRA paper No. 67901, posted 16 November 2015 18.32 UTC.

Bhue, C. and Kikon, Renbeni (2020), "Issues and challenges of MSP as an income enhancement approach in India", *Indian Economic Journal*, 68(2), 290–295.

Bhue, C. and Vijay, R. (2016), "Importance of landowning non-cultivating households some more evidence", *Economic and Political Weekly*, 51(25), 19–21.

Bhue, C., and Vijay, R. (2017). "Occupational diversification in the rural sector between 2003 and 2013: some more observations", *Indian Journal of Labour Economics*, 60, 663–670.

Binswanger-Mkhize, H. P. (2013), "The stunted structural transformation of the Indian economy agriculture, manufacturing and the rural non-farm sector", *Economic and Political Weekly*, 48(26–27), 5–13.

Chadha, G. K. (1993), "Non-farm employment for rural households in India: Evidence and prognosis", *The Indian Journal of Labour Economics*, 36(3), 296–327.

Chand, R. (1999), "Emerging crisis in Punjab agriculture", *Economic and Political Weekly*, 34(13), A-2–A-10.

Chand, R. and Parappurathu, S. (2012), "Temporal and spatial variation in agricultural growth and its determinants", *Economic and Political Weekly*, 48(26 & 27), 55–64.

Dandekar, A. and Ghai, R. (2020), "Migration and reverse migration in the age of Covid-19", *Economic and Political Weekly*, 19, 28–31.

Dev, Mahendra S. (2012), *Small Farmers in India: Challenges and Opportunities, WP-2012–014*, Mumbai, Indira Gandhi Institute of Development Research, pp. 1–37.

Eswaran, Mukesh, Kotwal, A., Ramaswami, B. and Wadha, W. (2009), "Sectoral labour flows and agricultural wages in India, 1983–2004: Has growth trickled down?" *Economic and Political Weekly*, 44(2), 46–55.

Gulati, A., Devesh, K. and Bouton, M. M. (2020), "Reforming Indian agriculture", *Economic and Political Weekly*, LV(11), 35–42.

Himanshu, Lanjouw P., Mukhopadhyay, A. and Murgai, R. (2011), *Non-Farm Diversification and Rural Poverty Decline: A Perspective From Indian Sample*

Survey and Village Study Data, Working Paper 44, Asia Research Centre, London School of Economics and Political Science, London, UK, pp. 1–41.

Jha, Brajesh (2006), *Rural Non-Farm Employment in India: Macro-Trends, Micro Evidences and Policy Options*, New Delhi, Agricultural Economics Unit Institute of Economic Growth University Enclave, pp. 1–66.

Ministry of Agriculture and Farmers' Welfare (2017), *Doubling Farmers' Income Post-Production Intervention: Agricultural Marketing, Department of Agriculture, Cooperation and Farmers' Welfare*, Ministry of Agriculture and Farmers' Welfare, New Delhi, Vol. 4, p. 2.

Ministry of Finance, Government of India (2017), "Economic survey 2016–17", *Department of Economic Affairs Economic Division*, 2, 177.

Raju, S. (2020), "Meerut mandi closed for 3 days", *Hindustan Times*, 6 May, https://bit.ly/2XphB8d.

Rawal, V., Kumar, M., Verma, A. and Pais, J. (2020), *COVID-19 Lockdown: Impact on Agriculture and Rural Economy*, SSER Monograph 20/3, Society for Social and Economic Research, New Delhi, pp. 1–39.

Samal, K. C. (1997), "Features and determinants of rural non-farm sector in India and Orissa", *Journal of Indian School of Political Economy*, 9(1), 65–93.

Singh, S. (2000), "Crisis in Punjab agriculture", *Economic and Political Weekly*, 35(23), 188–189.

The Hindu. (2020, June 15), 16 lakh migrants took 4,450 Shramik special to reach their home States: Railway. *The Hindu*. Special Correspondent. https://www.thehindu.com/news/national/60-lakh-migrants-took-4450-shramik-specials-to-reach-their-home-states-railways/article31834747.ece

Unni, J. (1998), "Non-agricultural employment and poverty in Rural India", *Economic and Political Weekly*, 33(13), A-36–A-44.

Vijay, R. (2012), "Structural retrogression and rise of 'new landlord' in Indian agriculture: An empirical exercise", *Economic and Political Weekly*, 47(5), 37–45.

Vijay, R. and Sreenivasulu, Y. (2017), *Nature and Extent of Tenancy arrangement in Godavari and Kaveri Delta Zones: A Comparative Study*, Hyderabad: NIRD CAS&DM research project for 2012–13.

2 Migration, Informality, and COVID-19 Pandemic in India

Debdulal Saha

Introduction

Migration has been discussed in development theory and policy discourse mainly in the context of understanding structural changes and dualistic nature of economy. Various socio-economic, demographic, political, cultural, spatial, and others have been identified as push and pull factors as explanations to cause and effect of migration. However, push and pull factors are very blurred in the present context. Both internal and international migration has been a subject of discussion at the global level. But the debate over migration in India is mostly limited to understanding the processes of urbanisation and urbanism. In fact, not much discussion on migration policy has been deliberated at both the international and national levels.

Rather, we can say that it is a new domain for exploration. At the global level (America, Europe, South and Southeast Asia), we have been witnessing growing policy-related concerns on migration since the last couple of years. At the national level, issues pertaining to migration are drawing attention in academic as well as in policy-making. In fact, there is no proper enumeration of migrants and no clear methodology as to how one should understand 'migration' in India. The ongoing pandemic and the lockdown in 2020 owing to COVID-19 have unfolded these gaps and raised issues.

India has witnessed humanitarian crisis in terms of hunger, poverty, labour migration, and loss of livelihoods across rural and urban areas due to the COVID-19 pandemic. In response to the most devastating pandemic – comparable in scale only to the 1918 Spanish-flu – India, like many other countries resorted to a nationwide lockdown to arrest the spread of the Coronavirus infection. In India, the lockdown, in fact, was the most comprehensive in the world – harsher than that in Italy, the United States of America, and even China. Once the lockdown was imposed, the economy came to a standstill, and millions of jobs became redundant overnight. In India, the first positive case of COVID-19 was reported from Kerala on 30 January 2020. With about 240 cases, the Government of India declared a complete lockdown in the country for 3 weeks owing to the contagiousness nature of the disease. Further, on 14 April, the lockdown was extended for

DOI: 10.4324/9781003282815-4

another 19 days due to the continuous increase in the number of active cases in major states. Phase-wise agricultural activities and small- and medium-scale industrial activities were allowed to restore.

While the exodus of migrants from the urban economy has become the central point of debate, how will rural economy absorb reverse migrants – which largely suffer from open unemployment and labour surplus – is one of the major concerns in the policy discourse. Two types of dominant narratives have been going around on how India as a nation-state will absorb the COVID-19 shock. While some have predicted that the eventual lack of jobs in the rural sector would compel the reverse migrants to migrate back to the cities; others have opined that this time around they would also factor in future COVID-like situations and reassess their options and decisions. It is evident that the labour market, mainly the informal workforce, was the worst hit due to the lockdown. This warrants a detailed discussion. In the process of shock absorption, India like many other countries faced the second wave of Coronavirus infections in 2021. The speculations were: will the government again impose lockdown as a measure? Will the economy and the workers undergo a similar situation? In other word, could we afford another lockdown in 2021? The Prime Minister of India addressed the nation for the first time after the second wave on 20 April 2021. Besides indicating nationwide health crisis, there were two important takeaways from his speech as far as migrants and people's mobility were concerned. Firstly, lockdown would be the last resort amidst the second wave of coronavirus. Secondly, there was no need of people leaving their place of destination. It might create crisis after crisis. Further, he mentioned that vaccination drives can be organised for the workers especially for those who are engaged in the urban economy. This indicates how the lockdown failed and was poorly managed in 2020, resulting in migrant crisis in India. Against this backdrop, this essay intends to discuss issues pertaining to migration with special focus on the informal labour market in India during the lockdown.

The essay is synthesised into eight sections. Why did the debate over migration and labour market become the central discussion point amidst global health crisis has been addressed in the introductory section? Conceptualisation of the book and data sources is mentioned in the second section. Before discussing the impact of COVID-19 on migration and labour market in India, migration pattern is discussed in the third section, whereas employment pattern is discussed in the fourth section. In neoliberal development, one of the major discussions is on labour market vulnerability and precarity. Poor social security and weak employment relations are briefly discussed in the fifth section. Impact of the pandemic on gender is inevitable. Thus, the recent time use data (NSSO, 2020) across gender is discussed in the sixth section. On the basis of various surveys conducted by various institutions and organisation, the impact of COVID-19 and nationwide lockdown on labour market and migrants have been examined in the seventh section. Plausible policy measures to safeguard the labour market and migrants are discussed in the concluding section as a way forward with discussions on how we should be better prepared for any such humanitarian crises arising in the future.

Conceptualisation and Data Sources

Migration and informal economy are interrelated and connected. Traditional models and theories of migration were viewed from dualism (Harris and Todaro, 1970; Fields, 1975; Gang and Gangopadhyay, 1987a, 1987b). The two-sector model believed that developing societies would be transformed from traditional economy to industrial/modern economies by absorbing surplus labour from the rural areas. This became an illusion. Later, duality of formality-informality was established to understand the transient employment phenomenon (Hart, 1973; Guha-Khasnobis and Kanbur, 2006). Migration has become an outcome of the urbanisation process; and informal sector complements to migration. Thus, in the development process, informal sector work and migration are complementary. Informal sector is considered to be a comfortable recourse for migrants, and in fact, it plays as a buffer ground for those trying to get into the formal sector jobs. The current pandemic has compelled us to rethink/question beyond the linear/traditional relationship between migration and informality. Looking at the current scenario, we intend to revisit the fundamental question posed by Jan Breman through his seminal work on *Footloose Labour* (1996: 1): "what was the destination of those workers who left or who were pushed out of agriculture?" In addition, we also intend to address the questions of the state's role in managing migrants and informality of the labour market?

We have not come out from the ongoing pandemic. The argument of this article is developed based on case studies and narratives from earlier surveys and studies conducted by various organisations and institutions such as Azim Premji University (APU), ActionAid, Stranded Workers Action Network (SWAN), and Indian Institute for Human Settlements (IIHS). The observation and facts have also been made from national news channels, newspapers and my day-to-day interaction with service providers and workers during the lockdown period. Secondary data sources have been presented from Period Labour Force Surveys (2017–18, 2018–19) and Centre for Monitoring Indian Economy (CMIE). Quarterly data released by the CMIE has been analysed to elucidate pre-lockdown period and post-lockdown period of the labour market.

Migration Pattern

Data from the population census since 1991 shows that the rate of migration went up among male, female, and total population (see Table 2.1). Further, data indicates that intra-state migrants are more as compared to inter-state migrants (Table 2.2). A closer look at the source of migration reveals that

Table 2.1 Percentage Share of Migrants in the Population

Category	*1991*			*2001*			*2011*		
	M	*F*	*T*	*M*	*F*	*T*	*M*	*F*	*T*
Rural	10.2	43	26.1	11.5	46.1	28.3	13.5	52.6	32.5
Urban	27.6	37.5	32.3	32.9	40.3	36.4	42.6	54.6	48.4
Total	14.8	41.6	27.7	17.5	44.6	30.6	22.6	53.2	37.5

Source: Kundu, 2018 (p. 636) based on various rounds of Census

Table 2.2 Migration by Source (in Million)

Non-migrants	755
Migrants From Other States	54
Migrants From Same Districts	278
Migrants From Other Districts but Same State	118

Source: Revi et al. (IIHS) 2020 based on Census 2011

Table 2.3 Mobility of People (in Million)

Urban to Rural	27
Urban to Urban	78
Rural to Urban	78
Rural to Rural	214

Source: Revi et al. (IIHS) 2020 based on Census 2011

when we compare rural to urban migration, a significant amount of migration took place as rural to rural migration (see Table 2.3). We can argue that urbanisation is not driven by traditional ways of thinking on rural-urban migration. Rather, it is due to natural population growth within urban areas and reclassification of urban areas (Revi et al., 2020).

Employment Scenario in India

The nationwide lockdown has severely affected the Indian labour market, mainly those who are engaged in manufacturing and service sectors. A few essential services were allowed during the first phase of lockdown. As we know, services sector contributes over 55% to the national GDP and almost one-third of workforce is engaged in the service sector. Therefore, shutting down service sector has cost both on the growth and employment levels. We also need to understand that manufacturing and service sectors are the house for semi-skilled and skilled labour force. Therefore, before critically analysing the impact of lockdown on the Indian labour market, we need to understand the conditions of the Indian labour market.

Table 2.4 Percentage Share of Employment Across Sectors

Share of Employment Across Sector	*2004–05*	*2011–12*	*2017–18*	*2018–19*
Agriculture	58.5	48.9	44.1	42.4
Industry	18.1	24.3	24.8	25.2
Services	23.4	26.8	31.1	32.4

Source: NSSO (2006, 2013) and PLFS (2019, 2020)

Table 2.5 Employment Trends in Major Activities Across Sectors

Sector	*2004–05*	*2011–12*	*2017–18*	*2018–19*
Agriculture	58.5	48.9	44.1	42.4
Mining and quarrying	0.6	0.5	0.4	0.4
Manufacturing	11.7	12.6	12.1	12.1
Electricity, water, and gas	0.3	0.5	0.6	0.6
Construction	5.6	10.6	11.7	12.1
Trade, hotels, transport, communication, and services related to broadcasting	17.7	16.7	19	18.6

Source: NSSO (2006, 2013) and PLFS (2019, 2020)

Although the share of the agricultural sector to the Indian GDP has been declining over a period of time, labour force is still engaged in the sector (see Table 2.4). Thus, agricultural sector in India is still a 'surplus sector' with disguised unemployment. On the other hand, engagement of workforce in the service sector has been slowly increasing. If we consider PLFS (2018–19), trade, hotel, and transport services (18.6%) and construction sector (12.1%) contributed a significant share in the service sector. Share of both these sectors has been steadily increasing over a period of time (see Table 2.5).

There are three broad categories of employment status such as self-employment, regular wage/salaries person, and casual workers. If we look at the status of employment, self-employment in rural areas declined from 2017–18 to 2018–19, whereas it marginally increased in the urban areas from 2017–18 to 2018–19. Notably, employment categories under wage/salaried person in both the rural and urban areas have marginally decreased. On the other hand, casual employment in both the rural and urban areas has increased from 2017–18 to 2018–19 (see Table 2.6). This is an alarming concern. Increasing causal employment indicates "job insecurity" as compared to "regular/salaried employment". Nature of casual workforce is also attached to "informality". If we look at gender-segregated

Table 2.6 Percentage Share of Workers in Usual Status (ps+ss) by Status in Employment During PLFS (2017–18) and PLFS (2018–19)

Employment Category	*Self-employment*			*Regular Wage/Salary*	*Casual Labour*
	Own Account Workers and Employer	*Helper in Household Enterprise*	*All Self-employed*		
	PLFS 2018–19				
	Rural				
Male	*48.2*	*9.2*	57.4	14.2	28.3
Female	*21.8*	*37.9*	59.6	11	29.3
Total	*41.4*	*16.7*	58	13.4	28.6
	Urban				
Male	34.6	4.1	38.7	47.2	14.2
Female	24.9	9.6	34.5	54.7	10.7
Total	32.6	5.3	37.8	48.7	13.5
	PLFS 2017–18				
	Rural				
Male	48	9.8	57.8	14	28.2
Female	19	38.7	57.7	10.5	31.8
Total	41	16.9	57.8	13.1	29.1
	Urban				
Male	34.9	4.3	39.2	45.7	15.1
Female	23.7	11	34.7	52.1	13.1
Total	32.6	5.7	38.3	47	14.7

Source: NSSO (2006, 2013) and PLFS (2019, 2020)

data in rural areas, male wage/salaried persons in rural areas has reduced by 0.2% from 2017–18 to 2018–19, whereas female wage/salaried person has reduced by 0.5% during the same period. Likewise, in the urban areas, female wage/salaried persons reduced by 2.6%, whereas male salaried/wage persons reduced by 1.5%. If we look at casual workforce, casual workers among rural female workforce increased by 2.5% while male casual workers reduced by 0.1%. In the urban areas, causal workforce among females increased by 2.4%, whereas male casual workforce increased by 0.9% (see Table 2.6).

Issues of Social Security

Poor social security model in India makes workers vulnerable particularly those who are engaged in the informal sector. The following table shows that workers are working without contract and without any basic social security benefits. In rural areas, 67.8% workers (reduced by 1.4%) work without any written job contract, whereas 70.5 person of the urban workforce

Table 2.7 Percentage Share of Regular Wage/Salaried Employees Working Without Job Contract and Social Security Benefits Among Employees (ps+ss) in Non-agricultural Sector

	% Share of Regular Wage/Salaried Employees Work Without Job Contract		*% Share of Regular Wage/Salaried Employees Work Without Social Security Benefits*	
	PLFS (2018–19)	*PLFS (2017–18)*	*PLFS (2018–19)*	*PLFS (2017–18)*
Rural				
Male	70.4	71.7	55.4	51.9
Female	58.2	58.5	57.7	55.1
Total	67.8	69.2	55.9	52.5
Urban				
Male	70.3	72.7	48.5	47
Female	71.2	71.4	52.6	50.1
Total	70.5	72.4	49.4	47.7

Source: PLFS (2019, 2020)

(reduced by 1.9%) work without job contract (see Table 2.7). The trend is similar in both male and female workers. This indicates that formal contract between "employer-employees" has reduced over time.

However, comparing PLFS 2017–18 and 2018–19, it is seen that workers (male and female) in the formal sector receive little more social security benefits from their employers in both rural and urban areas. Needless to mention, casual workers and self-employment work outside the purview of "social protection model". Over 55.9% and 49.4% of regular/salaried workforce work without any social security benefits in rural and urban areas, respectively. This indicates labour market insecurity.

From the labour market discussion, we can bring two important issues. Firstly, nature and status of employment clearly show that female workers are "disadvantaged" and "vulnerable" as compared to their male counterparts. Therefore, in case of crisis or job losses, women are more prone to face job loss compared to their male counterparts. Secondly, significant share of workers work without 'social and economic protection'. This makes labour market vulnerable and uncertain especially at the time of crisis.

Migration and Labour Market During COVID-19 Pandemic

Migration

We witnessed that the abrupt and unplanned announcement of the lockdown not only created panic among the poor, vulnerable, illiterate workers, and their dependants but also affected the general population. Migrant workers were not accepted by their urban counterparts. Migrant workers were also not given wage/salary, which raised concerns on sustenance in the urban areas. Data shows that a large number of migrant workers are short-term, seasonal, and cyclical migrants. Therefore, with uncertainty, these workers returned to their homes from urban centres. The initial phase of lockdown was more dehumanising. The most enduring images of the post-COVID-19 lockdown in India have been that of migrant labourers fleeing the urban spaces to return home, situated hundreds and even thousands of kilometres away, on foot. This led to a chain of events that eventually led to the crises unfolding on the streets in India. While the more fortunate could somehow find their way home, there were others who met with tragic death. There were 378 deaths as on 14 May 2020. Of these deaths, the highest number of 58 deaths were due to starvation and financial distress, 29 were due to exhaustion, 12 because of police brutality and state violence, road or train accidents involving migrants were put at 91, and 83 died by suicide because of lockdown-induced mental health conditions amongst other deaths. To state an instance, a 12-year-old child of a migrant labourer's family died due to exhaustion after walking for 100 kilometres with her parents (The Wire, 2020a). After the news of these deaths started grabbing headlines, the government decided to start what they called "shramik" or "labour" trains. People were crammed up in the coaches with no provision for water or food throughout the journey in the excruciating summer heat. A video that piqued the conscience of the entire nation was that of a migrant woman lying lifeless on a railway platform while her toddler was playing with the sheet covering her dead body. She died of extreme exhaustion and hunger after travelling for two days in the "shramik" trains (The Hindu, 2020).

While in most cases, the tacit support of the state in labour exploitation is unheard and goes unnoticed, the lockdown brought this inherent nature of the state into the open. The state of Karnataka cancelled all special "shramik" trains in a bid to force the labour to stay amidst concerns and representations made by prominent builders and real estate firms to the government. While the concerns are well founded but the denial of a choice to the migrants to return home reminds one of "bonded labour". The All India Central Council of Trade Unions described this move as a violation of the fundamental right of the freedom of movement and promotion of forced labour (The Wire, 2020b).

According to the Ministry of Railways (2020a, 2020b), 4,277 special Shramik trains brought back 6 million workers to their home states by 12 June 2020. A vast majority (68%) of these trains originated in Gujarat (24%), Maharashtra (19%), Punjab (10%), Uttar Pradesh (7%), and Bihar (7%) and overwhelmingly ended up in Uttar Pradesh (41%), Bihar (36%), Jharkhand (5%), Odisha (5%), and West Bengal (4%). The COVID crisis unfolded the extreme vulnerabilities faced by India's migrant population.

Labour Market

One needs to understand that the Indian labour market was not doing great even before the pandemic started since early 2020. The data shows how Indian labour market is volatile. We have considered four quarter data to

Table 2.8 LPR and UR Across Gender and Region During Lockdown and Post-lockdown Period

	Sept–Dec 2019	*Jan–April 2020*	*May–Aug 2020*	*Sept-Dec 2020*
LPR (Urban)	40.7	38.3	37.7	37.8
LPR (Rural)	43.7	42.4	41.5	41.9
LPR (Male)	68.8	68.8	64.3	67.9
LPR (Female)	9.5	11.1	7.8	9.5
UR (Urban)	9	12.4	12.7	7.8
UR (Rural)	6.8	9.5	11	6.7
UR (Male)	7	10.8	10.9	6.1
UR (Female)	26	25.9	17.1	15.1
LPR (Urban Male)	68.8	65	64.3	64.7
LPR (Urban Female)	9.5	8.5	7.8	7.4
UR (Urban Male)	7	10.8	11.7	6.5
UR (Urban Female)	26	25.9	21.9	20.8

Source: CMIE (Sept-Dec2019), CMIE (Jan-April 2020), CMIE (May-Aug 2020), CMIE (Sep-Dec 2020)

show how labour market was during the pre-lockdown stage, during the lockdown and the post-lockdown periods (see Table 2.8). The objective of considering September–December 2020 period is to show how the labour market is absorbing the shock and how fast the labour market is recovering. Labour force participation rate (LPR) has fallen from 40.7% (September–December 2019) to 38.3% (January–April 2020) in urban areas. Trend among LPR is similar in the rural areas. However, falling rate in rural LPR is less as compared to urban areas. Recovery period shows a very marginal impact on LPR in both urban (by 0.1%) and rural (0.4%) areas.

If we compare LPR between male and female, labour force participate rate is significantly low between male and female. In fact, during the lowdown, female LPR increased as compared to the male LPR and the gap between male and female LPR reduced from 7.6% to 6.1%. Surprisingly, data shows that during unlock period, both male and female LPR have been reducing. Comparing male and female LPR, recovery rate among female workers is slower than that among male workers. The gap between male LPR and female LPR has been wide. For instance, during January–April 2020, female LPR was 6.1 times lower than that of male LPR. However, female LPR further dropped in May–August 2020 and increased slightly in the period of September–December 2020. Not surprisingly, unemployment rate (UR) is low in rural areas as compared to urban areas. Female UR is higher than that of male. Female workers in urban areas faced more volatility as compared to rural areas. Female UR in urban areas is higher than that of male UR (see Table 2.8).

Time Use and Gender

The latest time use data released by the National Sample Survey Office (NSSO) shows how female workforce has been deprived during the ongoing pandemic. Working age group of 15–59 years between male and female workers shows that male workers (73.1%), not surprisingly, are engaged more in the economic and related activities as compared to the female workforce (22.6%). The male workforce in the employment activities is higher than that of female workers (see Tables 2.9 and 2.10). However, when we see unpaid and care giving domestic services for the household members, the share of female workers (89.4%) is much higher than that of male workers (24.1 percent). Females of working age group 15–59 spend more time in unpaid and care giving domestic services for household members while spending less time for leisure and other sport practices as compared to male. Although time use data during lockdown is yet to be released, one can anticipate from the following tables (2.9 and 2.10) based on time use survey collected during January–December 2019 that conditions of female workers will be even more deplorable during the lockdown.

Table 2.9 Percentage Share (%) of Persons Participating in a Day in Activities of Major Divisions of TUS Activity Classification Irrespective of Whether It Is a Major Activity or Not (Considering All the Activities in a Time Slot)

	Male (15–59)	*Female (15–59)*
Employment and related activities	73.1	22.6
Unpaid domestic services for household members	24.1	89.4
Unpaid caregiving services for household members	14.7	30.7
Culture, leisure, mass media, and sports practices	90.7	91.9

Source: NSSO, 2020.

Table 2.10 Minutes spent in a Day on an Average per Participant in the Activities of Major Divisions of TUS Activity Classification Irrespective of Whether It is a Major Activity or Not (Considering All the Activities in a Time Slot)

	Male (15–59)	*Female (15–59)*
Employment and related activities	521	385
Unpaid domestic services for household members	93	306
Unpaid caregiving services for household members	72	142
Culture, leisure, mass media, and sports practices	147	168

Source: NSSO, 2020

Facts and Findings From Ground Reality During Lockdown

A survey with over 16,900 workers across 402 districts conducted by Action Aid (2020) shows that during lockdown, 78% of workers lost their jobs and 48% of workers did not receive wages. About 17% of workers partially received wages across sectors. Since the lockdown, 57% of workers fell into debt trap. Only 45% of workers availed benefits under public distribution system (PDS). Interestingly, 39% of households lacked sufficient water supply. After lockdown, the plight of the workers did not show significant improvement. Although UR has reduced by 30%, it is still high at 48%. Surprisingly, 64% workers did not receive wages as compared to 48% during the lockdown. During the lockdown, 82% of workers had insufficient food. Although it is reduced during post-lockdown period to 68%, food insufficiency during the post-lockdown is very high.

Another study conducted by Azim Premji University (APU) during lockdown in 2020, covering about 5,000 workers, shows that 77% of households have been consuming less food than before. It shows 64 percent of workers received less earnings than before and 47 percent of households did not have enough money to purchase essential consumable (APU 2020). Another survey of 16,863 workers led by Stranded Workers Action Network (SWAN) during 2020 reveals that about 50% of the workers had rations of only one day and 72% for a maximum of two days in a week. About 82% had not received any support from the government in any means (SWAN, 2020).

Data and fact check unfold beyond labour market volatility and migrant crisis. It shows hunger and humanitarian crisis during pandemic. It is evident that female workers were more vulnerable and the condition of the urban workforce is even more precarious. Migrant workers including female workers in the category of urban working poor, in particular, were at risk and insecure. Post-lockdown recovery rate has been very slow. Therefore, it will take time to restore the economy including the labour market. Informal sector workers are, indeed, badly hit by the pandemic in both the urban and rural areas. Workers in the supply chain including garment workers and home-based workers were affected. One of the other vulnerable and disadvantaged groups in urban informal sector is domestic workers who lost their job or were unpaid immediately after the announcement of the lockdown. Notably, most of these workers are migrants, illiterate, and also gendered.

Discussion and Conclusion

The current pandemic and lockdown not only unfolded many questions on the weak Indian labour market but also raised questions on the role of state, institutional framework, and poor public policy system. However, it is important to remember that the Indian economy was not doing well even before the pandemic. For several quarters, the gross domestic product (GDP) recorded deceleration in output growth accompanied by fall in capacity utilisation ratio, marked by decline in investment-output ratio and slowdown in credit off-take. In the labour market, Periodic Labour Force Survey (PLFS) 2017–18 figures showed the highest UR in 45 years, as well as significant slowing down or negative real wage growth. As the lockdown significantly dismantled economic activities, UR soared as high as 23.5% in May 2020.

Discussion shows that the labour market is vulnerable and highly insecure. Poor nation state's social protection model makes it even more vulnerable. Workers lack social security with poor social security resulting in weak employer-employee relations. In other word, we can say that weak employer-employee relations lead to lack of social security benefits. It also shows workers are not only "footloose" (Breman, 1996) but also "unfree" and "bonded" (Breman, 2007, 2013). Besides, this unfolds labour market inequality and regional disparities. Guy Standing's (1997) seven forms of labour market insecurities shows that all the indicators are interrelated. If the labour market lacks one form of security, it might be trapped in other forms of insecurities. We witnessed the same during the pandemic. Not many organisations including trade unions and other membership-based organisations could come together and bargain over wages on behalf of the workers. Voices were raised about future course of action but not many organisations stood by these workers and for their workers' rights. The reasons could be many. Most of them are involved in informal nature of employment and thus, traceability of these workers during lockdown was difficult. Informal sector workers have weak collective bargaining. This is perhaps one of the main reasons why workers witnessed hunger and job-losses owing to the health crisis. Urban working poor (mainly those who are informally engaged) were the worst hit. They suffered from absolute poverty. They lost their shelter and lacked food.

One can argue that the migrant crisis is a result of state, policy, and institutional failure. Therefore, we need to relook at the role of the state, existing public policy, and institutional framework. State governments and urban areas will need to improve welfare and social protection measures and secure work opportunities in order to get this workforce to return to the cities. Minimum days of employment in urban areas mainly for seasonal and cyclical migrants could be guaranteed along with state-assisted social security. It is to be noted that most of the migrant workers are engaged in construction sector, rickshaw pullers, street vendors among others. They occupy the bottom of the informal employment pyramid – making them a sizable vulnerable group in the informal sector. Further, they are vulnerable in terms of low wage/income and security. Therefore, host state should provide all the basic socio-economic securities to the migrants as they are one of the most important service providers to the city. This will assure workers with basic needs. At least workers will be protected against facing homelessness in the urban areas.

NITI Aayog, a think tank of the Government of India, along with working subgroup and civil society prepared a draft national migrant labour policy in 2021. This was much needed. However, it took a nationwide lockdown during the COVID-19 pandemic to recognise the plight of an invisible workforce that contributes in no small measure to the nation's economy. A number of recommendations have been drafted in the draft policy. These are central database of internal migration, increases of minimum wages for migrant workers, skill-building among migrant workers, and grievance redressal mechanism among others. These are important points that are raised but one should realise that we have a number of policies and acts. What we need is amendment. For instance, the Inter State Migrant Workers Act, 1979, is already in place but it is not amended. One should remember that migrant workers are vulnerable to various health risks in the urban areas. Ensuring minimum wage will not help much. Cost of living in the urban areas is more as compared to rural areas. Therefore, living wage needs to be calculated and universal health insurance coverage should be introduced for the migrant workers in the city.

Informal sector is the worst hit by the pandemic as about 91% workforce are engaged in this sector. Within informal economy, migrant and female workers are the most vulnerable. As compared to men, women always become the first victim to any crisis. In COVID-19 pandemic, women working in retail, hospitality industry including hotels and restaurants, domestic work, and manufacturing industries went through job losses. Further, several reports unfold that domestic violence against women has significantly increased globally during lockdown as women co-share the space with the abusers. However, we witnessed that women were tirelessly involved in the care economy as frontline workers, healthcare providers, community workers, and volunteers at the ground during the pandemic. Therefore, it becomes even more pertinent to have gender equality while restoring the economy.

Equal opportunity in the job market and equal payment should be provided. Informal sector workers are engaged at the workforce without any social protection. Thus, there is a need for tailor-made social assistance and social insurance schemes for all categories of workers in the informal economy. There should be universal insurance provided by employers, especially for migrant workers. Equal amount of ration for both male and female workers should be arranged for and vaccination drives should be organised for migrant workers (male and female) in cities. National urban employment guarantee scheme should also be introduced like national rural employment guarantee scheme but with greater emphasis on increasing gender parity and representation.

References

Action Aid India (2020), *Workers in the Time of COVID-19, Round II of the National Study on Informal Workers*, India, Action Aid Association.

APU (Azim Premji University) (2020), *COVID-19 Livelihoods Survey, Early Findings From Phone Surveys*, Bengaluru: Azim Premji University.

Breman, Jan (1996), *Footloose Labour: Working in India's Informal Economy*, Cambridge: Cambridge University Press.

Breman, Jan (2007), *Labour Bondage in West India: From Past to Present*, New Delhi: Oxford University Press.

Breman, Jan (2013), *At Work in the Informal Economy of India. A Perspective From the Bottom Up*, New Delhi: Oxford University Press.

CMIE (Centre for Monitoring Indian Economy) (2020), *Unemployment in India: A Statistical Profile*, January–April, Mumbai: Centre for Monitoring Indian Economy Pvt. Ltd.

CMIE (Centre for Monitoring Indian Economy) (2020), *Unemployment in India: A Statistical Profile*, May–August, Mumbai: Centre for Monitoring Indian Economy Pvt. Ltd.

CMIE (Centre for Monitoring Indian Economy) (2019), *Unemployment in India: A Statistical Profile*, September–December, Mumbai: Centre for Monitoring Indian Economy Pvt. Ltd.

CMIE (Centre for Monitoring Indian Economy) (2020), *Unemployment in India: A Statistical Profile*, Mumbai: Centre for Monitoring Indian Economy Pvt. Ltd.

Fields, Gary S. (1975), "Rural-urban migration, urban unemployment and underemployment, and job-search activity in LDCs", *Journal of Development Economics*, 2(2), 165–187.

Gang, Ira N. and Gangopadhyay, Shubhashis (1987a), "Employment, output and the choice of techniques: The trade-off revisited", *Journal of Development Economics*, 25(2), 321–327.

Gang, Ira N. and Gangopadhyay, Shubhashis (1987b), "Optimal policies in a dual economy with open unemployment and surplus labour", *Oxford Economic Papers*, 39(2), 378–387.

Guha-Khasnobis, Basudeb, Kanbur, Ravi and Ostrom, Elinor (eds) (2006), *Linking the Formal and Informal Economy: Concepts and Policies*, New York: Oxford University Press.

Harris, John R. and Todaro, Michael P. (1970), "Migration, unemployment and development: A two-sector analysis", *American Economic Review*, 60(1), 126–142.

Hart, Keith (1973), "Informal income opportunities and urban employment in Ghana", *Journal of Modern African Studies*, 11(1), 61–89.

Kundu, Amitabh (2018), "Mobility in India: Recent trends and issues concerning database", *Social Change*, 48(4), 634–644.

Ministry of Railways (2020a), "Indian railways operationalizes 4197 Shramik special trains", https://pib.gov.in/PressReleasePage.aspx?PRID=1629043, accessed 6 April 2021.

Ministry of Railways (2020b), "Indian railways continue to give Shramik special trains to states as demanded", https://pib.gov.in/PressReleasePage.aspx?PRID=1631092, accessed 6 April 2021.

National Sample Survey Office (NSSO) (2006), *Employment and Unemployment Situation in India, 61st Round*, New Delhi: Ministry of Statistics and Programme Implementation.

National Sample Survey Office (NSSO) (2013), *Employment and Unemployment Situation in India, 68th Round*, New Delhi: Ministry of Statistics and Programme Implementation.

National Sample Survey Office (NSSO) (2020), *NSS Report: Time Use in India – 2019*, New Delhi: Ministry of Statistics and Programme Implementation.
Periodic Labour Force Survey (PLFS) (2019), *Annual Report, PLFS 2017–18*, New Delhi: Ministry of Statistics and Programme Implementation.
Periodic Labour Force Survey (PLFS) (2020), *Annual Report, PLFS 2018–19*, New Delhi: Ministry of Statistics and Programme Implementation.
Revi, A., Ray, M., Mitra, S., Anand, S., Sami, N. and Malladi, T. (2020), *Report to the XV Finance Commission on the Potential of Urbanisation to Accelerate Post-COVID Economic Recovery*, India, Indian Institute for Human Settlements.
Standing, Guy (1997), "Globalization, labour flexibility and insecurity: The era of market regulation", *European Journal of Industrial Relations*, 3(1), 7–37.
Stranded Workers Action Network (SWAN) (2020), *To Leave or Not Leave? Lockdown, Migrant Workers, and Their Journeys Home*, Stranded Workers Action Network (SWAN) (2020), "Migrant workers", *The Hindu*, 27 May, www.thehindu.com/news/national/other-states/migrant-workers-video-of-baby-with-dead-mother-in-bihar-railway-station-goes-viral/article31685803.ece/amp/, accessed 20 September 2020.
The Wire (2020a), "Not just the Aurangabad accident, 383 people have died due to the punitive lockdown", 10 May, https://m.thewire.in/article/rights/migrant-workers-non-coronavirus-lockdown-deaths/amp.
The Wire (2020b),"To appease builders' lobby, Karnataka cancels trains for migrant workers", 6 May, https://thewire.in/government/karnataka-trains-migrant-workers, accessed on 6 May 2020.

3 Effect of COVID-19 on the Economy of North Eastern Region of India

An Assessment

Rajdeep Singha

Introduction

The COVID-19 outbreak in many ways is a distinctive shock to the whole world. It is not only a health crisis but also an economic disaster for most of the economies around the world. One of the most prominent responses among the countries to stop the spread of the virus has been the lockdown of economic activities. India announced a nationwide lockdown on 24 March 2020. The urban centres of India were hit the hardest with very low economic activity in comparison to the rural areas (Dev and Sengupta, 2020). Rural areas opened up relatively quickly. The impact of this virus has varied between countries and has even varied among the different regions of the same country. From cross-country evidence, it was very clear that the poor and the marginalised regions have been the worst affected. Within India, the North Eastern region is one of the long-neglected backward regions. This chapter tried to understand the economic impact of COVID on the North Eastern region of India.

The World Bank predicted that the impact of COVID on annual world GDP is around –2 to –4% (Maliszewska et al., 2020). According to IMF (2021), projected India's GDP growth rate for the year 2021 is 11.5%, which is significantly higher than the emerging market and developing economics, that is 6.3%. Among the developing economies, India is worst hit by the pandemic. In 2020, the annual real GDP growth rate of India was negative 10.3 (IMF DataMapper, 2020). This pandemic hit India when GDP was growing slowly and unemployment was very high. The situation of the economy worsened due to the COVID shock. According to the Oxfam report, global inequality has increased manyfold due to the pandemic. It was predicted that India's inequality levels would fall back to the pre-independence level. India was able to reduce a significant amount of inequality till the 1980s but it has been on the rise since then (Chancel and Piketty, 2019). COVID is now popularly cited as the "pandemic of inequality" or as Oxfam said "The inequality virus" (Berkhout et al., 2021) An estimate by the Food and Agriculture Organization (FAO) suggests that COVID-19 may cause a rise

DOI: 10.4324/9781003282815-5

in each country's Gini by at least two per cent. António Guterres, Secretary-General of the United Nations, said:

> The COVID-19 pandemic has played an important role in highlighting growing inequalities. It exposed the myth that everyone is in the same boat. While we are all floating on the same sea, it's clear that some are in super yachts, while others are clinging to the drifting debris.
>
> (Guterres, 2020)

The chapter is organised into three sections. The first section has tried to assess/evaluate the magnitude of the effect of the Coronavirus on the economy of North East India by using a high-frequency variable, that is electricity consumption. The second section is about the pre-COVID economy of the North Eastern states. The impact on government finance, banking sector, and labour market is discussed in the third section followed by the conclusion.

Understanding the Magnitude of the Impact

Understanding the shock of this magnitude needs longitudinal data. In the absence of longitudinal data, this section accesses the impact through high-frequency data like demand for electricity or demand for consumable goods. It is assumed that economic growth and electricity demand are positively correlated. With an increase in economic activity, there is always an increase in energy demand. It is true since the time of the industrial revolution. The energy demand can broadly be segregated into two parts; first is the household consumption and second is the demand for production. Within last few decades, the access to modern appliances has increased many folds and the energy demand will continue to increase. On the other hand, one of the significant demands comes from business. It is true for inter-temporal as well as inter-region. The developed region of the country demands more energy compared to the less-developed region. For example, according to the Power System Operation Corporation (POSOCO), Government of India's data, in January 2019, out of a total of India's electricity demand, 60% was from the northern and western regions, whereas the demand of the North East was only about 1.5% (POSOCO, 2020).

In the same logic, demand for electricity can be used as a very important indicator of economic activities. At the all-India level, demand declined to 30% below last year's levels (Dev and Sengupta, 2020). In Figure 3.1, it is clear that there are similar impacts on the North East region also. In comparison to March 2019, the demand for electricity decreased by 68 MW in March 2020. The highest dip was recorded in April 2020, that is 368 MW. The economy started recovering slowly from July 2020 (Figure 3.1).

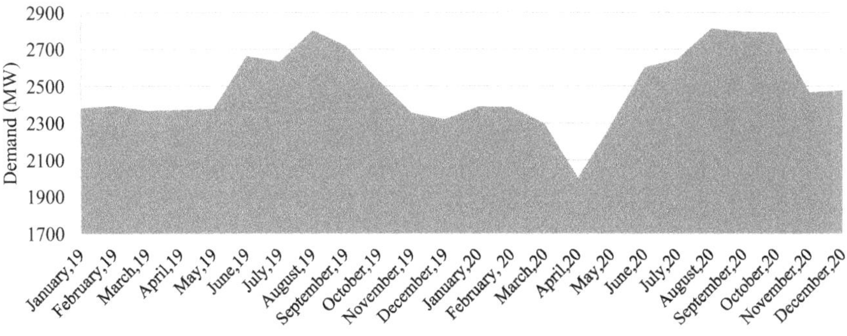

Figure 3.1 Evening Peak Hour Electricity Demand in North East

Source: Various monthly reports, POSOCO (*Sikkim is not included)

The Economy of North East India

Since 2015–16, the Indian economy was primarily experiencing a slowdown. The growth rate of GDP was reported at 4.2% in the year 2019–20, which is low since 2002–03. The pandemic disrupted both demand and supply. The GDP performance of individual states varies due to various region-specific variables. Between 2017–18 and 2018–19, except Meghalaya and Nagaland, the growth rate of all the North Eastern states was on the downwards trend. For example, in the same periods, the growth rate of Manipur decreased from 9.77% to 2.93%. The data for 2019–20 is only available for Meghalaya, Sikkim, and Tripura. Other than Sikkim, which shows slightly positive growth, the other two are again negative for that period. Agriculture is the only sector which shows some positive outcome during COVID crisis. According to the Central Statistics Office (CSO) data, except for the states of Sikkim and Manipur, there is a downward trend of value-added which was observed in agriculture (Table 3.1). It is important to note here that the activities, which were disrupted due to the lockdown, are contributing around 30% to 50% of the total value added (only Sikkim is below 30%) (Table 3.1).

The per-capita GSDP growth rate is another indicator to understand the signs of progress of a state. Similar to GSDP, Meghalaya's per-capita growth rate increased from 2% in 2017–18 to 7% in 2018–19. The per capita GSDP of Sikkim dropped by 9% in 2018–19 and Tripura is constantly growing at a 9% rate. From Table 3.2, it is clear that as a region, there is a decreasing trend in the last few financial years. At the all-India level and at the regional level, almost all sectors of the economy, except agriculture, posted a decline. GDP growth is necessary to generate virtuous circles of prosperity and opportunity. There are enough cross-country shreds of evidence that

Table 3.1 Net State Value Added by Economic Activity (in %) (At Constant Prices 2011–2012)

State /Year	*Agriculture, Forestry, and Fishing*	*Mining and Quarrying*	*Manu-facturing*	*Electricity, Gas, Water supply, & Other utility Services*	*Constru-ction*	*Trade, Repair, Hotels, and Restaurants*	*Transport, Storage, Communi cation, & Services Related to Broadcasting*	*Financial Services*	*Real Estate, Ownership of Dwelling & Professional Services*	*Public Adminis-tration*	*Other Services*
ARUNACHAL PRADESH											
2015–16	39.80	3.11	3.24	5.58	10.88	3.94	2.46	2.32	2.61	12.04	14.02
2016–17	33.38	4.27	3.64	6.32	11.11	5.41	2.42	2.07	2.66	12.60	16.13
2017–18	31.43	3.32	3.40	6.68	11.37	5.16	2.21	2.09	2.45	13.90	17.99
2018–19	30.04	3.32	4.23	6.37	11.89	5.12	2.52	2.00	2.35	13.66	18.51
ASSAM											
2015–16	19.69	13.38	13.36	1.21	9.03	13.57	5.91	3.74	5.52	6.57	8.02
2016–17	19.45	12.59	15.71	1.29	9.87	12.44	5.07	3.65	5.21	4.90	9.83
2017–18	18.20	12.59	16.34	1.75	9.52	12.50	4.59	3.69	4.82	6.15	9.86
2018–19	17.32	13.65	16.56	1.60	10.28	11.79	4.19	3.50	4.62	5.68	10.82
MANIPUR											
2015–16	17.46	NA	3.04	2.57	13.21	16.12	6.32	2.42	7.66	15.44	15.76
2016–17	18.21	NA	3.10	3.23	10.79	17.05	6.96	2.42	7.16	14.06	17.03
2017–18	24.62	NA	2.65	2.78	10.13	16.91	6.23	2.26	6.08	11.77	16.57
2018–19	22.05	NA	2.59	3.27	9.47	18.01	6.15	2.30	6.41	12.97	16.80
MEGHALAYA											
2015–16	20.28	6.35	6.65	1.59	7.06	23.43	5.51	3.88	6.43	9.29	9.53
2016–17	20.29	4.05	8.23	1.13	6.06	25.55	5.19	3.81	5.62	9.48	10.60
2017–18	19.15	3.37	9.97	1.06	6.18	26.64	4.48	3.76	5.26	9.31	10.83
2018–19	17.49	3.58	9.54	1.70	6.94	26.75	3.84	3.46	4.84	11.64	10.23
2019–20	16.31	3.55	10.34	1.73	7.22	28.16	3.88	3.28	4.47	11.32	9.75

MIZORAM											
2015–16	30.74	0.40	0.80	6.66	10.74	11.71	3.74	2.90	3.38	14.53	14.40
2016–17	29.80	0.26	0.80	7.39	10.81	13.45	3.48	2.27	3.21	14.25	14.30
2017–18	25.79	0.34	0.71	9.48	11.48	15.08	3.31	2.17	3.21	13.87	14.56
2018–19	24.55	0.35	0.67	9.57	11.34	15.12	3.41	2.26	3.14	15.04	14.55
NAGALAND											
2015–16	29.11	1.34	1.45	1.70	7.99	9.96	5.00	3.99	7.87	16.53	15.06
2016–17	30.23	0.29	1.65	1.71	7.97	9.27	5.09	3.75	7.19	16.79	16.07
2017–18	27.13	0.17	1.60	2.37	8.39	11.12	4.97	3.77	6.82	16.90	16.77
2018–19	25.31	0.14	1.64	2.36	8.13	11.99	5.22	3.45	6.27	18.71	16.79
SIKKIM											
2015–16	7.49	0.09	46.90	10.58	5.66	4.65	3.07	3.08	3.25	5.85	9.39
2016–17	7.72	0.09	49.79	9.98	4.76	4.64	3.27	1.88	3.16	5.50	9.22
2017–18	8.28	0.09	50.45	10.36	4.62	4.88	2.91	1.70	2.95	5.17	8.60
2018–19	8.02	0.08	49.02	11.07	4.60	5.02	2.71	1.61	2.86	6.74	8.30
2019–20	8.03	0.08	49.38	11.00	4.45	5.09	2.67	1.52	2.75	7.02	8.01
TRIPURA											
2015–16	30.20	12.97	4.31	3.13	6.73	9.24	3.77	5.02	4.60	10.03	10.00
2016–17	28.13	12.56	5.24	3.51	7.46	9.59	3.58	3.60	4.86	12.09	9.38
2017–18	25.83	10.96	4.05	4.11	6.77	12.73	2.93	3.97	6.39	10.67	11.59
2018–19	25.05	11.68	4.04	3.79	7.60	12.54	2.63	3.36	6.03	13.22	10.05
2019–20	24.23	11.37	4.09	3.87	7.96	12.39	2.54	3.19	5.70	13.80	10.86

Source: Handbook of Statistics on Indian States 2019–20, RBI

Table 3.2 Year-on-Year Growth Rate of per Capita GSDP (in per cent) 2011–12 Series

Year	*ARUNACHAL PRADESH*	*ASSAM*	*MANI-PUR*	*MEGHA-LAYA*	*MIZO-RAM*	*NAGA-LAND*	*SIK-KIM*	*TRI-PURA*
2012–2013	0	2	-2	0	5	5	1	8
2013–2014	7	4	6	0	14	6	5	8
2014–2015	14	6	6	-5	23	3	7	17
2015–2016	-3	14	5	0	8	1	9	-2
2016–2017	2	4	2	3	8	7	6	13
2017–2018	6	8	7	2	8	5	14	9
2018–2019	3	5	1	7	1	6	5	9
2019–2020	NA	NA	NA	6	NA	NA	6	9

Source: Handbook of Statistics on Indian States 2019–20, RBI

the insufficient growth coupled with the lack of demand has led to lowering of the living standards of the common people. The lack of demand reduces the average income of businesses, which then signals a plunge in job opportunities. A fall in GDP affects the poor more, and inequality becomes inevitable. According to a global baseline scenario, the impact of the pandemic on Gross Domestic Product has fallen by 2% below the benchmark. The impact on GDP is more for the developing countries, that is 2.5% compared to the industrial countries, that is 1.8%. Tables 3.1 and 3.2 suggest that at the time when COVID hit the North East economy, the health of the economy was already not in a sound position.

Effects of COVID

Government Finance

COVID presented many problems for the Government then they had ever faced. On the one hand, it has increased the government expenditure; on the other hand, it has lowered the government income. Globally, in the first three months of the pandemic, government expenditure in terms of the intervention was around US$9 trillion. As per estimates of the multilateral lender, the fiscal deficit of India in the year 2020–21 will increase to 13.1% from 8.2% of GDP in 2019–20, that is increase of 4.9% points. According to the International Monetary Fund (IMF), the Government of India's financial support to the COVID crisis can be divided into two parts:

(i) "Above-the-line measures": Government spending of around 3.2% of GDP, of which 2.2% of GDP is expected in the current fiscal year and foregone or deferred revenues of about 0.3% of GDP.
(ii) "Below-the-line measures": To support businesses, about 5.2% of GDP is channelisation for loans to different economic activities.

The above-the-line measure responses are mainly of two types: (a) transfer of kind (food, cooking gas) and (b) transfer of cash to the low-wage households, insurance for health workers. The IMF data shows that the Indian fiscal response has been more about the second type (IMF, 2021).

The fiscal impulse of the first type was around 1.8% of the GDP, whereas the second type of financial support was amounting to 5.2% of the GDP. Therefore, India's fiscal response looks more like the developed economies rather than the developing countries. The central government allocated Rs. 350 billion as budget allocation for health and well-being, including a provision for the country's COVID-19 vaccination programme in the financial year 2021–22. According to the Economic Survey 2021, the capital expenditure between April and December 2020 was Rs. 3.17 lakh crore, which was 24% higher than the capital expenditure between April and December 2019 (Economic Survey, 2021).

The Central Bank of India has also made available relief measures for both the borrowers and the lenders and for the Securities and Exchange Board of India (SEBI) by temporarily relaxing the norms and regulations concerning debt defaults on rated instruments and reduced the requirements for the market capitalisation of shareholding and the period of listing.

The state of the financial institutions leaves very little policy space available to the government to deal with the economic crisis. At the time of the Global Financial Crisis of 2008, India was also impacted but due to the better performance of the domestic economy, government was able to adopt and implement both monetary and fiscal stimulus measures.

This section analyses the finances of the North Eastern states as reflected in their budgets for 2020–21. It is important to note that most states brought

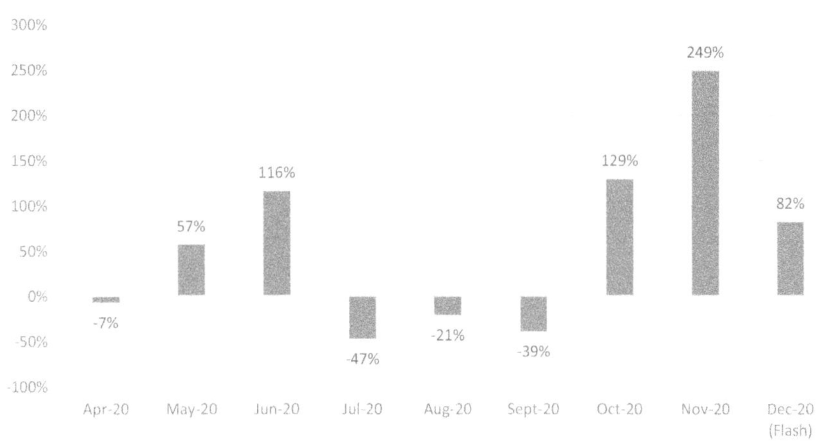

Figure 3.2 Growth (YoY) in Monthly Expenditure During FY 2020–21

Source: Economic Survey, 2021

out their respective budgets in February-March 2020, that is before the outbreak of COVID-19 in India. Hence, it is accepted that the budget estimates (BE) are very likely to get revised. However, the analysis assumes that the budgets were prepared to keep the crisis in mind as an early warning started coming from different parts of the world in January 2020 itself. It is needless to say that the state governments are in the front line of the fight against the pandemic (RBI, 2020).

The North Eastern states mostly budgeted gross fiscal deficit (GFD) as a percentage to GSDP (below 3%) except Manipur (6.6%) and Meghalaya (3.6%). Other than Mizoram, the ratio of gross fiscal deficit (GFC) to GSDP of all the North Eastern states is above the all-India average. Between 2018–19 and 2019–20, the GFD-GSDP ratio worsened for Tripura, that is increase from 2.1 to 2.8.

Since the data of the financial year 2020–21 is not available, to understand the probable impact of COVID, it will be fascinating to compare pre-COVID and the global financial crisis data. Indian economy began to slow down in 2007–08 (April–March) after reaching a GDP growth of 9.8% in the last quarter of 2006–07. The Indian economy grew at an annual average rate of 8.8% during the five years ending 2007–08. On the contrary, the growth rate of GDP growth slowed down to 4.2% in 2019–20. Indian economy performed relatively well during the crisis due to the good performance of the Indian economy before the financial crisis. The economy not only did good performance at the central level but many states also performed well during the same time. In other words, there were fiscal spaces available with the central as well as the state governments to deal with crisis.

The average data of 2003 to 2006 suggests that the median value of revenue surplus to GSDP ratio rose from 3.2% to 5.4% for the special category states.[1] Sikkim had the highest revenue surplus-GSDP ratio of 23.4% in 2006–07 (RE), but at the same time had the highest GFD-GSDP ratio of 10.5%. For the entire special category states among which majority are the North Eastern states, the median value of the GFD-GSDP ratio declined from 8.1% to 5.8% during the above period. The primary revenue surplus[2] remained adequate for all the North Eastern states, except Assam in 2006–07 (RE).

The financial health of many of the North Eastern states was better before the global financial crisis hit India (Table 3.3). In all the states except Assam, the revenue surplus was more than 5% of the GSDP. Sikkim and Manipur were in much better position with almost 15 and 30% revenue surpluses.

Labour Market

The COVID crisis, which initially began as a health crisis, quickly turned into a labour market crisis with an unprecedented magnitude. An initial estimate by ILO suggests that globally there were 7% losses in working hours but within a month, the loss increased to 14%. These losses of the labour

Table 3.3 Deficit Indicators of State Governments

	2006–07 (RE)			*2018–19 (RE)*			*2019–20 (BE)*		
	RD/ GSDP	*GFD/ GSDP*	*PD/ GSDP*	*RD/ GSDP*	*GFD/ GSDP*	*PD/ GSDP*	*RD/ GSDP*	*GFD/ GSDP*	*PD/ GSDP*
Arunachal Pradesh	−12.5	7.7	1.4	−26.5	4.3	2.0	−29.1	2.0	−0.4
Assam	1.2	7.2	3.0	−2.4	3.0	1.7	−0.9	3.1	1.7
Manipur	−14.8	4.3	−0.9	0.0	11.9	9.5	−1.3	6.6	4.3
Meghalaya	−5.4	1.4	−2.0	−1.5	3.5	1.5	−2.0	3.6	1.6
Mizoram	−5.1	8.3	1.8	−2.4	7.6	5.8	−5.6	2.1	0.7
Nagaland	−5.5	5.3	1.6	−2.0	5.1	2.1	−1.8	3.0	-0.1
Sikkim	−23.4	10.5	4.4	−3.3	3.4	1.7	−0.9	2.8	1.0
Tripura	−5.3	4.6	0.7	−3.2	2.1	0.5	−1.6	2.8	1.2
All States	**0.1**	**2.8**	**0.4**	**0.1**	**2.9**	**1.2**	**0.0**	**2.6**	**0.9**

Source: RBI (2020)

RE: Revised Estimates, BE: Budget Estimates, RD: Revenue Deficit, GFD: Gross Fiscal Deficit PD: Primary Deficit, GSDP: Gross State Domestic Product.

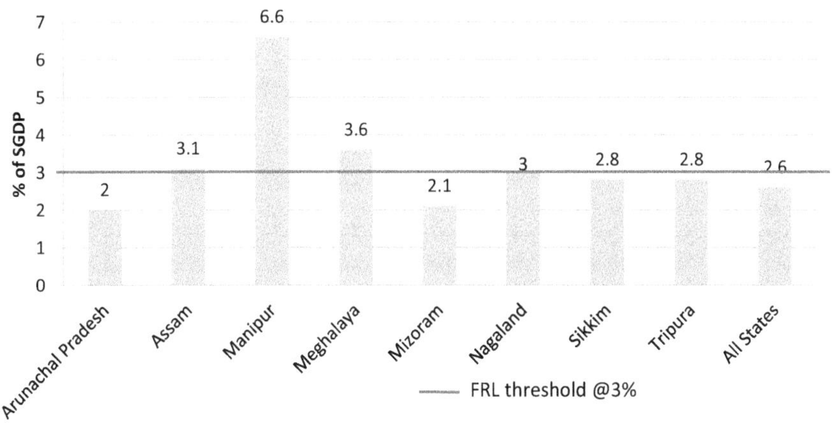

Figure 3.3 State-Wise GFD-SGDP Ration in 2019–20 (BE)

Source: RBI (2020)

market are measured by inactivity, unemployment, temporary suspension of work, or shorter hours. According to estimates, the loss was equivalent to 400 million full-time jobs (assuming a 48-hour working week). There are regional variations but all regions in the globe saw more than 10% losses (Lee, 2020)

India is no exception to global trends. According to the Centre for Monitoring Indian Economy (CMIE) data, close to 10.9 million jobs were lost across sectors and the year was termed the worst-ever year for the job

Table 3.4 Distribution of North Eastern States by the level of Gross Fiscal Deficit/GSDP Ratio

Range (%)	*2003–06 (Avg.)*	*2006–07 (RE)*
1 to 3	Nagaland, Assam, Tripura	Meghalaya
3 to 6	Meghalaya	Nagaland, Manipur, Tripura
6 to 9	Sikkim, Manipur	Assam, Mizoram, Arunachal Pradesh
Above 9	Mizoram, Arunachal Pradesh	Sikkim

Source: Author's calculation

Table 3.5 Labour Participation Rate and Unemployment Rate of Some of the North Eastern States

State	*Jan–April, 2019/ Jan–April,2020*			*May–August, 2019/ May–August, 2020*			*Sept-Dec, 2019/ Sept-Dec, 2020*		
	Total	*Urban*	*Rural*	*Total*	*Urban*	*Rural*	*Total*	*Urban*	*Rural*
LPR[3]									
Assam	−1.27	−2.89	−0.96	−6.91	−5.15	−7.25	−1.44	−4.64	−0.83
Meghalaya	0.01	−1.78	0.54	−1.63	−4.22	−0.86	17.59	7.68	17.38
Sikkim	−4.81	−7.23	−3.44	−2.93	−6.76	−0.6	−1.85	−5.84	0.66
Tripura	0.8	−0.86	1.51	−8.08	−9.21	−7.6	−12.26	−13.22	−11.86
India	**−1.87**	**−2.6**	**−1.5**	**−2.64**	**−3.13**	**−2.38**	**−2.19**	**−2.86**	**−1.84**
UER[4]									
Assam	−1.18	0.82	−1.52	−0.06	−1.48	0.19	−1.52	−5.25	−0.87
Meghalaya	−0.19	−0.63	−0.05	0.09	−0.33	0.26	−1.07	0.69	−0.26
Sikkim	−2.29	4.86	−6.68	1.46	4.53	−0.38	−3.78	−3.42	−3.97
Tripura	5.36	2.57	6.47	−4.06	−3.52	−4.24	−13.02	−14.85	−12.28
India	**3.53**	**4.86**	**2.93**	**4.09**	**4.26**	**4.02**	**−0.44**	**−1.2**	**−0.05**

Source: CMIE various reports

market in India since Independence. CMIE showed that the unemployment rate rose sharply to 9.1%, in December 2020 at the all-India level (CMIE, 2020)

The CMIE gives data for four North Eastern states, that is Assam, Meghalaya, Sikkim, and Tripura, and therefore the analysis of this section is based on these four states. The two most popular indicators to understand the labour markets are the Labour Participation Rate (LPR) and the Unemployment Rate (UER). In terms of LPR, the urban labour market was disrupted more than the rural labour market by the lockdown if one evaluates all the quadrimester of Meghalaya, Sikkim, and Tripura. For example, between May and August 2020, the LPR decreased by 4.22 in urban Meghalaya against May–August 2019 although the decrease in rural Meghalaya was 0.86. In the context of Assam, the impact of Corona is higher in the rural areas than in the urban areas but in the third quadrimester, the recovery is faster in the rural than in the urban areas. Among the four states of the North East, the worst affected state in terms of employment is Tripura. Between September and December 2020, the contraction of the unemployment rate was 14.85 in urban Tripura and 12.28 in rural Tripura. The unemployment rate in Tripura has been always high in comparison to the rest of the North East (Singha, 2018). During the same period, the labour force participation rate of rural Meghalaya was more than 17, which is the highest among all the North Eastern states.

Banking Sector

The banking sector plays a vital role in any economy and development economics in particular. A bigger role is assumed in the time of crisis. The quality performance of the banking sector helps an economy to recover quickly and can boost sustainable economic performances. At the macro level, loans disbursed[5] by banks in India as against deposits have constantly declined in 2020. The main reasons behind this decline are excess liquidity in the economy and lack of demand for credit. According to RBI data, the credit-deposit (CD) ratio has consistently declined from 75% to 71.3% between January and December 2020. As mentioned earlier, CD ratio falls due to excess liquidity and lack of alternatives in credit markets (Ghosh, 2020).

Historically the CD ratio is always less in North Eastern states compared to the rest of India. The impact started becoming clear in the month of April 2020 as credit growth dropped. The quarter-to-quarter comparison suggests that except for Nagaland, a declining trend was observed among the North Eastern states. Due to the sudden lockdown and insecurity about the future, the deposit rate to the bank increased significantly. In the whole North Eastern region, against the second quarter of 2019–20, rural and semi-urban CD ratio decreased from 53.43 to 49.71 and 44.71 to 43.03, respectively. On the contrary, the urban CD ratio increased from 35.45 to 36.82% in the same periods.

According to RBI, the purpose of credit is divided into two broad categories, that is food and non-food. The non-food categories include agriculture and allied activities, industry (micro and small, medium and large), services, and personal loans. Figure 3.4, at the all-India level, suggests that there was a rise in the credit for food purpose in 2020 in comparison to the last two years. In December 2020, the non-food credit was 99.01% of the total, which is the lowest in the last two years. It is expected that the broad all-India level trend is followed in the North Eastern region also.

According to the OECD data, since the end of December 2019, bank deposits have increased significantly in both developing and developed countries, far more than the average of the last five years. The same trend can also be noticed in the Indian context. Estimates by RBI indicate that household financial savings jumped to 21.4% of GDP in the first quarter (April–June) of 2020–21, up from 7.9% in the same period a year ago and

Table 3.6 C-D Ratio of North Eastern States (in per cent)

	2020–21:Q2			*2020–21:Q1*			*2019–20:Q2*			*2019–20:Q1*		
	Rural	*Semi-urban*	*Urban*	*Rural*	*Semi-urban*	*Urban*	*Rural*	*Semi-urban*	*Urban*	*Rural*	*Semi-urban*	*Urban*
ARUNACHAL PRADESH	21.78	24.63	0.00	21.35	23.62	0.00	24.73	27.65	0.00	20.22	25.03	0.00
ASSAM	54.43	48.12	37.71	52.85	46.99	35.93	59.27	49.83	36.36	57.10	48.91	38.45
MANIPUR	59.43	67.16	50.49	63.12	69.56	47.82	63.58	63.20	53.20	68.07	82.90	50.18
MEGHALAYA	41.77	32.89	35.42	43.51	34.40	33.34	45.46	33.85	24.18	43.35	32.70	22.40
MIZORAM	40.94	52.45	30.82	37.69	50.36	29.29	42.33	55.12	32.04	43.81	60.95	31.21
NAGALAND	67.87	32.58	35.41	66.06	30.61	34.70	68.23	34.35	39.01	65.89	32.90	37.15
TRIPURA	47.28	52.08	29.44	46.70	52.49	27.30	46.08	50.04	34.75	46.46	48.91	36.14
SIKKIM	29.61	27.39	31.00	29.61	32.00	30.00	32.00	41.00	31.00	32.00	38.00	27.00
NORTH EASTERN REGION	49.71	43.03	36.82	48.91	42.03	34.98	53.43	44.71	35.45	51.56	43.64	36.42

Source: Handbook of Statistics on Indian States 2019–20, RBI

Note: Q1= April to June & Q2= July to Sep

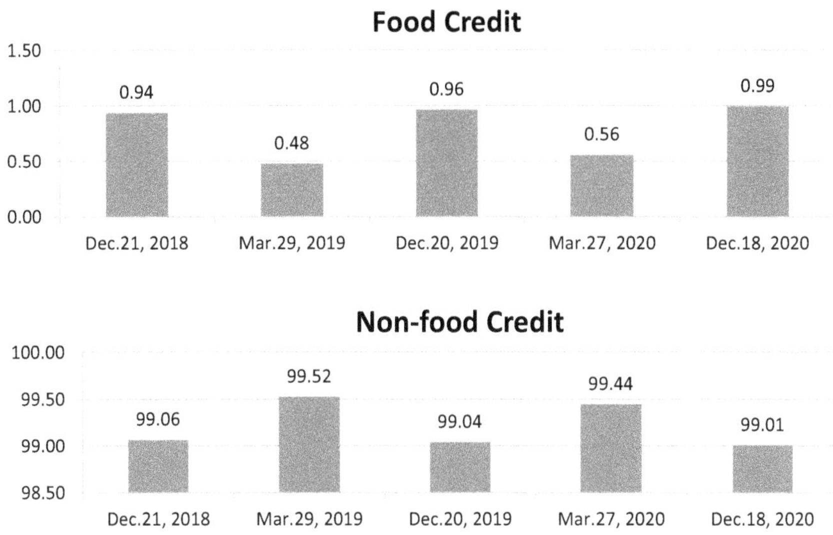

Figure 3.4 Food Credit and Non-Food Credit

Source: Handbook of Statistics on Indian States 2019–20, RBI (2020)

10% in the previous quarter (January–March) of 2019–20 (Nayak, 2020). One of the most popular views on why deposits surged during the COVID-19 pandemic is the precautionary savings view. This view suggests that as the pandemic deepened, concerns about economic disruptions and layoffs (Acharya and Steffen, 2020) led to households boosting savings as a precaution against declines in future income, and some of those additional savings flowed into bank deposits (Browning and Lusardi, 1996).

From Table 3.7, at the all-India level in comparison to the first quarter (April–June) 2019, in 2020, the saving rate increased. Rural saving increased more than in semi-urban or urban areas. One of the probable reasons was that the announcement of lockdown made purchases impossible and some relief measures by the government helped a household to increase savings and bank deposits. But this effect was temporary and as step-by-step containment measures were lifted gradually, the pent-up demand was satisfied in quarter two and the rate of savings decreased. But overall deposit rate remained above the average rate over the same period in 2020. State-wise analysis suggests that the saving rate increased among the North Eastern states except for rural Manipur and Mizoram.

It is also interesting to note that the current and time deposit is negative for most of the states. The negative growth rate current account reflects the poor performances of business sectors and negative terms deposit suggests people's liquidity preferences. Rural term deposits of Manipur, Mizoram,

Table 3.7 Percentage Change in Distribution of Deposits

	Rural			*Semi-urban*			*Urban*		
	Current	*Savings*	*Terms*	*Current*	*Savings*	*Terms*	*Current*	*Savings*	*Terms*
Between 2020–21:Q1 and 2019–20:Q1									
ARUNACHAL PRADESH	−3.16	3.44	−0.28	−3.16	2.51	0.64	NA	NA	NA
ASSAM	−0.07	2.18	−2.11	−0.15	1.13	−0.98	−0.06	0.02	0.05
MANIPUR	−2.24	−0.62	2.83	−0.50	4.22	−3.63	−0.21	5.81	-5.59
MEGHALAYA	−1.46	1.45	0.02	−1.08	1.67	−0.60	−0.33	4.84	-4.51
MIZORAM	−1.47	−5.66	7.13	−0.95	−2.38	3.29	1.23	-2.44	1.23
NAGALAND	−0.03	2.17	−2.23	−1.43	2.88	−1.44	0.80	1.62	-2.44
TRIPURA	0.73	1.68	−2.39	−2.35	0.59	1.76	0.94	2.22	-3.17
SIKKIM	−0.20	0.99	−0.81	−1.61	−2.12	3.79	0.01	-3.10	3.06
INDIA	0.04	1.31	−1.35	−0.19	0.81	−0.63	−0.04	0.24	-0.20
Between 2020–21:Q2 and 2019–20:Q2									
ARUNACHAL PRADESH	−0.84	3.12	−2.29	−1.18	1.00	0.19	NA	NA	NA
ASSAM	−0.31	1.02	−0.71	−0.28	0.12	0.16	−1.08	0.92	0.16
MANIPUR	0.12	1.04	−1.14	−1.99	12.44	−10.45	−0.22	2.97	-2.73
MEGHALAYA	0.07	0.91	−0.99	−3.42	2.53	0.89	2.65	4.13	-6.79
MIZORAM	−1.18	−1.62	2.86	0.74	−4.52	3.77	−0.07	-0.82	0.91
NAGALAND	−1.66	5.16	−3.48	0.83	4.36	−5.18	0.26	1.11	-1.38
TRIPURA	0.46	2.02	−2.47	−1.67	0.74	0.92	0.40	2.86	-3.26
SIKKIM	0.39	1.68	−2.05	9.19	−8.31	−0.95	−2.97	-1.72	4.70
INDIA	−0.05	0.97	−0.92	−0.28	0.85	−0.57	0.06	0.43	-0.50

Source: Handbook of Statistics on Indian States 2019–20, RBI

Note: Q1= April to June & Q2= July to Sep

and Meghalaya were positive in the first quarter but Manipur and Meghalaya's growth rate of term deposit became negative in the second quarter. It is quite clear from the table that the effect of lockdown varied between rural, semi-urban, and urban areas. The volatility and uncertainty of the pandemic and unclear future economic prospects have motivated individuals for precautionary saving, crowd out investment, and postpone purchases of durable goods. Theoretically, there is a positive correlation between changes in the uncertainty of income and precautionary savings of individual (Mody et al., 2012). The lockdown was also likely to change the consumption patterns of the non-poor households. Non-poor households generally tend to spend a higher share of their income on services that are heavily affected by containment measures such as international travel, restaurants, and cultural events. As the uncertainties are likely to persist for some time, so does this motive for saving.

On a year-on-year basis, the recent RBI's data on Sectoral Deployment of Bank Credit shows that the gross bank credit grew by only 5.8% in January 2021, lower than the growth of 8.5% in January 2020. Between

Table 3.8 Deployment of Gross Bank Credit by Major Sectors (All India)

Sector	*Variation (Year-on-Year)*		*Variation (Financial Year)*	
	31 Jan 2020/18 Jan 2019	*29 Jan 2021/31 Jan 2020*	*31 Jan 2020/29 Mar 2019*	*29 Jan 2021/27 Mar 2020*
I. Gross Bank Credit (II + III)	8.5	5.8	3.5	2.5
II. Food Credit	**11.3**	**10.4**	**89.7**	**68.3**
III. Non-food Credit (1 to 4)	**8.5**	**5.7**	**3.1**	**2.2**
1. Agriculture and Allied Activities	**6.5**	**9.9**	**3.8**	**9.5**
2. Industry	**2.5**	**−1.3**	**−2.4**	**−4.3**
3. Services	**8.9**	**8.4**	**0.7**	**1.6**
3.1. Transport Operators	8.1	8.9	6.6	8.1
3.2. Computer Software	-0.4	-0.2	1.3	-6.6
3.3. Tourism, Hotels, and Restaurants	17.4	8.9	16.4	7.5
3.4. Shipping	-10.9	7.5	-13.8	9.5
3.5. Aviation	-60.5	120.0	-64.5	91.0
3.6. Professional Services	1.9	-25.0	0.4	-27.1
3.7. Trade	4.8	15.7	-1.6	8.8
3.8. Commercial Real Estate	14.7	2.8	12.3	1.7
3.9. Non-Banking Financial Companies	35.8	6.6	17.3	-2.1
3.10. Other Services[3]	-15.4	17.5	-21.4	7.0
4. Personal Loans	**16.9**	**9.1**	**12.5**	**6.7**

Source: Handbook of Statistics on Indian States 2019–20, RBI (2020)

January 2020 and 2021, the credit growth to agriculture and allied activities accelerated to 9.9% from 6.5%.

Credit to industry contracted by 1.3% in January 2021 as compared to 2.5% growth in January 2020 mainly due to contraction in credit to large industries by 2.5% (2.8% growth in January 2020). Credit to medium industries registered a robust growth of 19.1% in January 2021 as compared to 2.8% a year ago and credit to micro and small industries registered a growth of 0.9% in January 2021 as compared to 0.5% a year ago. Within the industry, credit to "mining and quarrying", "food processing", "textile", "gems and jewellery", "petroleum, coal products and nuclear fuels", "paper and paper products", "leather and leather products, and vehicles, vehicle parts and transport equipment" registered accelerated growth in January 2021 as compared to the growth in the corresponding month of the previous year. However, credit growth to "rubber plastic and their products", "beverages and tobacco", "chemicals and chemical products", "basic metal and metal products", "construction" and "infrastructure" decreased.

The services sector saw a moderate fall to 8.4% from 8.9%, for the period. Credit to sectors like trade, aviation, shipping saw growth. The commercial real estate and tourism, hotels and restaurants, and professional services segment have been severely impacted due to the lockdown. As per the RBI

Table 3.9 Services Sector Performance in India's GVA (All India)

Sector	*Share in GVA (%)*	*Growth (% YoY)*					
	2020–21(AE)	*2218–19 (RE)*	*2019–20 (PE)*	*2020–21 (AE)*	*2020–21 (H1)*	*2020–21*	
						Q1	*Q2*
Trade, hotels, transport, communication, and services related to broadcasting	15.4	7.7	3.6	-21.41	-31.5	-47	-15.6
Financial, real estate, and professional services	22.2	6.8	4.6	-0.82	-6.8	-5.3	-8.1
Public administration, defence, and other services	16.7	9.4	10	-3.68	-11.3	-10.3	-12.2
Total services (excluding construction)	54.3	7.7	5.5	-8.8	-15.9	-20.6	-11.4

Source: Economic Survey, 2020–21

data, financing to professional services has decelerated to (–) 25% from 1.9% YoY basic. In the first advance estimate of 2020–21, the growth of the service sector is reduced by 8.8%, whereas the growth rate was 5.5% in 2019–20. The biggest losers among the three broad components of the service sector are trade, hotel, transport, and communication. The growth of this category decreased from 7.7 in 2018–19 to 3.6 in 2019–20 and according to the advance estimate of 2020–21, the downfall is around 21%.

The data mentioned earlier does not include the informal sector. While the informal economy now accounts for roughly half of India's GDP, the share of the private and public corporate sector accounts for 80–90% of the workforce with two out of every three jobs in India's informal being in businesses engaged in a trade or providing services. Like demonetisation, it is quite evident that the informal sector had more negative effects compared to the formal sector (Balamurugan and Hemalatha, 2017; Agrawal, 2018; Ghosh et al., 2017).

Conclusion

On 31 December 2019, for the first time, China reported the COVID virus from Wuhan. Almost after one month on 30 January 2020, India reported its first case of the virus. The Prime Minister of India declared a nationwide total lockdown on March 24. The impact of the lockdown was felt in every corner of the Indian economy from the time when all the economic activities were stopped. The lockdown was extended further with phasewise relaxations. The country was divided into three zones (red, orange, and green) and the degree of restriction was varied accordingly. Due to the very nature of the restriction, the impact was also varied between different sectors, different regions, and also different categories of households. It is evident from different regional-level studies that the less developing regions suffered more than the developed regions. This chapter focused on one of the backward regions of India, its North East, whose history and trajectory of development have been different from the rest of India. The analysis of public finance of different states of North East suggests that the impact has been far-reaching and it will take longer than expected to recover. During this difficult time, the government needs to balance between tackling the increasing gross fiscal deficit (GFC) and extending support (financial as well as kind) to the population. The non-rich households need more support now than ever.

The performance of the labour market in the North East has been very poor. The CMIE data of four states suggests that labour force participation decreased and unemployment increased. The rate of change was more in urban areas than in the rural areas. Tripura and Meghalaya are the worst performers with a significant rise in unemployment rate and fall of Labour Participation Rate. In the long run, there is a strong possibility that a discouraged worker effect will arise in the North East.

The chapter also found that the demand for credit decreased and the amount of deposits increased during this time. The general public did precautionary savings as they were in panic and also faced uncertainty regarding future income. Although there has been some support from the government in terms of food grains but the demand for credit for food purposes increased during COVID. The data also suggests that it is the service sector that took most of the hits. The service sector is one of the biggest employers not only in the formal sector but also in the informal economy.

In the time of the global financial crisis, the government played a very vital role; likewise similar role is expected in this crisis also. Many poor households are facing a huge crisis that they have never seen before. The job losses and unprecedented return migration from urban to rural played a catalyst role. The analysis of this chapter suggests urgent attentions form the governments of all the levels. The need of the hour in the North East is as follows: (i) support for poor households in terms of cash and non-cash, which requires a balancing act between government expenditure and income and (ii) the focus should be given to the labour market through standard job creation. In rural India, the Mahatma Gandhi National Rural Employment Guarantee Act (MGNREGA) has become the last resort of employment for millions of people including migrant workers and can also play a vital role in recovery (Vasudevan et al., 2020). Similar to MGNREGA, the government should think of a policy for urban areas also.

Notes

1 The Special Category States are Arunachal Pradesh, Assam, Himachal Pradesh, Jammu and Kashmir, Manipur, Meghalaya, Mizoram, Nagaland, Sikkim, Tripura, and Uttarakhand.
2 Revenue deficit minus interest payments.
3 LPR is the ratio of the labour force to the population greater than 15 years of age.
4 UER is the unemployed who are willing to work and are actively looking for a job expressed as a per cent of the labour force.
5 As per the Reserve Bank of India rules, a bank has to keep aside 3% of deposits as cash reserve ratio (CRR) and another 18% in statutory liquidity ratio (SLR) compliant holdings. The rest, along with other resources, can be used for lending.

References

Acharya, V. and Steffen, S. (2020), "Stress tests for banks as liquidity insurers in a time of COVID", *VoxEU. org*, 22 March, http://pages.stern.nyu.edu/~sternfin/vacharya/public_html/pdfs/bank-liquidity-stress-test-Acharya-Steffen-v20March2020-FINAL-2.pdf, accessed November 2020.

Agrawal, Abha (2018), "Demonetization and cashless economy", *ACADEMICIA: An International Multidisciplinary Research Journal*, 8(6), 73–80.

Balamurugan, S. and Hemalatha, B. K. (2017), "Impacts on demonetization: Organized and unorganized sector", *IOSR Journal of Humanities and Social Science*, e-ISSN(2017), 0837–2279.

Berkhout, E., Galasso, N., Lawson, M., Rivero Morales, P. A., Taneja, A. and Vazquez Pimentel, D. A. (2021), "The inequality virus: Bringing together a world torn apart by coronavirus through a fair, just and sustainable economy", www.oxfam.org/en/research/inquality-virus.

Browning, M. and Lusardi, A. (1996), "Household saving: Micro theories and micro facts", *Journal of Economic literature*, 34(4), 1797–1855.

Chancel, L. and Piketty, T. (2019), "Indian income inequality, 1922-2015: From British Raj to Billionaire Raj?" *Review of Income and Wealth*, 65, S33–S62.

CMIE (2020), *CMIE Statistics*, Centre for Monitoring Indian Economy. www.cmie.com/.

Dev, S. Mahendra and Sengupta, R. (2020), "Covid-19: Impact on the Indian economy", Indira Gandhi Institute of Development Research (IGIDR) Working Paper Series, WP-2020–013.

Ghosh, Jayati, C., Chandrasekhar, P. and Patnaik, Prabhat (2017), *Demonetisation Decoded: A Critique of India's Currency Experiment*, London and New York: Taylor & Francis.

Ghosh, Shayan (2020), "Credit-deposit ratio takes a hit in 2020", *Livemint*, 24 December, https://Credit-deposit ratio takes a hit in 2020 (livemint.com), accessed 10 January 2021.

Government of India (GoI) (2021), *Economic Survey 2020–21*, Vol. I, January, Department of Economic Affairs, Ministry of Finance Affairs, Government of India.

Guterres, Antonio (2020), "Nelson Mandela annual lecture 2020", www.nelsonmandela.org/news/entry/annual-lecture-2020-secretary-general-guterres-full-speech, accessed 31 May 2021.

ILO (2020), "COVID-19 and the world of work: Impact and policy responses", March, www.ilo.org/wcmsp5/groups/public/ – dgreports/ – dcomm/documents/briefingnote/wcms_738753.pdf, accessed 15 December.

IMF (2021), www.imf.org/en/Topics/imf-and-covid19/Policy-Responses-to-COVID-19#I, accessed March 2021.

IMF DataMapper (2020), "Real GDP growth", www.imf.org/en/Countries/IND#countrydata.

Lee, S., Schmidt-Klau, D. and Verick, S. (2020), "The labour market impacts of the COVID-19: A global perspective", *The Indian Journal of Labour Economics*, 63, 11–15.

Maliszewska, M., Mattoo, A. and Van Der Mensbrugghe, D. (2020), *The Potential Impact of COVID-19 on GDP and Trade: A Preliminary Assessment*, World Bank Policy Research Working Paper, 9211, World Bank.

Mody, A., Ohnsorge, F. and Sandri, D. (2012), *Precautionary Savings in the Great Recession*, IMF Working Papers, No. 42, International Monetary Fund. www.imf.org/external/pubs/ft/wp/2012/wp1242.pdf, accessed 10 January 2021.

Nayak Gayatri (2020), "COVID caution pushes household savings by more than two-fold in Q1'20–21", *The Economic Times*, 17 November, https://economictimes.indiatimes.com/news/economy/finance/covid-caution-pushes-household-savings-by-more-than-two-fold-in-q120–21/articleshow/79264627.cms?utm_source=contentofinterest&utm_medium=text&utm_campaign=cppst, accessed 15 December 2020.

NSSO (2019), *Periodic Labour Force Survey (2017–18)*, Ministry of Statistics and Programme Implementation, Government of India.

OECD (2020), "General assessment of the macroeconomic situation", Chapter 1 of *OECD Economic Outlook*, Vol. 2020, Issue 2, Paris: OECD Publishing, pp. 9–59.
POSOCO Monthly Report (2020), *Power System Operation Corporation Limited (POSOCO) National Load Despatch Centre*, New Delhi, December, https://posoco.in/download/monthly_report_december_2020/?wpdmdl=34420.
Reserve Bank of India (2020), "State finances: A study of budgets of 2020", www.rbi.org.in/scripts/AnnualPublications.aspx?head=State%20Finances%20:%20A%20Study%20of%20Budgets, accessed November 2020.
RBI, R. (2020), "Handbook of statistics on Indian states 2019–20", https://rbidocs.rbi.org.in/rdocs/Publications/PDFs/HS13102020_F947063857A8E4515A045CC91EE92BFAB.PDF.
Singha, R. (2018), "Employment diversification in Tripura", in *Employment and Labour Market in North-East India: Interrogating Structural Changes*, London and New Delhi: Routledge, pp. 369–389.
Vasudevan, G., Singh, S., Gupta, G., et al. (2020), "MGNREGA in the times of COVID-19 and beyond: Can India do more with less?" *The Indian Journal of Labour Economics*, 799–814.

Part II

Unforeseen Transformation

4 COVID-19 and Health Workforce in India

Time for Radical Change?

Ramila Bisht, Shaveta Menon, and Balakrishnan Nair

Introduction

The COVID-19 pandemic has transformed into more than a disease affecting the human body, confounded globally by enormous heterogeneity (Christopher et al., 2020), having transcended boundaries and affected both the diseased and those caring them, including the health workers (HWs) providing care to COVID-19 patients. Despite confronting several structural issues and real dangers, the HWs have continued to provide an unprecedented level of care during these times. Due to their dedicated services, the government and media gave them the title of "corona warriors". But these warriors have been struggling to protect themselves and their families (Basu, 2020) with apparently little help from the government. Although the WHO 2007 framework identifies health workforce as one of the crucial building blocks of the health system, it fails to locate the role of the HWs within this system. However, for effective health service delivery, it is essential to place the needs of health workforce at the centre of the healthcare strategies (Anand and Bärnighausen, 2012).

WHO has defined HWs as "all the people engaged in action whose primary intent is to enhance health". This includes workers such as health service providers, health management teams, and support workers (WHO, 2006). This health workforce is heterogeneous in nature and differentiated in its size, composition, and distribution, India being no different (Rao et al., 2009). This heterogeneity has been instrumental during the COVID-19 pandemic in exaggerating problems such as occupational hazards, workplace stresses, and other morbid conditions faced by them (Mohanty et al., 2019).

We trace various issues faced by the HWs during the COVID-19 pandemic, exacerbated due to the already present and ignored problems. Although most of these problems are common to all segments of HWs, a quick glance on the reporting of these problems reveals that the lower spectrum of the hierarchical medical system of the country has been largely ignored. In this chapter, we aim to elaborate on the role played by doctors, nurses, and the community HWs working in both public and private health centres and discuss the reporting of their problems. We exclude the health

DOI: 10.4324/9781003282815-7

management and support workers such as administrative staff and support staff in hospitals such as accountants, clerks, drivers, and painters.

Health Workers in India

Healthcare services in India are provided by a varied range of professionals trained in various specialities of medicine and healthcare. The formal healthcare providers, such as trained doctors (allopathic, ayurvedic, and homoeopathic) and dentists, form the upper segment of the pyramid of human resources for health. Among the subordinate HWs are the nurses, ANMs (Auxiliary Nurse Midwife), ASHA (Accredited Social Health Activist) workers, and other outreach staff (Karan et al., 2019). However, the derangement in the health workforce is observed at various levels of rural-urban gaps, public and private employment, different cadres of HWs, and their associated implications on the health of the population. On the basis of the National Sample Survey Office (NSSO) estimated from January 2016, the total size of the health workforce in India is 3.8 million. Out of these, 63% of the allopathic doctors and 88% of the AYUSH (Ayurveda, Yoga and Naturopathy, Unani, Siddha, and Homeopathy) practitioners are self-employed. It is surprising to note that while 71% of India's population is rural, only 36% of the HWs are in these areas. The percentage of doctors and nurses in the rural areas is 34% and 33%, respectively, which presents a dismal picture (Karan et al., 2019).

Also, in a country with a population of 1.3 billion, around 20,000 doctors out of 9.26 lakh are trained in critical care, pulmonology, and emergency medicine. These specialists are deemed necessary while addressing the critical caseload due to COVID-19 (Radhakrishnan and Bhan, 2020). In addition, an acute shortage of specialists in government hospitals due to promotion, retirement, termination, resignation, non-availability of suitable candidates, and low rates of joining at initial levels (PTI, 2014) has created a multitude of problems for the HWs while also compromising the quality of care.

Problems Faced by Health Workers in India During COVID-19

Work conditions are important in determining the level of stress and rate of infectivity, which is further determined by their placement in the spectrum of health system during the pandemic (Behera et al., 2020). Several reports highlight the issues faced by the HWs in the country. However, a search of media and published literature reveals that most of the writings are concentrated on HWs occupying higher positions in the ladder of the health system. Therefore, highlighting the problems and issues faced by the HWs *vis-a-vis* their placement in the health system becomes crucial.

Morbidity and Mortality in Health Workers

HWs worldwide have been at the forefront fighting the virus and risking lives while saving others. Out of all the COVID-19 cases, 14% of those reported to the WHO were related to the HWs. This figure could run to as high as 35% in low- and middle-income countries, where the HWs represent only 2% of the total population. According to the data released by the Health Ministry of India in September 2020, Telangana (18%), Maharashtra (16%), Delhi (14%), Karnataka (13%), Puducherry (12%), and Punjab (11%) reported high COVID-19 infection rates among HWs. However, the government argued that the limited availability of data makes it impossible to establish whether the HWs got infected at the workplace or from the community (Sharma, 2020). For those availing relief, the government has given provisions under the "*Pradhan Mantri Garib Kalyan Insurance Package for Health Workers fighting COVID-19*" maintained at the national level. Nonetheless, the central government had very conveniently stated that since health is a state subject, it has not maintained any data on the HWs' mortality. In September 2020, the Government of India reported that 155 HWs had lost their lives due to the virus, out of which 64 were doctors (PTI, 2020).

On the contrary, the Indian Medical Association (IMA) rebuked the government for washing off its hands. It released the statement that 515 doctors working for COVID patients lost their lives to this deadly disease. It becomes very significant to note that of these, 201 doctors were in the age group of 60–70 years, and 171 in the age group of 50–60 years. In addition, 66 doctors who died were in the age group exceeding 70 years (The Wire, 2020). Updates on data by mid-December 2020 by IMA revealed that 2,784 doctors were infected with the virus and 728 died because of it. Among those infected, 1,471 were practising doctors, 930 were resident doctors, and 383 were house surgeons. On similar lines, the Trained Nurses Association of India estimated that by mid-October, 47 nurses lost their lives (Rana, 2020). The latest analysis of the number of deaths due to Coronavirus in India showed that people in the age group of 50–59 years were the worst hit as far as deaths and disease were concerned (Dutta, 2020a). It is interesting to note that, even with their usual stressful and hectic lifestyles, the average age of death in doctors under normal circumstances is 55–59 years that is ten years less than the general population (Jacob, 2017). Most deaths were due to cardiac arrests (Sayyed, 2010), showing increased susceptibility towards stress, an ailment commonly seen in health sector during COVID-19 pandemic.

Additionally, the poor coordination between the government and the private sector hospitals also came to light. The private hospitals alleged of harassment at the hands of the government over COVID-19 guidelines. Private sector practitioners were forced to give services in the dedicated COVID centres chosen by the government, leading to neglect of their own patients.

Furthermore, the insurance plan does not cover the HWs working in the private sector (BMJ, 2020), making it difficult for them to engage with the government in treating patients infected with COVID-19.

Apart from the private-government demarcations, it is also disturbing to note that the morbidity and mortality data of those working at the lower rung of the occupational hierarchy, such as community HWs, has not been reported. Additionally, there are regional reports on the level of dissatisfaction felt by the contractual healthcare employees. Various HWs employed on a contract did not have access to COVID incentives, compensation, or health insurance. Besides, the mismatch in pay parity between the regular and the contractual HWs and stressful working conditions in COVID-19 has widened the differences and difficulties associated with a contractual work. For instance, in Karnataka, a regular AYUSH doctor earns Rs. 56,000 per month, while an outsourced or contractual one only earns Rs. 17,000 to Rs. 25,000 per month.

Similarly, a staff nurse earns Rs. 34,000 per month while a contract nurse earns Rs. 12,000 to Rs. 13,000 per month. Likewise, an ANM earns Rs. 30,000 while a contract ANM earns Rs. 8,000–Rs 10,000 per month (Express News Service, 2020). In August 2020, more than 3.5 million HWs launched a two-day strike to express their discontent with the wages and supply of PPE kits. Many protests by temporary contractors brought to light the step-motherly treatment meted out to them due to their job contracts (Jamkhandikar, 2020).

Predominant reasons for the increased morbidity and mortality among HWs have been the insufficient availability of Personal Protective Equipment (PPE). Previous studies have revealed the inadequate availability of N95 masks in high-risk zones of Indian hospitals even before the advent of a pandemic (Raj et al., 2019). This shortage of PPE led to staff using less protective mask or masks made of cloth or rainwear material, which on continued use and reuse increased their chances of infection (Behera et al., 2020).

Fatigue or Burnout

Fatigue or burnout among HWs is due to "professional burnout", a significant global health concern which results from an increased workload, insufficient time to cope with occupational challenges, and a lack of interpersonal support in everyday life. During the COVID-19 period, the fear of being infected, social disruptions, and quarantine have been additional factors that affected the workers' psychosocial well-being (Sultana et al., 2020). Burnout has been categorised by International Classification of Disease (ICD) as an "occupational phenomenon" because of chronic workspace stress that has not been successfully managed (WHO, 2019).

This burnout increased during the COVID-19 period, leading to several healthcare positions lying vacant, overwhelming the already stressed workforce, and resource crunched the work environment. In pre-COVID India, there was a shortage of six lakh doctors and two million nurses. This understaffing increased the workload on the existing workforce and made the situation graver. This exposed the lack of respect by the establishments for the healthcare profession (Wallen, 2020). The medical system throughout the globe needs nurses in far greater number than the doctors. While WHO recommends three nurses for 1,000 people, India has only 1.7 nurses for 1,000 people (Rana, 2020).

The excessive workload due to less workforce has been an essential determinant in exacerbating the already stressed workforce. Of all the HWs, nurses have been seen to report a higher prevalence of burnout (Lasebikan and Oyetunde, 2012). This is due to their caring role that leaves them more vulnerable to psychological and physical stressors arising from the holistic patient care (Boyle, 2011). In fact, those working in the emergency and the intensive care units were disproportionately affected when they were the ones who needed PPE the most (Nagesh and Chakraborty, 2020). The workers who faced resistance from the communities due to fear, mistrust, and poor communication due to the outbreaks also suffered with burnout. The problem of irregular pay, lack of family support, and personal time emerged as pressing issues among outreach workers (Bisht and Menon, 2020) during COVID-19.

Mental health issues among HWs occur when they are expected to work mandatorily and are at the same time devoid of a therapeutic support system. This leads to a feeling of despair and helplessness, exaggerating the work pressures and leading to suicide (Dutta, 2020b). These issues are common among the doctors and the nursing staff due to their jobs, while suicides among doctors are becoming a public health crisis (Perapaddan, 2018).

A study conducted in PGIMER, Chandigarh, concluded that of the total of 445 doctors who participated in the survey, 30% were depressed and 17% thought of ending their lives (Grover et al., 2018). There were also reports on the nurses committing suicide facing mental repercussions from COVID-19 (Sensharma, 2020). Although the National Crime Records Bureau (NCRB) regularly reports on the number of suicides and evaluates the variables linked to them (Joseph, 2020a), there has been a lack of data on suicides among HWs during the time of the pandemic especially those at the lower rung of the health system.

Stigma and Violence

In addition to the challenges mentioned earlier, the HWs throughout the country have faced stigma and ostracisation at the hands of the local community. Spread of misinformation through social media termed as a "virtual infodemic" was instrumental in tagging the HWs as potential carriers of the virus, which made them easy targets of the already frustrated community. Also, during initial stages, the pandemic was labelled as the disease of the rich and doctors who are mostly perceived as the affluent lot in

India were stigmatised (Menon et al., 2020). This associated stigma led to violent attacks against HWs, adding to their agony of being recognised as the "newer untouchables". There have been scattered reports of violence against HWs, although congregated data on the same could not be obtained (Iyengar et al., 2020).

This violence against doctors and other medical professionals has increased in the past decade with almost 75% of the doctors facing it. Emergency and ICU physicians face violence while dealing with the relatives of patients, mostly in the public hospitals that boast of free treatment. The major reason behind these attacks is the shortage of workforce, improper infrastructure, and increased patient load (Kapoor, 2017). At the same time, the private hospitals withdrew from the fight against COVID-19 making it increasingly difficult for patients to access medical care leading to panic among people (Yamunan, 2020) making HWs more prone to such violent attacks.

Politics of Policy and HWs in COVID-19

The society increasingly relies on health and medical science to contain such outbreaks. This requires the diverse nature of the engagements of the government at various levels with citizens and organisations involved in the process of policy-making and implementation (Weible et al., 2020). India's skeletal health system finds its root in the federal nature of the country's system, the centralised schemes and policies, and the intergovernmental transfer system. The subject of healthcare falls under the purview of state responsibilities. However, the states are not vested with adequate financial powers to meet the responsibility of associated expenditure. States raise 38% to 40% of the total revenues from taxes, spending 58–60% of this revenue on a range of items including health and family welfare. The dominance of the centre stems from the fact that while public health, sanitation, and hospitals are under the state jurisdiction, the legal medical and other professions fall in the concurrent list, meaning that they are controlled by the central government. In contrast to the response of most federal countries, the key policies and planning framework in the health sector in India has been provided by the centre (Sahoo, 2016).

There have been various instances of demands being made by the states to the centre for receiving PPE, testing kits, and financial aid (Atreya, 2020). Initially, when an early analysis exposed a disruption in the health services, the data was retracted by the central government. The doctors and nurses critical of the government's response to the crisis were apparently harassed (Dreze, 2020). Due to increasing financial strain, the states deferred salaries or cut funds (Sikarwar, 2020) leading to discontent in its health workforce. Also, small hospitals and healthcare facilities downsized on staff due to decreased revenues and uncertainties, leading to a shortage of HWs when they reopened. Besides, the ancillary workforce was not ready to join hospitals due to fear of COVID, low wages, short-term contracts, and poor working conditions. This created an uproar among the HWs, and there were reports of those working on contracts going on strike in some states.

For instance, in Bihar, 700 contract nurses working in AIIMS Patna went on strike demanding the same treatment as provided to 120 regular nurses in the facility. This meant higher remuneration and provision of similar leaves (Jacob et al., 2020). However, it is interesting to note that the institutes that are of national importance and provide professional training and research come under the purview of the Union list. The central government is responsible for converting the contractual workers into permanent workers. However, the state health services were affected due to the unrest in the HWs working in central government-controlled institutions in the state, bringing to light the divide of power. As already mentioned, the Indian health system is facing a shortage of healthcare professionals. Various strategies were roped in during this time, including new recruitments to handle the increasing workload in government hospitals. For example, in Punjab, the recruitment saw most previously vacant posts advertised ranging from doctors and specialists to the lower rung workers such as multipurpose HWs male and females (Kumari, 2020)

Lack of Training and Infection Control Among Health Workers

Training of the HWs on use of PPE and ensuring the infection control measures is of utmost importance. The shortage of PPE during COVID was a global phenomenon caused due to its increased demand, panic buying, and irrational use (WHO, 2020). This shortage was also experienced during the Ebola virus outbreak in 2014–16, resulting in many infected HWs. The WHO reported that during January 2014 and March 2015, HWs had 21 to 32 times greater chances of contracting Ebola due to failure of infection prevention and control which also included the lack of PPE (WHO, 2015b).

Despite having access to PPE, several HWs were not trained on its usage; thus, they ended up using them incorrectly. Doubts and confusion were also raised on the safety and quality of PPE received by the HWs. An online survey in the country that was carried out by independent public health researchers revealed a lack of appropriate training on the use of PPE in HWs and a perceived discrimination in its supply. Of all the 392 respondents approximately, 90% did not know which PPE to wear in which settings, more than 50% had not received any training on the proper use of PPE, and 20% had learnt how to use PPE through YouTube videos or from their colleagues. Another important revelation in the survey was that 37% of all the respondents perceived discrimination in distribution of PPE according to the workplace hierarchy (Joseph, 2020b).

This lack of timely training can be related to the time constraints and excessive workloads due to shortage of HWs, which leads to suboptimal knowledge and lack of infection control by the workers (Behera et al.,

2020). Along with the chronic shortage of the HWs, proper implementation of policies concentrating on infection control and practices also remains poor in Indian healthcare facilities. In 2010, National Airborne Infection Control (AIC) guidelines were adopted in India, which included various policies for TB prevention and control. However, a study found that these AIC systems were poorly developed and implemented (Parmar et al., 2015). During COVID-19, this lack of infection control has mostly been witnessed in hospitals (Nandi, 2020). In other words, the infection control measures for various communicable diseases have been in place but not properly implemented. Another study showed that the primary health centres were constrained in their functioning due to poor infrastructure, which led to sub-optimal infection control measures (Garg et al., 2020) exposing the HWs to an infection escalated environment.

Solutions and Way Forward

As mentioned in the previous sections, the problems faced by the HWs especially those working in the public sector have been largely due to an overwhelmed health system. To reduce the stressors on the health workforce and improve the health service delivery, various practical and cost-effective solutions have been offered.

Community Engagement

As mentioned in the earlier sections, mistrust and fear among the community regarding providing health services were brought to the surface during COVID-19. This led to a violent behaviour towards the HWs temporarily stagnating the health service provisioning and increasing stress among the HWs. In case of Ebola, the negative community response witnessed in the early stages was high level of fear along with confusing communication approaches asking them to seek diagnosis and treatment, when services were not in place causing significant level of distrust between the community and the HWs. However, proper training and communication helped bridge the gap between HWs and communities in a positive manner (WHO, 2015a).

WHO has defined community engagement as "a process of developing relationships that enable stakeholders to work together to address health related issues and promote well-being to achieve positive health impact and outcomes". As mentioned earlier, the health workforce is a vital asset of the health system of the country. However, while considering the issues of empowerment and community engagement, the HWs are overlooked. The preparedness of the health workforce to engage with other professionals, patients, sectors, and local communities will determine how well the trust is built. It is imperative to note that the poor engagement knowledge and competencies of HWs have long-term effects on the performance of the health system (morale of the staff, burnout, and stress). However, the "soft skills" of engaging more in dialogue with the community are not taught in professional health education, which focuses more on building the technical competencies (WHO, 2017).

Since most of the Indian population lives in the rural areas that is already short of HWs, community engagement by engaging with the local panchayats and stressing the role of civil society is important to enjoy the community's confidence. Bridging the gap between the trust deficit present between HWs and the public (Bhaduri, 2020) can help alleviate stressors of the HWs too. An independent WHO panel in its second report has lauded the community engagement by ASHA workers in India highlighting community engagement as a successful strategy in enhancing the nation's response to COVID-19 (Dasgupta, 2021).

Technological and Other Solutions for the Post-COVID World

Before COVID-19 pandemic, the Indian health-seeking behaviour involved visiting specialists for every minor or major health ailments. This behaviour had led to the underutilisation of primary health centres and resulted in overwhelmed tertiary hospitals and their outpatient clinics. It is highly unlikely that a caring and compassionate workforce will flow out of the health systems with fragmented infrastructure (WHO, 2017). During COVID-19, the hospitals only carried out emergency consultations while halting all other outpatient clinics to avoid congregation of people, thus reducing infections in HWs (Hollander and Carr, 2020).

Due to lockdowns, intense screening for COVID-19 before hospitalisation, non-entertainment of minor ailments at the tertiary hospital clinics, and even closure of many outpatient clinics forced residents to use home remedies, adopt AYUSH methods of treatment, consult local physician, or even use telemedicine facilities (Chaturvedi et al., 2020). Continuing this strategy in post-COVID India will allow people to control their health by practicing an individualised healthcare plan guided remotely by healthcare professionals. It will also help in coping with shortage of healthcare personnel because of spiking demand, illness among HWs, and a high rate of absenteeism, which is common during crisis (Damery et al., 2009).

Another key suggestion for effective COVID-19 prevention and treatment has been considering remote operations through electronic medical devices. Besides COVID-19 tracking apps and other surveillance tools to monitor the spread of epidemic, several healthcare operations can also be conducted remotely through computer programs and mobile applications (Bassi et al., 2020). These technological advances can be helpful in near future to reduce the workload of the HWs and can close the distance between a patient and a healthcare provider with minimal cost and devices.

Indian primary care has adopted many such "point of care" devices, for instance "*Swasthya Slate*", that has the potential to undertake more than 30 doorstep lab investigations at a negligible cost. These devices have the capacity to store data offline and upload it to the central electronic healthcare data repositories when they get access to the Internet. These devices operate at a basic digital wireless network generation like 2G, which are easy to introduce even in far-fledged rural areas (Sittig et al., 2013). Such devices can help reduce the waiting time in the public hospitals and hence promote better interaction with the HWs.

Motivation in Health Workers and Managerial Considerations

Our country can do better by practicing more effective management in healthcare, which in turn affects service quality and the organisational culture. Effective management plays a critical role in supporting the professional needs of HWs. For instance, job satisfaction stems from complex interactions between the organisational environment, on the job experience and motivation. Job satisfaction is linked to motivation, which is crucially linked to retention and performance of the HWs (Tzeng, 2002). Nonetheless, in India, job satisfaction in the HWs is low (Peters et al., 2010), which is evident from the rates of absenteeism seen during the spread of COVID-19. Shortfall of trained healthcare managers has been exhibited as a felt need in India (Tiwari et al., 2018).

Several health management models advocate empathy between team members, non-invasive ways of performance management, and quality control. When operating remotely, the manager and the healthcare team can adopt better management models to avoid conflicts and confusion especially when they can't see each other in person. Some key strategies relate to better accountability, feeling of stewardship, regular support, enhancing productivity, knowledge sharing, and congruent work environment. When working remotely, it is always a struggle to measure the amount of work done by each staff member. Managers should have a general idea of the time taken to complete a task using strategies like daily reporting and regular communication (Nair and Krishnamurthi, 2020).

Managers should always remind their staff not to overwork and ask for their needs regularly. The staff should be encouraged to talk about progress and issues and create a knowledge-sharing environment while inculcating a feeling of empathy and belongingness within the team. As the patient data is also collected remotely in these scenarios, the team must be careful and responsible for its managing. Finally, a respectful, appreciative, and motivating environment must be created where recognition and gratitude are conveyed to the team members in everyday conversations (Nair and Krishnamurthi, 2020).

Conclusion

An effective healthcare system plays a critical role in supporting the healthcare needs of reducing the risks of morbidity and coping with stress. The uncertainty associated with the pandemic of COVID-19 has not only exposed the vulnerabilities of the HWs but also revealed the slow approach of the system to resolve their issues. Strengthening and revisiting the infection control measures in the public health infrastructure will prevent the rapid spread of infections among HWs. The addressal of these issues at the earliest will help place the HWs at the centre of the health systems. Further, research on policy and locating the HWs in the policy process can be helpful in providing a conducive work environment. For India, the need of the hour is to come up with innovative solutions while engaging with the community and bridging trust deficits. In addition, building resilient health systems can help ease the burden off the HWs during such uncertain working conditions of the pandemic and the like in unforeseeable future. Strategies that provide socio-techno-managerial and workable explanations to assist in easing the grievances of the HWs might act as saviours. For these solutions to see the light of the day, the problems of the HWs must be brought from the political backburner to the forefront in India.

References

Anand, S. and Bärnighausen, T. (2012), "Health workers at the core of the health system: Framework and research issues", *Health Policy*, May, 105(2–3), 185–191. Doi: 10.1016/j.healthpol.2011.10.012.

Atreya, S. (2020), "Health a state subject but Covid proved how dependant India's states are on centre", *The Print*, 18 June, https://theprint.in/opinion/health-a-state-subject-but-covid-proved-how-dependant-indias-states-are-on-centre/442602/, accessed 25 December 2020.

Bassi, A., Arfin, S., John, O. and Jha, V. (2020), "An overview of mobile applications (apps) to support the coronavirus disease 2019 response in India", *Indian Journal of Medical Research*, May, 151(5), 468–473.

Basu, S. (2020), "COVID-19 health facility preparedness for protecting healthcare workers: Designing a tool for rapid self-assessment", *Indian Journal of Medical Sciences*, 21 August, 72(2), 83–87.

Behera, D., Praveen, D. and Behera, M. R. (2020), "Protecting Indian health workforce during the COVID-19 pandemic", *Journal of Family Medicine and Primary Care*, 30 September, 9(9), 4541–4546.

Bhaduri, S. D. (2020), "The criticality of community engagement", *The Hindu*, 6 April, www.thehindu.com/opinion/lead/the-criticality-of-community-engagement/article31264494.ece, accessed 25 December 2020.

Bisht, R. and Menon, S. (2020), "ASHA workers are indispensable. So why are they the least of our concerns?" *The Wire*, 1 May, https://thewire.in/rights/asha-workers-coronavirus, accessed 25 December 2020.

BMJ (2020), "Covid-19: India's private doctors and government clash over pandemic response", *British Medical Journal*, 22 September, 370–371. https://doi.org/10.1136/bmj.m3711.

Boyle, D. A. (2011), "Countering compassion fatigue: A requisite nursing agenda", *The Online Journal of Issues in Nursing*, 31 January, 16(1). https://doi.org/10.3912/OJIN.Vol16No01Man02.

Chaturvedi, S., Kumar, N., Tillu, G., Deshpande, S. and Patwardhan, B. (2020), "AYUSH, modern medicine and the Covid-19 pandemic", *Indian Journal of Medical Ethics*, 13 May, 32546457.

Christopher, D. J., Isaac, B. T., Rupali, P. and Thangakunam, B. (2020), "Health-care preparedness and health-care worker protection in COVID-19 pandemic", *Lung India: Official Organ of Indian Chest Society*, June, 37(3), 238–245.

Damery, S., Wilson, S., Draper, H., Gratus, C., Greenfield, S., Ives, J., Petts, J. and Sorell, T. (2009), "Will the NHS continue to function in an influenza pandemic? A survey of healthcare workers in the West Midlands, UK", *BMC Public Health*, 14 May, 9(1), 1–13.

Dasgupta, S. (2021), "Community engagement by ASHA workers behind India's successful Covid-19 response – WHO panel", *The Print*, 19 January, https://theprint.in/india/community-engagement-by-asha-workers-behind-indias-successful-covid-response-who-panel/588374/, accessed 25 January 2021.

Dreze, J. (2020), "India is in denial about Covid-19 crisis", *Scientific American*, 25 August, www.scientificamerican.com/article/india-is-in-denial-about-the-covid-19-crisis/, accessed 25 January 2021.

Dutta, S. S. (2020a), "50–59 age group worst hit by Coronavirus", *New Indian Express*, 3 November, www.newindianexpress.com/nation/2020/nov/03/50-59-age-group-worst-hit-by-covid-2218623.html, accessed 25 December 2020.

Dutta, S. S. (2020b), "Along with Covid-19, healthcare sector deals with another crisis: Doctors' suicides", *New Indian Express*, 24 August, www.newindianexpress.com/nation/2020/aug/24/along-with-covid-healthcare-sector-deals-with-another-crisis-docs-suicides-2187397.html, accessed 25 December 2020.

Express News Service (2020), "Contract, outsourced health workers strike, ask for pay parity", *New Indian Express*, 25 September, www.newindianexpress.com/states/karnataka/2020/sep/25/contract-outsourced-health-workers-strike-ask-for-pay-parity-2201564.html, accessed 25 December 2020.

Garg, S., Basu, S., Rustagi, R. and Borle, A. (2020), "Primary healthcare facility preparedness for outpatient service provision during the COVID-19 pandemic in India: Cross-sectional study", *JMIR Public Health and Surveillance*, 7 May, 6(2), e19927. http://dx.doi.org/10.2196/19927.

Grover, S., Sahoo, S., Bhalla, A. and Avasthi, A. (2018), "Psychological problems and burnout among medical professionals of a tertiary care hospital of North India: A cross-sectional study", *Indian Journal of Psychiatry*, June, 60(2), 175–188.

Hollander, J. E. and Carr, B. G. (2020), "Virtually perfect? Telemedicine for COVID-19", *New England Journal of Medicine*, 11 March, 382(18), 1679–1681.

Iyengar, K. P., Jain, V. K. and Vaishya, R. (2020), "Current situation with doctors and healthcare workers during COVID-19 pandemic in India", *Postgraduate Medical Journal (BMJ)*, 18 August, 1–2. http://dx.doi.org/10.1136/postgradmedj-2020-138496.

Jacob, G. (2017), "Do doctors die young, and why?" *The Hindu*, July, www.thehindu.com/opinion/open-page/do-doctors-die-young-and-why/article21381601.ece, accessed 25 December 2020.

Jacob, N., Inamdar, V., Saha, A. and Bhardwaj, S. (2020), "Low salaries, poor facilities deter health workers from COVID-19 care", 30 July, www.indiaspend.com/low-salaries-poor-facilities-deter-health-workers-from-covid-19-care/, accessed 25 December 2020.

Jamkhandikar, S. (2020), "Covid-19: Angry health workers launch a strike", 8 August, https://science.thewire.in/health/covid-19-angry-health-workers-in-india-launch-a-strike/, accessed 25 December 2020.

Joseph, J. P. (2020a), "Suicides among doctors were too common in India. Then the Pandemic came", *The Wire*, 19 August, https://thewire.in/health/suicides-among-doctors-covid-19-pandemic, accessed 25 December 2020.

Joseph, J. P. (2020b), "India Covid-19: Online survey shows not all is well on PPE availability front", 5 July, https://science.thewire.in/health/india-covid-19-online-survey-ppe-availability-training-containment-zones/, accessed 25 December 2020.

Kapoor, M. C. (2017), "Violence against the medical profession", *Journal of anaesthesiology, clinical pharmacology*, June, 33(2), 145–147. Doi: 10.4103/joacp.JOACP_102_17.

Karan, A., Negandhi, H., Nair, R., Sharma, A., Tiwari, R. and Zodpey, S. (2019), "Size, composition, and distribution of human resource for health in India: New estimates using National Sample Survey and Registry data", *BMJ Open*, 27 May, 9(4), e025979. Doi: 10.1136/bmjopen-2018–025979.

Kumari, A. (2020), "Punjab to recruit over 2900 medical staff to handle increase in Covid-19 patients", 7 August, www.ndtv.com/jobs/punjab-government-invites-application-on-2-984-posts-of-health-department-2275958, accessed 25 December 2020.

Lasebikan, V. O. and Oyetunde, M. O. (2012), "Burnout among nurses in a Nigerian general hospital: Prevalence and associated factors", *International Scholarly Research Notices*, 29 April 2012, epub, 402157–402156. https://doi.org/10.5402/2012/402157.

Menon, V., Padhy, S. K. and Pattnaik, J. I. (2020), "Stigma and aggression against healthcare workers in India amidst COVID-19 times: Possible drivers and mitigation strategies", *Indian journal of psychological medicine*, 7 July, 42(4), 400–401. https://doi.org/10.1177/0253717620929241.

Mohanty, A., Kabi, A. and Mohanty, A. P. (2019), "Health problems in healthcare workers: A review", *Journal of Family Medicine and Primary Care*, August, 8(8), 2568–2572. Doi: 10.4103/jfmpc.jfmpc_431_19.

Nagesh, S. and Chakraborty, S. (2020), "Saving the frontline health workforce amidst the COVID-19 crisis: Challenges and recommendations", *Journal of Global Health*, 24 April, 10(1), 1–4. Doi: 10.7189/jogh-10-010345.

Nair, B. and Krishnamurthi, R. (2020), "Conducting a large stroke epidemiological study during the COVID pandemic", in *Novel Approaches to Research During the COVID-19 Pandemic*, 2 December, New Zealand: AUT's School of Clinical Sciences.

Nandi, J. (2020), "Lack of PPE, poor infection control put medical staff at risk of Covid-19", *Hindustan Times*, 4 April, www.hindustantimes.com/india-news/lack-of-ppe-poor-infection-control-put-medical-staff-at-risk-of-covid-19/story-5jmeJgwUAaFuu4wfiCu8XN.html, accessed 25 December 2020.

Parmar, M. M., Sachdeva, K. S., Rade, K., Ghedia, M., Bansal, A., Nagaraja, S. B. and Dewan, P. K. (2015), "Airborne infection control in India: Baseline assessment of health facilities", *Indian Journal of Tuberculosis*, 23 January, 62(4), 211–217. Doi: 10.1016/j.ijtb.2015.11.006.

Perapaddan, B. S. (2018), "Suicide among doctors a public health crisis, says IMA", *The Hindu*, 31 March, www.thehindu.com/news/cities/Delhi/suicide-among-doctors-a-public-health-crisis-says-ima/article23396037.ece, accessed 25 December 2020.

Peters, D. H., Chakraborty, S., Mahapatra, P. and Steinhardt, L. (2010), "Job satisfaction and motivation of health workers in public and private sectors: Cross-sectional analysis from two Indian states," *Human Resources for Health*, 25 November, 8(1), 1–11.

PTI (2014), "Acute shortage of doctors and specialists in government hospitals across India", *Economic Times*, 11 July, https://economictimes.indiatimes.com/industry/healthcare/biotech/healthcare/acute-shortage-of-doctors-and-specialists-in-government-hospitals-across-india/articleshow/38218775.cms?from=mdr, accessed 25 December 2020.

PTI (2020), "Data on health workers infected or who died during Covid duty not maintained at the Central level: Govt", *The Times of India*, 19 September, https://timesofindia.indiatimes.com/india/data-on-health-workers-infected-or-who-died-during-covid-duty-not-maintained-at-central-level-govt/articleshow/78194741.cms, accessed 25 December 2020.

Radhakrishnan, R. and Bhan, A. (2020), "Indian doctors on how hospitals should handle Covid-19", 24 March, www.ndtv.com/opinion/indian-doctors-on-how-hospitals-should-handle-covid-19-2200095, accessed 25 December 2020.

Raj, A., Ramakrishnan, D., Thomas, C. R. M. T., Mavila, A. D., Rajiv, M. and Suseela, R. P. B. (2019), "Assessment of health facilities for airborne infection control practices and adherence to national airborne infection control guidelines: A study from Kerala, southern India", *Indian Journal of Community Medicine: Official Publication of Indian Association of Preventive & Social Medicine*, October, 44(1), S23–S26.

Rana, C. (2020), "In 2020, health workers counted their Covid-19 causalities because the government did not", *Caravan*, 31 December, https://caravanmagazine.in/health/health-workers-counted-their-covid19-casualties-because-the-government-did-not, accessed 25 January 2021.

Rao, K. D., Bhatnagar, A. and Berman, P. (2009), "India's health workforce: Size, composition, and distribution", *India Health Beat*, August, 1(3), http://documents1.worldbank.org/curated/en/928481468284348996/pdf/702410BRI0P1020k0Final000Vol010no03.pdf, accessed 25 December 2020.

Sahoo, N. (2016), "An examination of India's federal system and its impact on healthcare", *ORF Issue Brief*, October, 160, 1–12, www.orfonline.org/wp-content/uploads/2016/10/ORF_IssueBrief_160_HealthFederalism_FinalForUpload.pdf, accessed 25 December 2020. It seems the date is October 2016.

Sayyed, N. (2010), "Doctors have shorter life span that patients", *DNA India*, 1 February, www.dnaindia.com/lifestyle/report-doctors-have-shorter-lifespan-than-patients-1341722, accessed 25 December 2020.

Sensharma, A. (2020), " 'Extremely stressed' by treating coronavirus patients, nurse commits suicide in Ahmedabad's civil hospital", *Jagran*, 26 May, https://english.Jagran.com/india/extremely-stressed-by-treating-coronavirus-patients-nurse-commits-suicide-in-ahmedabads-civil-hospital-10012258, accessed 25 December 2020.

Sharma, N. C. (2020), "14% of the global Covid-19 cases are among health workers: WHO", *Live mint*, 18 September, www.livemint.com/news/india/14-of-global-covid-19-cases-are-among-health-workers-who-11600406028538.html, accessed 25 December 2020.

Sikarwar, D. (2020), "Covid-19 battle: Cash strapped states send SOS to Centre", *Economic Times*, 6 April, https://economictimes.indiatimes.com/news/politics-and-nation/cash-strapped-states-send-sos-to-centre/articleshow/74998913.cms?from=mdr, accessed 25 December 2020.

Sittig, D. F., Kahol, K. and Singh, H. (2013), "Sociotechnical evaluation of the safety and effectiveness of point-of-care mobile computing devices: A case study conducted in India", *Electronic Health Records: Challenges in Design and Implementation*, 115.

Sultana, A., Sharma, R., Hossain, M. M., Bhattacharya, S. and Purohit, N. (2020), "Burnout among healthcare providers during COVID-19 pandemic: Challenges and evidence-based interventions", *Indian Journal of Medical Ethics*, 4 July, 1, 1–4. https://doi.org/10.20529/IJME.2020.73.

Tiwari, R., Negandhi, H. and Zodpey, S. P. (2018), "Health management workforce for India in 2030", *Frontiers in Public Health*, 20 August, 6, 227. Doi: 10.3389/fpubh.2018.00227.

Tzeng, H. M. (2002), "The influence of nurses' working motivation and job satisfaction on intention to quit: An empirical investigation in Taiwan", *International Journal of Nursing Studies*, 4 June, 39(8), 867–878.

Wallen, J. (2020), "More than 80 per cent of newly qualified doctors in Indian state quit after Covid-19 wage cuts", *The Telegraph*, 2 September, www.telegraph.co.uk/global-health/science-and-disease/80-percent-newly-qualified-doctors-indian-state-quit-covid-19/, accessed 25 December 2020.

Weible, C. M., Nohrstedt, D., Cairney, P., Carter, D. P., Crow, D. A., Durnová, A. P., Heikkila, T. Ingold, K., McConnell, A. and Stone, D. (2020), "COVID-19 and the policy sciences: Initial reactions and perspectives", *Policy Sciences*, 18 April, 53(2), 225–241. https://doi.org/10.1007/s11077-020-09381-4.

WHO (2006), "Health workers: A global profile. World health report", *WHO*, www.who.int/whr/2006/06_chap1_en.pdf, accessed 25 December 2020.

WHO (2015a), "Enhanced capacity building. Training for frontline staff on building trust and communication", *WHO*, July, www.who.int/servicedeliverysafety/areas/qhc/trust-communication_training-guide.pdf?ua=1, accessed 25 December 2020.

WHO (2015b), "Health worker Ebola infections in Guinea, Liberia, and Sierra Leone: A preliminary report", 21 May, https://apps.who.int/iris/bitstream/handle/10665/171823/WHO_EVD_SDS_REPORT_2015.1_eng.pdf, accessed 25 December 2020.

WHO (2017), "WHO community engagement framework for quality people centred and resilient health services", March, https://apps.who.int/iris/bitstream/handle/10665/259280/WHO-HIS-SDS-2017.15-eng.pdf, accessed 25 December 2020.

WHO (2019), "Burn-out an 'occupational phenomenon': International classification of Diseases", *WHO*, 28 March, www.who.int/news/item/28-05-2019-burn-out-an-occupational-phenomenon-international-classification-of-diseases, accessed 25 December 2020.

WHO (2020), "Shortage of personal protective equipment endangering health workers worldwide", *WHO*, 3 March, www.who.int/news/item/03-03-2020-shortage-of-personal-protective-equipment-endangering-health-workers-worldwide accessed 25 December 2020.

The Wire (2020), "IMA says at least 515 doctors have died of Covid-19", 2 October, https://science.thewire.in/health/ima-515-doctors-covid-19-deaths-india-health-workers/, accessed 25 December 2020.

Yamunan, S. (2020), "Fear of Covid 19 spread makes private hospitals turn away patients or charge them with higher bills", *Scroll in*, 23 April, https://scroll.in/article/959727/fear-of-covid-19-spread-makes-private-hospitals-turn-away-patients-or-charge-them-higher-bills, accessed 25 December 2020.

5 COVID-19 and the Indian Health System

A Democratic Deficit

Ritu Priya and Mathew George

Introduction

The Indian Health System can be conceptualised as a complex mix of public and private sector health services and policies to address preventive, promotive, curative, and rehabilitative healthcare needs of people. It includes modern, conventional bio-medicine and seven other recognised systems (AYUSH – ayurveda, yoga and naturopathy, unani, siddha, sowa-rigpa, and homeopathy). Enabling sub-systems such as the human resource of doctors, nurses, and paramedics, their educational institutions, research and development institutions, and the medical-industrial complex of diagnostics, pharmaceutical, biologicals, and equipment industry, insurance companies and corporate hospitals are critical components. Public health and its health systems research component are meant to inform rational policy formulation and strategic planning for the health system.

Outside these formal components lie the non-formal practitioners of traditional medicine within homes and communities, as well as the non-MBBS *jhola-chhap daktars* using bio-medical therapies. The complexity is compounded by the users of these services, that is the heterogeneous people of the country, and their pluralistic health behaviours and perceptions (Das et al., 2020; Priya et al., 2019). Besides health care, a wide array of social determinants and their influence on human health are meant to be addressed by public health (WHO, 2008). Livelihoods, economic systems, and habitat have been closely linked to this pandemic (Prasad et al., 2020). This chapter will examine the responses to the COVID-19 pandemic by the state and the citizens with regard primarily to health services and public health measures.

The diversity in social, environmental, economic, political, and cultural spheres across states and districts as well as regional/religious/caste communities compounds the complexity of the system. Constitutionally, health service is a state responsibility while control of infectious diseases is a concurrent subject. It is within this backdrop that we will examine the COVID-19 responses across different components of the system – the state, the knowledge institutions, healthcare delivery systems, and the citizens.

DOI: 10.4324/9781003282815-8

The Indian State Response

The central government's acts of commission in the first wave and omission in the second wave have been the big picture over these 15 months. The central and state governments' responses exemplify Foucault's concepts of bio-politics and governmentality to their full. Biopolitics implies mechanisms through which human life is managed under processes of authority, knowledge, and power of subjectification (van den Berge, 2020; Lemke et al., 2011). This nature of power has transformed from that of a sovereign to that of the society and is more discursive, with professional knowledge being a significant contributor. The perspective underlying the handling of COVID-19 by the Indian state has elements of welfarism, public health, and political image-making as well as promotion of commercial interests, all combined to shape its responses.

There has also been a marked element of following Global Health institutions and researchers' prescriptions, to the detriment of local priorities and context specific strategies (Priya et al., 2020a). All the fault lines of society came into sharp focus through the responses to the pandemic, leading to what can also be examined using the concept of "necropolitics", which signifies processes that decide which social segments' lives are prioritised and who is left to die (Sandset, 2021). Underlying the responses is the politics of knowledge and political economy of the medical-industrial complex and public health, from global to local. Causality of the acts of commission and omission can be understood by analyses of the contemporary dominant approach to pandemic control and its science (Leach et al., 2021; Sathyamala, 2020; Priya et al., 2020b). While recognising the critical role of other spheres, we will focus primarily on the public health measures and analyse them through these lenses.

The Official Policy Response

The first case was detected in India on 29 January 2020 and two more in the first week of February, all students in Wuhan, China, who returned home to Kerala once the outbreak erupted there. The WHO declared it a Public Health Emergency of International Concern on 30th January. A Group of Ministers was set up at the centre to monitor the progression of the disease, who handed over charge to the Indian Council of Medical Research (ICMR). The ICMR scientists produced predictive models and recommended monitoring of all international travellers as well as their quarantine upon entry (Mandal et al., 2020). However, as per Directorate General of Civil Aviation data, over 78 lakh persons entered India in the months of February and March 2020 with lackadaisical checks of only 15.24 lakh passengers screened (Dasgupta, 2020).

Travel advisories on 5 February 2020 banned entry of foreigners only from China and other European countries from 3 March. Bans were strictly imposed for all international travellers and flights from 11 and 23 March 2020, respectively (MoHFW, 2020; MoHA, 2020). The visit of President Trump of the United States on the 24 and 25 February 2020 was a greater political priority than the emerging public health crisis, as may have the communal riots in east Delhi (23–29 February).

Seriousness of the pandemic was recognised by the political leadership only in mid-March when the WHO declared it as a "pandemic" on 11 March 2020, and various modelling exercises predicted unprecedented magnitude of cases, overwhelming of health services, and a large number of deaths (Ferguson et al., 2020). The disease had spread by then within the population, largely among the urban middle class and elite. Having lost time, the central government came into what seems like a panic reaction. It announced the largest and most comprehensive lockdown of social and economic activities across the entire country of 1.4 billion persons from 25 March, with a four-hour notice. There were then 536 confirmed cases and ten deaths reported in the country (Worldometer Coronavirus, 2020) largely from four cities. While the public was prepared for the lockdown through a 12-hour "Janata Curfew" on 22 March, inadequate planning before the drastic announcement was evidenced by the lack of attention to consequences for the majority of poorer sections, and without acknowledging the diversity in demography, nature of migration, and pattern of disease distribution across India.

The primary purpose of the lockdown, as internationally proposed, was to buy time to prepare health systems. Instead of focusing on strengthening health services as pandemic preparedness, the Ministry of Home Affairs and its Disaster Management Administration was given charge. From then on, much of the pandemic control became a centralised law-and-order issue. The negative impact of the hard lockdown on the urban poor who were unable to comply with the required "sit at home, wash hands frequently" prescription became evident on the streets of the metros and highways leading out from them. The migrant informal sector workers poured out to return to their native places for some assurance of a roof and food for survival. The macro-economic and social impacts were soon evident as well. So some loosening of the lockdown with a calibrated approach by labelling districts as red, orange, and green based on their case rates was instituted.

The disaster management response to COVID-19 was short term and was unable to sustain for long, as "natural" disasters are typically expected to last as short-lived events. The disaster management authority's limitations in addressing the technical knowledge necessary for dealing with a public health emergency and the failure to create effective inter-sectoral linkages with the health agencies, which have greater stake and experience in disease-related matters, led to several challenges for an effective pandemic response (Thomas, 2020; NDMA, 2020).

Once the lockdown was initiated and its calibrated application was instituted, with the pandemic hitting the people on a large scale, the centre left the states to respond as best they could, washing its hands off direct intervention. The states were now required to provide support to the migrant workers for food and deal with the ramping up of health services. The centre's responsibility of ensuring smooth inter-state movement of supplies and for people returning home or travelling for health care along with providing subsistence support required by a majority of citizens to tide over the economic lockdown came as measures that were too little, too late (Kumar, 2020). Not only did it not support States by ensuring funds for COVID healthcare, but it also did not release the GST fund share statutorily due to them.

Despite a stricter lockdown, sero-survey results showed that Indian cities reached higher infection rates than in other countries, indicating a limited slowing down of the pandemic (Priya and Chaudhary, 2021). This will be remembered in history as an example of how a solution can become worse than the problem.

One positive contribution of the lockdown was that it created basic awareness about a new disease in a short period of time across all sections. Supplementing this had been the mass messaging for preventive intervention.[1] However, the upsurge in cases during and after lockdown indicates limited impact. Understanding obtained from health-seeking behaviour studies tells us that coercion and fear do not lead to consistent change unless conducive conditions are created (Bandura, 1990).

Public Health Response

Tracking-tracing-testing-isolation is undoubtedly the most important public health intervention, which if carried out effectively on the ground can reduce spread of the disease in its early phases until community transmission sets in. Among those infected, deaths can be reduced if adequate treatment facilities are ensured. The ICMR, an agency under the Ministry of Health and Family Welfare largely for promoting and funding medical research in the country, was chosen to become the nodal health agency, putting aside the National Centre for Disease Control that is normally charged with investigation and control of infectious disease outbreaks/epidemics. The ICMR analysed possible strategies to control the spread and recommended identification of symptomatic travellers and their contacts for isolation.

> The critical concerns are the efficiency and timeliness of quarantine and isolation and the challenges of detection of COVID-19 with symptoms similar to many other lower respiratory tract infections. There is a need to engage community-based organizations that can take up the work of symptomatic surveillance, as well as raising awareness of the need for self-quarantine where possible, and referral to hospital where necessary, till infection is confirmed. Till that time, assurance of food and supplies should be given following examples of such practices in Kerala.
>
> (Mandal et al., 2020)

ICMR-supported research identified the virus strain, developed the RT-PCR test to detect cases with 70% accuracy, and required a minimum of 6–8 hours for results and special BSL2 and 3 laboratories to process the samples of nasal and throat swabs. This included the intensive task of upgrading laboratories from merely one available at the National Institute of Virology to 1,000 by June 2020 (DHR, 2020; ICMR, 2020). Despite the limitations of the technology, a positive test became the holy passport for accessing treatment. The choice of RT-PCR as the "gold standard test" despite knowledge of it giving 30% "false negative" results, thereby systematically missing 30% infected persons, added to the continuing spread.

The escalating spread provoked a debate about whether "community transmission" had started, but the government did not acknowledge its occurrence. While this may be an image-projecting issue for the political leadership, it has implications for epidemic control strategies. Once community transmission is reached, it requires a shift from the tracking-testing to a syndromic symptom-based management strategy (WHO, 2020), but the fetish of a positive test continued in the second wave.

It is well known that risk varies across social groups for most diseases and was unlikely to be any different for COVID-19. When we use the entire population as the denominator for estimating the problem, we assume that the problem is distributed evenly across the population with homogeneous distribution. Within the public health response, the "one-size-fits-all" approach and medicalised mindset become obvious with the series of nationwide guidelines[2] released by the ICMR. Most of these seem to be written more by an institution-centric "clinical logic" that expects suspected cases to come for diagnosis and treatment than by the "public health" approach of going to the people and identifying cases, motivating and providing services in their context. The classical primary healthcare approach of disease control, which envisages community-based interventions and community participation at every stage of control efforts, was conspicuously missing.

The approach adopted failed to understand and interpret the pandemic from people's lived experiences and excluded the most vulnerable and needy from the process of testing and treatment. This calls for knowledge about the societal dynamics of transmission of COVID-19 among people as related to their living and working conditions (Leach et al., 2021). Social and behavioural studies on COVID-19 transmission were completely missing in the Indian context, including from the containment zones and hotspots.

The testing guidelines fail to mention from where, how, and by whom the suspected patients of COVID-19 need to be identified in the population of a city, block, district, or state. This led to lack of clarity on the processes to be followed to identify suspected cases in the community and its failure to integrate this with the functions of the existing government health services, the only nationwide network that can be relied upon during epidemics despite all its shortcomings.

The Health Services Response

The health services response was a highly medicalised one, guided by the Hospital-ICU-Ventilator imagery, as emerging from the high-income western countries, and fed by the initial small fraction of infected persons who became moderately or seriously ill with COVID-19. Curative care for COVID-19 implies a continuum of care for those set of services that are necessary for treating and supporting all those detected positive – the 80% asymptomatic/with mild symptoms, 10–15% of those who go to the moderate category and those with co-morbidities who are at higher risk of becoming serious, and the roughly 5% who are severely affected. Since it is very difficult to predict the trajectory of the disease in an individual, support and monitoring are essential at all stages.

The central government, in its guideline[3] released on 7 April 2020, proposed a three-tier structure for treatment of COVID-19. COVID Care Centres (CCCs) were to handle mild cases and Designated COVID Health Centres (DCHC), the moderate cases needing medical attention and oxygen if necessary. Dedicated COVID Hospitals (DCH) were to cater to severe cases needing specialised medication, respiratory support, and intensive care. Unfortunately, these guidelines led to no effective integration of COVID-19 services into the existing health services of the states since they were mostly viewed as temporary stand-alone arrangements. With the already inadequate health services, this has meant a heavy toll during the first and second waves of the pandemic.

Primary Level Care

Primary level care for mild COVID cases required consultation, diagnostic services, and basic treatment to monitor for signs of escalation to a moderate stage, and provide necessary psychosocial support and allaying of anxieties. Hence it could be undertaken under medical supervision by paramedics, trained volunteers such as teachers, and interested youth. Unfortunately, this dimension did not get the attention it deserved.

The primary level functionaries were deployed largely for tracking-tracing-testing-isolation and no one was designated to provide care to mild positive cases. People resorted to various kinds of self-care and support, from home remedies and telephonic consultations to going to hospital. In the initial phase when the number of cases was low, in several cities, patients with a positive test result and mild symptoms were admitted in COVID-19 hospitals, which were otherwise well equipped to deal with tertiary level care facilities for COVID-19. Later, when increasingly serious cases started coming to the hospitals, there was triage and prioritisation of serious cases over the less serious ones.

In states like Kerala, Tamil Nadu, and Chhattisgarh, exclusive COVID first-line treatment centres (CFLTCs) were opened under the administrative support of local self-governments and district authorities with community volunteers being mobilised for additional hands. They were mostly developed in schools, colleges, or community centres and at times AYUSH hospitals with a 50-bed facility arranged under the administrative control of a nodal officer. A similar structure was established in several slums of Mumbai immediately after community spread of the disease was established for the first time in the city. Worth mentioning is the support these facilities offered for people who had difficulty in getting isolated in homes due to overcrowding, thereby curbing spread. However, what was found in Kerala's context was that they were utilised in the initial phase when there was ambiguity about diagnostic and treatment needs but, as people started preferring home isolation and care, acceptance of these centres soon waned (Ansina, 2021).

Failing to get integrated with other functions of the health department, as the first wave abated, many were shut down and hence were not available for the second wave. Data shows that in one of the districts of Kerala, the number of CFLTCS proposed during the month of July was 94 with a total bed capacity of 7,252. By August 2020, the number of functional CFLTCs reduced to 19 with 1,770 beds and reached the single digit of seven by February 2021. In the month of April 2021 during the second wave, only two centres were admitting patients with a total bed capacity of 200 beds (Ansina, 2021).

Telephonic monitoring and advice services were set up by most states for follow-up of all test-positive cases, but this was done perfunctorily and more as a ritual, not becoming a functional support system in most places. In Mumbai where a decentralised war room was made operational at the ward level, it appears to have been effective for referral coordination between citizens and hospital bed availability (Saigal, 2021).

The unmet need for consultation by even the mild cases was so glaring that a large number of doctors and civil society organisations and community networks initiated their own informal and formal support systems through call-in telephonic services. However, even in the second wave when cases had increased over fourfold and almost half were in rural areas, this was not in focus in the MOHFW-released Standard Operating Procedure for peri-urban, rural, and tribal areas (MoHFW, 2021). Given the shortage of personnel and level of community transmission, mobilisation of community volunteer teams trained to supplement the efforts of paramedics of the rural health services would have been essential. Training the *jhola-chhaap daktars*, the non-formal rural health practitioners on whom the majority in rural India rely for routine health care was another avenue that some civil society organisations and state governments, such as West Bengal, drew upon in this crisis.

Secondary Level Care

Secondary level care was required as an intermediate layer for those who escalated beyond the mild symptoms but not needing intensive care.

However, the DCHC ended up providing either primary level services or referral to specialised COVID hospitals. From the provider side, all medical personnel and other resources were concentrated in the state-of-the-art hospitals specially designated for COVID-19. Mass media attention too was focused on these hospitals. From the patient perspective, if they thought that the severity of the disease demanded institutional care, people were not willing to take a risk by getting admitted in a facility which did not have ICU or ventilator support. Thereby they resorted to tertiary centres that got unnecessarily overburdened or to private nursing homes.

In the peak of the second wave, community services again came forward, for instance with Gurudwaras setting up oxygen hubs (oxygen *langars)* in and around Delhi and Resident Welfare Associations of middle-class areas organising their own oxygen hubs. What this demonstrated was the unmet need of such close-to-community medical facilities for tiding over the stage of moderate disease.

Tertiary Level Care

Tertiary level COVID-19 care developed very dynamically through the pandemic. However, it had inherent difficulties, one of it was that the patient could not be accompanied by friends or family members during the treatment process, and during triage, hospitals prioritized higher risk patients while denying treatment to others. These led to high distrust towards the care rendered in both public and private hospitals. Failure to regularly update the relatives of patients about the disease situation may be explained by the high patient load under difficult conditions, but where addressed, this measure led to better mutual understanding.

Initial phases of tertiary care posed multiple challenges for the health professionals and patients. Infectiousness of the Coronavirus and high case fatality in the most advanced countries, the lack of protective equipment and uncertainty surrounding effectiveness of treatment protocols generated fear even among the healthcare professionals. The private sector shut down and it was only public hospitals that provided COVID-19 and non-COVID care during April and May 2020. The inadequacy of beds and other infrastructure, personnel, and drugs together resulted in a very difficult situation (BMJ 2020).

Bed availability was then ramped up in public facilities with additional space in hotels and community spaces, commandeering private hospitals with capacity to provide a large percentage of their beds for COVID-19 patients, and so on. Personal Protective Equipment (PPE) kits and ventilators were manufactured in the country on a large scale in a short period of time. A few months into the first wave, the private sector hospitals overcame their fear of the pandemic and realised that they could function with reasonable knowledge of medical protocols, even though constantly evolving and changing with new study results and experience coming in. Eventually all the beds mobilised were not used, as the first peak of cases and deaths in

May–June 2020 abated and had not reached the peak heights projected by several modelling exercises.

The tertiary care hospitals were further challenged by the second wave that started in late February 2021, initially in Mumbai and Delhi, with cases and deaths numbering more than four times that of the first wave. Both the public and private sectors again faced shortage of infrastructure and personnel. People dying at home, in ambulances, and hospital waiting rooms filled the mass media for about two months.

The constraint of health infrastructure got further fuelled by the shortage of medical oxygen, which was initially reported in Delhi, followed by the neighbouring states of Haryana, Uttar Pradesh, as well as the more endowed state of Goa in the west. This overlooking of the need for ramping up oxygen is unexplainable since the National Task Force and Empowered Group for Supplies had itself flagged the issue as had the Parliamentary Standing Committee on Health and Family welfare in 2020 with funds being allocated to set up oxygen production plants in hospitals across the country (Parliament of India-Rajya Sabha, 2020). Yet, little had moved till 31 March 2021 when a fraction of the funds was released by the central government with the shortage of oxygen already the alleged reason for many of the COVID-19 deaths happening then.

The Vaccine Crisis

With vaccines, poised as the biggest game changer in the pandemic, it was no mean achievement that the ICMR together with industry partner Bharat Biotech developed a COVID-19 vaccine indigenously and was ready to produce it for mass administration by January 2021. Another vaccine, developed by Oxford University and AstraZeneca, was being produced in India by private industry, the Serum Institute of India, and ready for supply. Being the producer of half the world's vaccine volume in pre-COVID times, it was expected that India's vaccine industry would have no problem in delivering on the scale required for India and the world. This was also the promise of the government. However, what transpired by April 2021 revealed the biggest fiasco of all.

The country was short by a long margin for the vaccines it needed. For the entire population above 44 years of age, that is about 300 million, 600 million doses would be needed, to be administered at the earliest, if they are to be able to protect from the second and subsequent waves of the pandemic. However, only a fraction of this was being ordered in tranches over the months. On 19 April 2021, the government devolved even this responsibility to the states, announcing a new "Liberalised Pricing and Accelerated National COVID-19 Vaccination Strategy" by which it will procure 50% of supplies directly and leave the other 50% for states and private hospitals.

It appears that the centre was ready to assure vaccination for half the identified priority sections and leave others to exclusionary processes. The vaccination programme was rolled out in a phased manner based on risk levels, which was the health professionals first, then the police and other front-line professionals, then the elderly who are the highest risk group for mortality due to COVID-19. All these were to be covered by the government free of charge. Before all those above 60 years could be covered, it was opened up also for the 45–59-year-old age group. Whatever doses were there largely remained in the urban areas, only an estimated 12–15% inhabitants of rural and semi-rural having received at least one dose of the vaccine by May 2021 (Radhakrishnan, 2021).

Further systematic exclusion occurred through the administering system adopted. The primary healthcare approach envisions vaccines to be given close to people's residences as done for the child immunisation programme. Instead, the CoWIN app was developed for COVID-19, a technology interface that has reversed the approach. Those who are eligible are expected to register for vaccinations on the CoWIN app and once they get an appointment, they are expected to reach the designated facility for the shot. As in the case of testing, here too, the digital divide and urban-rural divide have led to exclusions. The exclusionary process goes further against the poor and the rural when the private sector is allowed to purchase directly from the manufacturers and provide for its clients.

International Discourse, Political Imagery, and Political Economy of Health Care

Thus, the entire approach to pandemic management has been too centralised yet incoherent. Detailed examination of the major areas of commission such as the lockdown and healthcare provisions reveals major areas of omission. The lockdown is likely to have slowed down the spread of infection to some degree, yet the infection rate has been higher than any other country, as revealed by the sero-surveys (Murhekar et al., 2021). Death rate will only be known with any level of assurance after census data becomes available. It will show not only the direct COVID-19 deaths but also the extra deaths due to loss of economic viability of families and the citizens' lack of access to routine non-COVID healthcare.

The official response to the pandemic needs to be understood by situating it in the prevailing international and national discourse around health and healthcare. There is a continuation of the colonial legacy that all credible knowledge for policy-making comes from the West. We work with international analyses and prescriptions that are inherently reductionist since they consider only a limited set of variables that can be assessed and aggregated at global scale (Priya and Das, 2020). This has been compounded by the economic structural adjustment policies and globalisation initiated in the 1980s and 1990s with privatisation of health care in a corporate mould. The three-tier structure of rural health services could have served COVID-19 epidemic needs very well, if it had been robust and in full vigour in normal times. Unfortunately, it has not been developed as envisaged at the time of independence. What was developed went into a decline in the decade of the 1990s and beyond (Qadeer et al., 2019).

It bounced back to an extent after 2005–06 when the National Rural Health Mission (NRHM) was launched, with infrastructure, personnel, and medicines all being in better situation than before. OPD attendance at public facilities went up and public expenditure on health went up from 17% of total health expenditure on health in the country to 30%, with some relief to people (WHO, 2021). Unfortunately, instead of escalating this further, the National Health Mission (NHM) has seen decline in policy support since 2015–16, weakening the system at multiple levels (George, 2020).

The move from the Primary Health Care approach of the 1970s to the Universal Health Coverage slogan of the 2000s is indicative of this structural backlash to any questioning of the doctor-hospital-centred model, of attempts at its democratisation (Bisht, 2013). This shift has been promoted by the United States- and Europe-dominated international agencies such as the Rockefeller, USAID, and the philanthro-capitalism of the Gates and other Foundations as well as the medical-industrial complex of pharmaceutical and biological industries, insurance companies, and corporate hospital chains. With some recognition of market failure in the healthcare sector, these agencies allowed for public system strengthening to the extent that it can administer the immunisation schedule (for which a public provider is essential) and act as a demand creator for the private medical sector. The renewed decline in support to public systems since 2015–16 and a blatant pro-commercial interest policy thrust are reflected in initiatives such as the Ayushman Bharat scheme that relies on social insurance using public funds routed through private insurance firms and services provided by the empanelled private sector.

What the oxygen fiasco suggests is the lack of a grounded approach of analysing our own situation and pursuing solutions based on our priorities. The international discourse of the pandemic had set the tone for the lockdown and the hospital-centred approach. While PPEs and ventilators were concerns in the high-income countries, oxygen supply was not. Moreover, since medical use of oxygen is only a small fraction of the total oxygen produced, producers were not pro-active about the medical market. With neither the industry nor the international discourse pushing for oxygen, it dropped off the pandemic management radar at national level.

However, the vaccine fiasco remains unexplained. Part explanation can be the commercial interests of industry monopoly and international political image-making. However, ignoring the simple mathematics of India's numbers is inexplicable, unless one does not believe in the solution of vaccines per se or one apparently believes that "depopulation" is the only solution for a "sustainable" and "manageable" world.

Political image-making by the central leadership had it at its self-congratulatory best in January 2021, as evident in the Economic Survey

2020–21 (Priya and Chaudhary, 2021) and statements made by the Prime Minister and Union Health Minister right up to March 2021. Assembly elections across four states in March and April as well as the efforts to garner international mileage were on the immediate political agenda. The lull in COVID-19 cases between November 2020 and February 2021 allowed the central government to claim that "we have won the war" against the pandemic and a complacency seems to have set in for the believers of this claim. It allowed for unrestricted election rallies and the religious gathering of the Kumbh Mela. The complacency led to all emergency activities including ramping up of healthcare being put on hold or even abandoned (Jain, 2021). Health facilities created in 2020 were dismantled without any strengthening of the regular health infrastructure. Vacant posts of health personnel were not filled (Gokhale, 2021).

This politics of knowledge and political economy has combined with all the existing fault lines in society – class, caste, religious and gender divides, the power mongering and authoritarian thrust of those holding state power, and the attempt by national and international capital to further increase their profits using the pandemic as an opportunity. The best management skills, scientific and technological capacities, and all health service providers needed to be mobilised across the country for providing humanitarian care. For this, a well-coordinated "all of government" and a decentralised "all of society" response was essential to overcome the crisis. However, the approach adopted seems to have been that of centralised control and individualised leadership, to the detriment of a wholesome response, eventually leading to unnecessary compounding of national trauma and the loss of citizens' lives.

Conclusion

As a prime public health crisis, the pandemic called for a public health approach informing its politico-administrative measures. While recognising the severe constraints in effective handling of a new and evolving pandemic, this chapter locates limitations of the response in the politics of knowledge and its underlying dynamics of economic, political, and governance processes. A compromised set of public health approaches and tools were put to use and available public health capacities within the country were not adequately mobilised.

Evidently, there has been a failure in locating the pandemic within the lives of people and rolling out a successful public health response to COVID-19. The entire gamut of health care which would have offered some respite to those infected with the disease was mired within the larger politics of knowledge and political economy of a medical-industrial complex that prioritises commodification over everything else. This was a result of the dominant global health approach over the primary healthcare approach, coupled with the health system development policies of the government that have systematically weakened the public sector and favoured private sector growth specifically at the secondary and tertiary levels. This has not only resulted in the exclusion of the poor and the vulnerable but also became a complex machinery that renders possibilities of life and death of all people at all times as negotiated struggles rather than as processes with assured support systems.

Could we have done better? With a political vision of making maximum use of all resources and capacities within the country: of epidemic control science and its institutions, of all health infrastructure and delivery mechanisms, all forms of knowledge (public health, clinical, social science, and managerial; biomedicine, AYUSH, and local health traditions), and harnessed all public and private vaccine production units in the country, we would have done better. Democratisation of information, transparency about the basis for decision-making, would have minimised the insecurity and distrust between centre and state governments, between people and the health services. We may have done better with data transparency and sharing for wider use to understand challenges better and develop innovative solutions, decentralised planning of control activities, and their implementation so that it was suited to local context, with community members mobilised and allowed to undertake collective welfare activities with safeguards. Consultation and dialogue would be necessary at each step.

We argue through the narrative in this chapter that much suffering could have been prevented if such a holistic health system approach had been adopted. Experience from efforts within the country and outside, in this and previous epidemics, provides enough basis for this expectation. The role of the central government would still have been critical: for ensuring finances at all levels (national to state, district, and local), facilitating and mobilising all research institutions and industry, inter-sectoral coordination, inter-state movement, medical and food supplies to all, and so on. Instead of a law-and-order authoritarian exercise, it would then have been an "all of society" effort of caring and being cared for, individually and collectively. This is the difference a contextualised primary healthcare approach versus a medicalised global health approach can make in a public health crisis.

Notes

1 IEC material was propagated by MoHFW with toll free numbers; see the link www.mohfw.gov.in/pdf/ProtectivemeasuresEng.pdf. Another guideline specific to government employees is issued by DoPT, www.mohfw.gov.in/pdf/PreventivemeasuresDOPT.pdf accessed on 7 May 2020.

2 A series of guidelines was issued on testing during 17 March till 18 May 2020, with several modifications as newer experiences emerged about the disease. Inclusion of newer category of patients was based on as and when new categories of patients are identified in any of the known hospitals. Change of criteria in short duration is not a good practice for a large-scale programme as bringing in change requires a longer time among those who are implementing. For more details, see www.icmr.gov.in/cteststrat.html

3 www.mohfw.gov.in/pdf/FinalGuidanceonMangaementofCOVIDcasesversion2.pdf accessed on June 2020

References

Ansina, H. (2021), "Policy analysis of COVID 19 first line treatment centres (CFLTCs): Implementation and activities in Kerala", Unpublished Field Practicum report submitted to the School of Health Systems Studies, Tata Institute of Social Sciences Mumbai.

Bandura, A. (1990), "Perceived self-efficacy in the exercise of control over AIDS infection", *Evaluation and Program Planning*, 13(1), 9–17.

Bisht, R. (2013), "Universal health care: The changing international discourse", *Indian Journal of Public Health*, 57(4), 236.

BMJ (2020), "COVID 19: India's private doctors and government clash over pandemic response", *BMJ News*, BMI 2020 370:m3711. Doi: 10.1136/bmj.m3711.

Das, J., Daniels, B., Ashok, M., Shim, E.-Y. and Muralidharan, K. (2020). "Two Indias: The structure of primary health care markets in rural Indian villages with implications for policy", *Social Science & Medicine*, 301, 112799. Doi: 10.1016/j.socscimed.2020.112799.

Dasgupta, S. (2020), "India screened only 19% of inbound passengers for COVID until 23 March, RTI reply reveals", *The Print*, 15 March, https://theprint.in/health/india-screened-only-19-of-inbound-passengers-for-COVID-until-23-march-rti-reply-reveals/422140/, accessed 23 May 2021.

DHR (2020), *Enhance India's Testing Capacity, 21st May 2020*, Department of Health Research, Ministry of health and family welfare, GoI, www.icmr.gov.in/pdf/press_realease_files/Testing%20Capacity_22%20May%202020_v3.pdf, accessed 7August 2020.

Ferguson, N., Laydon, D., Nedjati-Gilani, G., Imai, N., Ainslie, K., Baguelin, M. and Ghani, A. C. (2020), "Report 9: Impact of non-pharmaceutical interventions (NPIs) to reduce COVID19 mortality and healthcare demand", *Imperial College London*, 10(77482), 491–497.

George, M. (2020), "The fragmentation and weakening of institutions of primary healthcare", *Economic & Political Weekly*, 55(42), 58–64.

Gokhale, O. (2021), "Enough steps haven't been taken to fill up vacant medical posts since last year: Bombay HC", *The Indian Express*, 15 May, https://indianexpress.com/article/cities/mumbai/enough-steps-havent-been-taken-to-fill-up-vacant-medical-posts-since-last-year-bombay-hc-7316462/ accessed 14 June 2021.

ICMR (2020), "Advisory newer additional strategies for COVID testing", pp. 1–7, www.icmr.gov.in/pdf/COVID/strategy/New_additional_Advisory_23062020_3.pdf, accessed 10 August 2020.

Jain, V. (2021), "Deep rooted health issues, Complacency behind second COVID 19 wave in India", *Business Standard*, 10 May, www.business-standard.com/article/current-affairs/india-s-deep-rooted-issues-behind-the-second-wave-of-covid-19–121051000161_1.html, accessed 6 June 2021.

Kumar, A. (2020), "What can be done to ensure the wheels do not come off the Indian economy?" *Wire*, 31 March, https://thewire.in/economy/indian-economy-covid-19-lockdown-policy, accessed 19 April 2020.

Leach, M., MacGregor, H., Ripoll, S., Scoones, I. and Wilkinson, A. (2021), "Rethinking disease preparedness: Incertitude and the politics of knowledge", *Critical Public Health*, 1–15.

Lemke, T., Casper, M. and Moore, L. J. (2011), *Biopolitics: An Advanced Introduction*, Vol. 5, New York: NYU Press, Chapter. 3, pp. 33–52.

Mandal, S., Bhatnagar, T., Arinaminpathy, N., Agarwal, A., Chowdhury, A., Murhekar, M., . . . Sarkar, S. (2020), "Prudent public health intervention strategies to control the coronavirus disease 2019 transmission in India: A mathematical model-based approach", *The Indian Journal of Medical Research*, 151(2–3), 190.

MoHA (2020), *Advisory: Travel and Visa Restrictions Related to COVID 19*, Bureau of Immigration, Ministry of Home Affairs, Government of India, https://boi.gov.in/content/advisory-travel-and-visa-restrictions-related-COVID-1, accessed 24 August 2020.

MoHFW (2020), "Travel Advisory, dated 05th March 2020", www.mohfw.gov.in/pdf/Traveladvisory05022020.pdf, accessed 24 August 2020.

MoHFW (2021), "SOP on COVID 19 Containment and management in Peri Urban", *Rural and Tribal Areas*, 16 May, www.mohfw.gov.in/pdf/SOPonCOVID19Containment&ManagementinPeriurbanRural&tribalareas.pdf, accessed 23 May 2021.

Murhekar, M. V., Bhatnagar, T., Selvaraju, S., Saravanakumar, V., Thangaraj, J. W. V., Shah, N. and Zaman, K. (2021), "SARS-CoV-2 antibody seroprevalence in India, August – September 2020: Findings from the second nationwide household serosurvey", *The Lancet Global Health*, 9(3), e257–e266.

NDMA (2020), *COVID 19 Impacts and Responses: The Indian Experience, January-May 2020*, India: National Disaster Management Authority.

Parliament of India- Rajya Sabha (2020), "Department-related Parliamentary Standing Committee on Health and Family Welfare", 123rd Report on the outbreak of Pandemic COVID 19 and its management, https://rajyasabha.nic.in/rsnew/Committee_site/Committee_File/ReportFile/14/142/123_2020_11_15.pdf, accessed 23 May 2021.

Prasad, V., Sri, B. S. and Gaitonde, R. (2020), "Bridging a false dichotomy in the COVID-19 response: A public health approach to the 'lockdown' debate", *BMJ Global Health*, 5, e002909. Doi: 10.1136/ bmjgh-2020-002909.

Priya, R., Acharya, S., Baru, R., Bajpai, V., Bisht, R., Ghodajkar, P., Guite, N. and Reddy, S. (2020a), "Indian public health associations on COVID-19 the politics of knowledge", *Economic & Political Weekly*, August 8, IV(32 & 33), 19–22.

Priya, R., Acharya, S., Baru, R., Bajpai, V., Bisht, R., Ghodajkar, P., Guite, N. and Reddy, S. (2020b), "Beyond biomedical and statistical approaches in COVID-19: How shoe-leather public health works", *Economic & Political Weekly*, 31 October, IV(44), 47–58.

Priya, R. and Chaudhary, K. (2021), "COVID-19 cases and deaths, lessons from the first wave", *The Frontline*.

Priya, R. and Das, S. (2020), "The blind spots of public health", *The India Forum*, 25 August, www.theindiaforum.in/article/blind-spots-public -health.

Priya, R., Singh, R. and Das, S. (2019), "Health implications of diverse visions of urban spaces: Bridging the formal-informal divide", *Front Public Health*, 7, 239. Doi: 10.3389/fpubh.2019.00239.

Qadeer, I., Saxena, K. B. and Arathi, P. M. (2019), *Universal Healthcare in India from Care to Coverage*, New Delhi: Sage.

Radhakrishnan, V. (2021), "Vaccination in rural India trails urban areas even as cases surge", *The Hindu*, 18 May 2021, www.thehindu.com/news/national/vaccination-in-rural-india-trails-urban-areas-even-as-cases-surge/article34589734.ece, accessed 12 June 2021.

Saigal, S. (2021), "Beating back the pandemic in Mumbai", *The Hindu, Ground Zero*, 15 May 2021, www.thehindu.com/news/national/ground-zero-beating-back-the-pandemic-in-mumbai/article34561408.ece, accessed 15 May 2021.

Sandset, T. (2021), "The necropolitics of COVID-19: Race, class and slow death in an ongoing pandemic", *Global Public Health*, 1–13.
Sathyamala, C. (2020), *COVID-19: A Biopolitical Odyssey*, Working Paper No. 667, Erasmus International Institute of Social Studies.
Thomas, C. (2020), "COVID 19: Lessons for disaster management", *Down to Earth*, 11 June.
van den Berge, L. (2020), "Biopolitics and the coronavirus: Foucault, Agamben, Žižek", *Netherlands Journal of Legal Philosophy* (1).
WHO (2008), *Closing the Gap in a Generation: Health Equity Through Action on the Social Determinants of Health: Commission on Social Determinants of Heath Final Report*, World Health Organization, Geneva.
WHO (2020), *Preparing for Large Scale Community Transmission of COVID-19: Guidance for Countries and Areas in the WHO Western Pacific Region*, 28 February, World Health Organization, Geneva.
WHO (2021), *Global Health Expenditure Database, National Health Accounts Indicators*, World Health Organization, https://apps.who.int/nha/database/ViewData/Indicators/en, accessed 14 June 2021.
Worldometer Coronavirus (2020), "Country: India", www.worldometers.info/coronavirus/country/india/, accessed 23 May 2021.

6 COVID-19 Pandemic and Its Impact on the Indian Education System

Chandan Kumar Sharma and Angel Habamon Syiem

Introduction

The situation arising out of the COVID-19 pandemic wreaked havoc among all sections of humankind. The prolonged lockdown and the norms of physical distancing imposed by governments around the world to stem the spread of the virus created serious challenges for normal social practices and processes. India has also borne the brunt of the pandemic. Various sectors and sections of the Indian society have been seriously affected, one of the worst casualties being its education system.

With the closure of the educational institutions in the country in the third week of March 2020, online education system has been promoted to ensure the continuity of the teaching-learning process. However, it has been found that this system, which requires paraphernalia such as smart phones, laptops, internet connectivity, and continuous electricity supply at both ends, has left out a large number of students from the economically marginal classes or those from the geographically remote areas. The online education has thus proved to be an exclusionary system. Since most of the economically marginalised section hail from the socially marginalised groups such as the Scheduled Castes and the Scheduled Tribes, the online education system created, nay perpetuated, what has been described as the "digital divide" between the marginalised sections and the more privileged sections of the Indian society. Poor parents faced great hardship to provide the necessary paraphernalia to their children to take part in the online classes. Not only the students but the teaching community has also had to face much adversity in conducting the classes.

This chapter seeks to shed light on these adversities that the online education posed. It is clear that inadequate infrastructure on account of prolonged neglect of the education sector has exacerbated the problems inflicted by the pandemic. However, it is also a matter of concern that without addressing this, there has also been a campaign to shift to online education system (Singh, 2020), although the positive dimension of online education needs to be emphasised. The essay also highlights the perils of this on the basis of the experience during the pandemic. It further argues that this deprivation

DOI: 10.4324/9781003282815-9

of education of students from marginal sections contravenes the right to education that our children are guaranteed by the Indian Constitution. The essay, however, identifies the positive lessons from our experience of online education during the pandemic, which could be used in our teaching-learning process in the future.

Indian Education Sector: A Brief Overview

For a long time, under the Constitution of India, school education was a state subject, and the only role that the Union Government played was that of coordination and checking the standards of higher education. Forty-second Constitutional Amendment, 1976 made education a subject under the concurrent list empowering the Union Government to legislate or promulgate policies on education periodically.

The Indian education system has three broad levels: primary, secondary, and higher. National organisation such as the National Council for Educational Research and Training (NCERT) plays an important role especially in the preparation of a National Curriculum framework for schools. At the level of the state, the State Council for Educational Research and Training (SCERT) implements the guidelines set forth by the NCERT. School education in India is regulated by mainly three boards. While school education at national level is under the purview of the Central Board of Secondary Education (CBSE) and Indian Certificate of Secondary Education (ICSE), at state level, it is under the purview of various state boards. Among them, the CBSE and state boards are government bodies and ICSE is a non-government body. As far as higher education is concerned, universities and colleges are regulated by the University Grants Commission (UGC). Technical education, however, is regulated by the All-India Council of Technical Education (AICTE). Similarly, Medical Council of India (MCI) and Bar Council of India (BCI) regulate medical and legal education.

With the insertion of Article 21 A of the Constitution by the 86th Amendment Act of 2002, Right to Free and Compulsory Education became part of the fundamental rights of its citizens. In the year 2009, a legislative step was taken through the passing of the Right of Children to Free and Compulsory Education Act (RTE), 2009. This guaranteed free and compulsory education of satisfactory quality for all children below 14 years. As India has been engaged in taking steps towards implementing this after dealing with challenges such as financial gap, corruption, equality, and lack of infrastructure for a long time, one can easily guess what kind of implication an unexpected disaster like the COVID-19 pandemic can spell out for the Indian education scenario. While there are studies showing the impact of the shift from classroom to online lectures, the budget allocation of the 2020–21 for education, however, reduced by Rs. 4,971.34 crore for school education and Rs. 1,115.87 crore for higher education (Mehra, 2021) earmarking only 3.5%

(Sarkar and Mitra, 2021) of the GDP, which is way below the recommended 6% even in the National Education Policy (NEP) 2020.

The Digital Divide

It is to be noted that even prior to COVID-19, at least in higher education, there has been constant effort to introduce the blended mode of education. To this end, some of the initiatives that the Union Ministry of Education introduced were SWAYAM, which provides for a massive open online course (MOOCS), and SWAYAMPRABHA, which makes available quality educational programmes on television. Several digital contents are made available also through initiatives such as National Digital Library, e-PG Pathshala, Shodhganga, and e-ShodhSindhu. Accelerated hands on learning are also provided through e-Yatra, FOSEE, Spoken Tutorial, and Virtual Labs. At school level, primary and secondary, Diksha portal provides for multi-lingual e-learning content for students and teachers where content have been created by around 250 teachers. Similarly, other initiatives such as National Repository of Open Educational Resources (NROER) are also relevant. The Bharatnet project launched in the year 2012 with the aim of providing broadband connectivity to around 2,50,000 Gram Panchayats if implemented effectively would help students in the rural areas for online education.

When India was hit by COVID in March 2020, both union and state governments came up with several initiatives to boost up online learning. The Ministry of Education, for example, came up with initiatives with mottos such as "One nation, one digital platform" and "one class-one channel". Further, the ministry announced a week-long campaign called, "Bharat Padhe Online" to seek suggestions and "ideas" from mainly teachers and students to improve already functional online learning (Hindustan Times, 2020). In order to ensure equity in digital learning, TV and radio have been used to reach out to the students.

At the state level, Chhattisgarh initiated *Padhai Tuhar Dwar* (education at your doorsteps) portal. Delhi came up with a plan on how to make the classes available for each level under "Learning with Human Scheme" (Parul, 2020). One mechanism implemented in the state of Kerala was by broadcasting free-to-air television channel. In collaboration with UNICEF, the Odisha government started an initiative for the children enrolled in Anganwadi centres, by the name *Ghare Ghare Arunima* (dawn at every home) (Orissa Diary, 2020).

Notwithstanding such initiatives by the government, one of the most prominent fallouts of the online teaching-learning process has been that it immediately became clear that it deprived a large section of students who had very limited or no access to the relevant technologies required for the online mode, a phenomenon that came to be described as the digital divide.

It is to be noted that only 8% of India's students have a laptop with Internet connection. The rest cannot look beyond a smartphone – a clumsy means of accessing study material, let alone writing exam answers (Chaudhuri, 2020). In the state government schools attended by the mass of students, even this support is enjoyed by only 56%, the figure being 74.2% in private schools, according to the Annual Status of Education Report (ASER) 2020.

Further, in a 2017–18 survey, the Ministry of Rural Development found that only 47% of Indian households receive more than 12 hours of electricity and more than 36% of schools in India operate without electricity. Again, as per the Key Indicators of Household Social Consumption on Education in India report, based on the 2017–18 NSSO, fewer than 15% of rural Indian households have Internet access (as opposed to 42% urban Indian households). Only 13% of people surveyed (aged above 5) in rural areas – just 8.5% of females – could use the Internet. Thus, students from families with better living standard shift to online education with relative comfort, while students from underprivileged backgrounds are likely to suffer because of either the inaccessibility of the technology or the low education of their parents to guide them through tech-savvy applications (Modi and Postaria, 2020).

NSSO 2014–2015 data suggests that economic factors are critical to children dropping out of school in India. The pandemic and lockdown have affected 1.4 million migrant workers and others working in the unorganised sector (90% of India's population is engaged in disorganised work). The migrant workers either have moved back home along with their children or are unable to send remittances home this season. In such a situation, the emphasis on technology-driven education has prevented many children from continuing school education (Ibid.).

This situation worsened further in geographically difficult regions of the country such as hilly or riverine areas where the availability of power and mobile or Internet connectivity is often a luxury. Our personal experience as teachers serving in North Eastern India, characterised by hilly as well as flood-prone areas, has shown that students living in such areas experienced serious problem in accessing online education. Students pursuing higher education who were asked to vacate their hostels and attend classes from their homes after the pandemic broke out often had great difficulties in attending their classes and uploading their answer scripts after taking their online examinations during the period. When floods came with the arrival of the rainy season after just a couple of months after the pandemic broke out in India, many students of the flood-ravaged areas had to leave their homes and take shelter in relief camps, which turned their class schedule upside down. Further, the students of Jammu & Kashmir had been at the receiving end during the pandemic as the Internet service in the state was banned since 2019 which continued till February 2021.

Such disparity in access to education raise important questions as was observed by the Supreme Court (SC) in the year 2011 that the responsibility of the state does not end with providing free and compulsory education. It is important for the state to also extend the right and make sincere effort to have education of quality without any discrimination (2011 8 SCC 737). In 2019, the Kerala High Court observed that the right to Internet access is also an integral part of right to education, which assumes even more significance with schools closed down for months and education continuing online (W.P (c). No. 19716/2019-L).

Gender Divide

Online education also had a much severe effect on the girls rather than on the boys. With limited financial resources for education, more often than not, families choose to educate their sons rather than daughters. Additional burdens on girls in terms of household chores, taking care of the sick in the family have also affected their accessibility to education. It was estimated by the Malala fund that globally more than 20 million girls would be out of school due to COVID-19 and the majority of them would be from developing countries like India (Malala Fund, 2020).

It was observed that the female students from poor Indian families were further constrained because of inadequate access to the Internet and gadgets or because the male child and his education are prioritised. Several cases of suicides of female students from marginal background have been reported in the national media from various parts of the country. On 1 June 2020, B. Devika, a class ten Dalit student of Malappuram district of Kerala, committed suicide over not having access to a laptop or a smartphone because of which she was unable to attend online classes (Philip, 2020). On 7 September 2020, Jayanti Bauli, 20, a B.A. first-year student of Mal College of Jalpaiguri District, West Bengal, hung herself for not getting a smartphone for her online classes. Her father was a daily wage worker (Agarwal, 2020). Another suicide that received wide publicity was the case of Aishwarya Reddy from Telangana on 2 November 2020. She was a B.Sc. second-year student in Mathematics at Delhi University's prestigious Lady Shri Ram College for Women. In a suicide note she had left, she wrote, "because of me, my family is facing many financial problems. My education is a burden. If I can't study, I can't live" (Baruah, 2020). These are only some of the select cases after online education started during the first few months of the pandemic. These cases clearly bring forth the pressure that the online education created on female students.

When hostels were closed down and students were asked to leave, many female students would plea that they should be allowed to stay in the campus. During our conversation, they confided that at the hostels, they experienced independence and personal space for the first time in life that was lacking at their homes. The environment at home, they said, was not conducive for studying and completing their academic work during the pandemic.

Further, balancing work and life in times of COVID where household chores and professional work take place from the same space has become particularly challenging for female teachers. While dealing with the very uncertainty of the virus, female teachers had to juggle between work pressure and familial responsibilities, including online classes of their children, which has been mentally and physically exhausting.

Challenges in Conducting Examinations

With the pandemic hitting states and areas in different degrees and at different times in a country as large and diverse like India, the academic calendar went haywire. There were schools, colleges, and universities, which could manage to complete the academic period on time while others were totally off the mark. CBSE, ICSE, and state boards had to drastically reduce their syllabi to cope with the situation. Considerable differences were also seen in the conduct of school board examinations under the CBSE, ICSE, and the respective state boards. Assignments and tests took place on online mode. Students were expected to scan the scripts, and then mail them to the course instructors or upload them through the given online portals.

There have been great uncertainties in the conduct of examinations. While the mode of conduct of examinations was seen to be flexible across schools, boards, and higher educational institutions, there was a need for some form of uniformity in the completion of the academic calendar. To this end, the SC directed the school boards to declare the class 12 final results by 31 July 2021 based on internal assessments. In 2020 too, class 10 and class 12 finals had been cancelled and final results were declared based on internal assessments. However, unlike in 2021, the internal assessments in 2020 were already completed on regular mode, while no classes or examinations on regular mode could take place for almost a year for the final-year students of 2021. In 2020, CBSE could conduct only a couple of examinations for 12th final and the students were evaluated only on the basis of these examinations and the internal assessments resulting in abnormal inflation of marks (Sindwani, 2020). Many state boards, however, conducted final written examinations amidst considerable uncertainty and the results showed that students of state boards scored relatively less than the CBSE and ICSE students. In 2021, however, after long dithering, following the SC directive, CBSE and ICSE evaluated their final-year students only on the basis of internal assessments. In the absence of any such internal assessment mechanism among the state boards, they resorted to other methods to evaluate final examinations, and such evaluation this time around has witnessed abnormally high scores as well as pass percentages in state boards. This has created further complications in the admission process for the 2021–22 session including rationalisation of marks across boards and shortage in seats in higher educational institutions.

As for entrance examinations for entry into engineering and medical institutions, originally scheduled for April 2020, the second round of Joint Entrance Examination (JEE) Main 2020 was held in September 2020 after the SC cleared the way for it despite widespread protest. Similarly, National Eligibility Entrance Test (NEET), after several postponements, was finally held on September 2020 with states taking measures to facilitate the process (NDTV Education, 2020). For 2021, after a lot of delays, JEE & NEET Main were conducted in August and September 2021, respectively.

For higher education, UGC notified guidelines for the final-year examinations to be conducted by 31 August 2021 and resume new academic sessions from 1 October. In the meantime, from the first week of September 2021, educational institutions have been opened all over India following COVID protocols. However, it is anybody's guess how the situation unfolds in near future amidst the talk of the arrival of new wave of COVID.

Education Beyond Classroom Teaching

Way back in the year 1968, Elizabeth Drews proposed what could be seen as a new direction in education, that is "focusing on the creative growth of the self and the synergic relationship of the individual with society" (Drews, 1968). Education has an impact on a child's physical, psychosocial, and cognitive needs. It is true that the advancement in science and technology and the ability of continuing education with the help of digital devices and Internet access have been a blessing during emergency such as the pandemic. Other than the valuable educational resources, it did serve as a source for recreation in the absence of peers and outdoor activities (Pathak, 2020). The closing of schools and educational institutions along with social distancing has, however, adversely impacted the socialising ability of children and their overall development. The effect is also seen among the college and university students, who benefit much from their peers as well as from the overall academic and extra-curricular environment beyond the classrooms. While this may affect creative and critical faculties of all students in general, those from under-privileged background seem to be at the receiving end.

Further, fieldwork/field experiences are an important component in various branches of higher education and research, especially in social sciences. Although some institutions have adopted precautionary measures or alternate method of data collection and fieldwork, these obviously cannot be a substitute for the experiences gained through physical visits.

Mental Health of Students

While studies are yet to reveal, from the ongoing situation, it is seen that the uncertainty caused by the pandemic has also had a significant effect on the mental health of young individuals. There is an overall anxiety about the virus and confinement including on measures such as quarantine and closures of educational institutions. Along with that, as mentioned earlier, the uncertainty with regard to conduct of examination has impacted students at all levels. Adding to it, prolonged use of electronic devices, which has become a necessity for the continuation of teaching-learning process, has also led to stress among the students. Besides, with the employment market running low during the pandemic, there is also a constant fear among the final-year students, especially of marginal background, of not getting employment.

Further, increased use of unsupervised Internet has also maximised the cases of sexual exploitation and cyberbullying of children. Parents' supervision is not always feasible especially when both parents are working and even more difficult as some schools instruct parents to leave their children so that they can learn on their own. A study (Jain et al., 2020) shows that there is a growth in the factors affecting cyberbullying susceptibility during the COVID-19 pandemic as a result of an increase in social media and online gaming activity.

Rise in Drop-outs

Encouraging children and youth to study entails a struggle for parents; the online education further burdened them with not only providing their children with smartphones and laptops but also ensuring that children follow their lessons. It was reported that on account of the pandemic, 320 million learners in India have been adversely affected and transitioned to the e-learning industry, which comprises a network of 1.5 million schools. An NSSO 2014 report highlights that 32 million children were already out of school before the pandemic – the majority of them belonging to the socially disadvantaged class in the country (Modi and Postaria, 2020). The situation unfolded during the pandemic indeed exacerbated this.

The ASER 2020 survey conducted during the end of September 2020 on children between the age of 5 and 16 in 8,963 schools to study the accessibility of digital content to children and their engagement with the content and its impact unravelled the lack of quality education and infrastructure in the rural areas. Besides others, one of the issues that was highlighted by the survey was that of the number of possible school drop-outs when schools start functioning normally in the future. According to UNESCO estimates, 23.8 million children, adults, and youth are at risk of not returning to educational institutions, globally (United Nations, 2020). This although is an anticipation, it is something that needs to be paid attention to for preparedness to mitigate such occurrence. Such anticipation may be because of several reasons. A large number of children from underprivileged background already had to be engaged in employment for survival of their family as their parents either have lost their jobs or are not earning as in the pre-pandemic times. Many children of such background also lost either one or both of their parents during the pandemic. This drew curtains on their education as they have been pushed to earning their livelihood.

Impact on Teachers

Reaching out to low-tech students was not an easy task for the teachers who more often than not were dealing with their own crisis. Creative pedagogical tools had to be adopted that would serve the needs of a mixed classroom. Using voice messages, text messages, and even phone calls for the low-tech students and making pre-recorded videos and creating Google classrooms and WhatsApp groups for mid- to high-tech students were commonly seen. Starting from the fear of privacy in the initial stage of online classes, they have come a long way, to many adopting Zoom, Google Meet, and similar platforms for online live classes at least at the university and private school levels.

Teachers, however, are over-burdened with unreasonable expectation of being well versed in online teaching without proper training and lack of technical infrastructure at home. Training is not very common, especially at school level particularly in the rural areas and in many colleges too. An online survey reveals that 84% of the teachers are experiencing challenges in dealing with the transition from traditional to online or remote learning pedagogy (India Today, 2021). It is also important to note that the country's education system also has large number of contractual teachers, many of whom lost their jobs during the pandemic or have not been paid their salaries for months.

Other than teaching what was on the syllabus, teachers in such situation also had to focus on spreading information about the pandemic, in order to dispel myths and diffuse panic among students many of whose families had been affected by it. Therefore, they had to be transformed from mere knowledge providers to counsellors and caregivers. This was quite difficult as they themselves were struggling with their own health and family problems.

Takeaways and Way Forward

The pandemic caught us by surprise. There was lack of preparedness for such an emergency and hence its negative impact became all the more severe. However, the shift from offline to online mode of teaching-learning process has also ushered many opportunities. Online teaching system has facilitated the continuation of teaching-learning process, notwithstanding all the problems associated with it. It has allowed the teachers and students alike to get acquainted with the digital platforms for learning and communication. This has made possible the organisation/conduct of the much-needed academic activities like seminars, talks, interviews, and Ph.D. viva voce examinations in short notice with limited use of resources. The situation arising out of the pandemic has also led to the production of better quality online learning materials. All these can go a long way in complementing the normal education system in future.

It, however, needs to be emphasised that addressing the digital divide is the foremost task before the government. Smartphones are now no longer a luxury but a necessity. Hence, state governments should work on providing basic technology as part of necessary infrastructure in schools in order to meet the need of social equity. Along with digital infrastructure, empowering and training teachers in adopting creative methods of teaching is necessary. Proper methods must be devised to encourage poor parents to enrol their children in schools after the pandemic through scholarships and awareness programmes. Blended mode of education is here to stay as is emphasised also by the NEP 2020. Hence, proper mechanism for imparting quality education across all sections of students needs to be ascertained by urgent government action.

Conclusion

It is true that the social and pedagogical requirements can seldom be achieved through remote or online mode of learning. It was, however, the best alternative that was available when the pandemic hit the country. There are indeed short- and long-term implications of the pandemic on education. Short-term effects are the concerns of accessibility and affordability for the marginalised section of the society along with long-term implications like increase in the number of school drop-out, educational gaps between the haves and the have nots, mental health of both students and teachers, and lack of employment opportunities that needs to be addressed immediately. The possibility of online education needs to be explored to expand the scope of our education system keeping in mind the principle of non-discrimination.

References

Agarwal, P. (2020), "West Bengal: 20-year-old dies by suicide for not having smartphone to attend online classes", 10 September, https://thelogicalindian.com/education/20-year-old-woman-dies-by-suicide-for-not-having-smartphone-to-23623, accessed 1 August 2021.

Baruah, S. (2020), "LSR student suicide: No laptop to hostel stay, key concerns were flagged to college admin by students", *Indian Express*, 10 November, https://indianexpress.com/article/cities/delhi/lsr-student-suicide-no-laptop-to-hostel-stay-key-concerns-were-flagged-to-college-admin-by-students-7034481/, accessed 3 June 2021.

Chaudhuri, S. (2020), "The network problem", *The Telegraph*, Calcutta, 27 November.

Drews, E. M. (1968), "Beyond curriculum", *Journal of Humanistic Psychology*, 8(2), 97–112.

Faheema Shirin R.K. v. State of Kerala W.P (c). No. 19716/2019-L.
Hindustan Times (2020), "Union HRD minister launches 'Bharat Padhe online' campaign to invite ideas to improve online education ecosystem", 10 April, www.hindustantimes.com/education/union-hrd-minister-launches-bharat-padhe-online-campaign-to-invite-ideas-to-improve-online-education-ecosystem/story-w9Bw2e3jZKuhkgVamav8zH.html, accessed 19 July 2021.
India Today (2021), "84% of teachers facing challenges during online classes: Survey", 18 March, www.indiatoday.in/education-today/latest-studies/story/84-of-teachers-facing-challenges-during-online-classes-survey-1780816-2021-03-18, accessed 11 August 2021.
Jain O., Gupta M., Satam S., & Panda S. (2020), Has the COVID-19 pandemic affected the susceptibility to cyberbullying in India?, 28 September, https://www.ncbi.nlm.nih.gov/pmc/articles/PMC7521933/, accessed 13 August 2021.
Malala Fund (2020), "Malala Fund releases report on girls' education and COVID-19", 6 April, https://malala.org/newsroom/archive/malala-fund-releases-report-girls-education-covid-19, accessed 20 July 2021.
Mehra, A. (2021), "Education budget 2021–22: Ministry of education gets Rs 93,224 crore, Rs 8,100 crore more than revised estimates", 2 February, www.shiksha.com/articles/education-budget-2021-22-ministry-of-education-gets-rs-93-224-crore-rs-8–100-crore-more-than-revised-estimates-blogId-54023, accessed 23 July 2021.
Modi, S. and Postaria, R. (2020), "How COVID-19 deepens the digital education divide in India", 5 October, www.weforum.org/agenda/2020/10/how-covid-19-deepens-the-digital-education-divide-in-india/, accessed 2 August 2021.
NDTV Education (2020), "From JEE, NEET to boards: How India held exams in 2020 amid COVID-19", 21 December, www.ndtv.com/education/from-jee-neet-boards-how-india-held-exams-in-2020-amid-covid-19, accessed 28 July 2021.
Orissa Diary (2020), "Ghare Ghare Arunima – Continued activities based learnings for over 16 lakh Anganwadi children of Odisha at home during lockdown", 21 April, https://orissadiary.com/ghare-ghare-arunima-continued-activities-based-learnings-for-over-16-lakh-anganwadi-children-of-odisha-at-home-during-lockdown/, accessed 3 June 2021.
Parul (2020), "How Covid-19 pandemic affects the Indian education system?" 4 July, www.inventiva.co.in/stories/parul/how-covid-19-pandemic-affects-the-indian-education-system/, accessed 18 July 2021.
Pathak, A. (2020), "Rethinking education in the age of the coronavirus", *The Wire*, 2 April, https://thewire.in/education/education-modernity-coronavirus, accessed 28 June 2021.
Philip, S. (2020), "Kerala Dalit student kills herself, parents say upset over not being able to attend online classes", *The Indian Express*, 3 June, https://indianexpress.com/article/education/kerala-dalit-student-kills-herself-parents-say-upset-over-not-being-able-to-attend-online-classes-6439682/, accessed 19 August 2021.
Sarkar and Mitra (2021), "Education budget 2021–22 is out of sync with NEP", 17 February, www.newsclick.in/Education-Budget-2021-22-Out-Sync-NEP, accessed 12 August 2021.
Sindwani, P. (2020), "Here's how the marks for CBSE class 10 and 12 students will be calculated", *Business Insider*, 26 June, www.businessinsider.in/education/news/checkout-how-the-marks-will-be-calculated-for-cbse-class-10th-and-12th-result-will-be-declared-by-15-july/articleshow/76637634.cms, accessed 28 June 2021.

Singh, D. (2020), "Covid-19: How education can be the silver lining in pandemic cloud", *Daily O*, 29 April, www.dailyo.in/variety/covid-19-coronavirus-pandemic-school-college-university-education-research/story/1/32790.html, accessed 20 December 2020.

State of Tamil Nadu v. K. Shyam Sunder (2011) 8 SCC 737.

United Nations (2020), "Policy brief: Education during COVID 19 and beyond", August, www.un.org/development/desa/dspd/wp-content/uploads/sites/22/2020/08/sg_policy_brief_covid-19_and_education_august_2020.pdf, accessed 23 June 2021.

7 NGOs in the Times of COVID-19

Namami Sharma

Introduction

In June 2020, the Supreme Court (SC) of India, while taking up the Suo moto case of stranded migrants during the COVID-19 lockdown, acknowledged the work of the NGOs in dealing with the crisis. The Bench comprising Justice Ashok Bhushan, S. K. Kaul, and M. R. Shah had stated:

> (Although) it is the responsibility and duty of the States and Union Territories to take care of the needs of the migrant labourers, in this difficult time non-governmental organisations and individuals have also contributed and played an important role in extending a helping hand to the migrants.
>
> (PTI, The Hindu, 2020)

Barely six months back, Indians had read and heard about the COVID-19 virus that had a catastrophic impact on the population of Wuhan in China. The virus was known to have a very high infection rate. Governments across the globe were clueless about the extent of the impact. No one had imagined that in no time this virus was going to affect governments and personal lives alike. The multifarious impact of the virus was unprecedented. It was not only fatal to human beings but also about to create conditions that were never seen before.

For the next few months, the news reports across the globe were reporting the high incidence of COVID and COVID-related casualties. Countries in Europe, the United Kingdom, and the United States of America declared lockdown, barring people from socialising and venturing out of their homes. COVID cases gradually found its way to India, beginning from Kerala. On 25 March 2020, three months after the virus was reported, the Prime Minister of India announced a countrywide complete lockdown for 21 days. People were barred from stepping out of their homes. All public and private services were restrained from operation. Only the health services and a few essential services were allowed to function.

DOI: 10.4324/9781003282815-10

The most affected population during the lockdown was the migrant population in different cities. This constituency of people had migrated mostly under distress and was working in urban centres away from their hometowns. In my mind, the situation was analogous to the children's game "statues", where the appointed "curator" turns his back while the participants race across the field. The curator suddenly turns around and says "statues" and everyone must freeze in their position and hold on for as long as the curator keeps looking at them. Here, the state acted as the "curator" while the citizens were the "statues" and the state had its "gaze" held firmly on the citizens. When the lockdown was announced, the migrants found themselves under the unmoving gaze of the Indian state, curtailing their movement too, just like in statues. On account of the increasing fear of infections and the varied repercussions of the infection, the Indian state had no choice but to shut down. The earlier statement of the SC upheld the contribution of the NGOs in helping them move and return to their native places. This statement was flashed in several popular dailies. The spotlight came upon the NGOs and the media began reporting about their work.

The entity of an NGO has always been there, working in a microcosm, contributing in its own way to society. Though the NGOs have contributed immensely across various developmental sectors, their presence and work seem to be not adequately noticed. Besides, the challenges faced were also no less. The intent of this chapter is to examine the work of NGOs during the time of COVID-19. I have drawn examples to highlight the points based on various news reports, web sources, and my personal interactions with NGOs and Civil Society organisations across the state of Assam. I have used the term organisation and NGO simultaneously throughout the chapter.

What Are NGOs?

The not-for-profit or the non-governmental organisations, popularly known as the NGOs, are autonomous agencies, drawing funds from different sources and working largely towards the welfare of society. The NGOs work across sectors like education, health, livelihood generation, environmental conservation, and in achieving social justice in all these sectors. In the COVID-19 situation, the NGOs worked with a two-pronged approach. On one hand, it attended to the immediate problem, while on the other hand, they also worked towards realising the full potential of the circumstances by highlighting structural lapses in service delivery and subsequently filling up the gaps.

NGOs function through hired professionals, trained in various knowledge and skill sets. This makes the functioning often confined to fixed sectors. During the pandemic, an alternate picture was witnessed where NGOs ventured out of their sectoral microcosms and worked in different capacities in combating various problems that had emerged. A solidarity was experienced by the NGOs while connecting and cooperating for a common cause.

One important constituent of NGOs are the volunteers. Apart from the hired executives, NGOs often have a wide network of volunteers. In the neo liberal era, volunteerism is often driven by factors other than the spirit to volunteer or the motivation to be a part of the change making process. Volunteerism in India is influenced by a constellation of factors like securing educational opportunities, influence of the peer, seeking employment, and exposure (Ghose and Kassam, 2012). This group is not paid and poses a minimal liability to the organisation. On the contrary to the usual, during the pandemic, volunteers who worked on the ground exhibited the true spirit of volunteerism. A survey conducted among 2,270 volunteers and 14 civil society leaders in China revealed the increased "value among local citizens, civil society including community-based groups, and regional government to fill gaps in public services" (Qing et al., 2021).

NGO volunteers in India also had taken up a myriad of works ranging from setting up help desks at hospitals to helping municipalities with funerals. The organisation Helping Hand Foundation (HHF) had established help desks at the District Hospital in King Koti, Government General and Chest Hospital in Erragadda, and Osmania General Hospital (Shanker, 2020). The Popular Front of India volunteers have helped the municipality to give a dignified farewell to all patients who have died of COVID-19. Till the month of August 2020, they had helped cremate or bury at least 1,117 people who had died of COVID. Their voluntary network is spread from the southern states till Bihar in the east and Goa and Maharashtra on the west (Kaur, 2020).

The times of COVID were unusual and there was a certain cluelessness that befell upon the state. The cascading effect that the lockdown had on the economy of the country was unforeseen. On the one hand, there were loss of livelihoods (Human Rights Watch, 2021), pushing families to poverty and despair; on the other hand, there were rising cases of mental health issues in the family set up. The State was overburdened with issues to handle. While the State was busy dealing with the rising cases and contemplating on ways to deal with the upcoming pressure on health services, the NGOs came forward to deal with the other emerging issues and fill in the gaps. NGOs went beyond their areas of engagement to contribute and help in whatever ways they could.

NGOs and Areas of Engagement

There were several emerging areas in which the NGOs were found to play an important role. A few of the highlighted areas of work were facilitating the migrants for passage, providing essential services, spreading information and awareness, addressing mental health issues, and assisting the state machinery in delivering the services. The NGOs ventured out of their respective sectors, rapidly shifting the focus from other causes to deal with the emergent issues raised by the Pandemic.

Working With the Migrants

The COVID lockdown declared in the month of March 2020 had created a widespread panic among the people. The most affected were the workers in the unorganised sector, especially the migrants. Due to lockdown, the work that they were engaged in had come to a halt and there was no income. In many cases, where employers had provided living quarters, the migrant workers were asked to vacate. With no income and an uncertain future in the expensive cities, they were forced to return back to their native places. With the public transport not functioning, the workers had no choice but to start their journey by foot. They had to negotiate with police and state machinery at the interstate borders while making the tumultuous journey.

The role of the NGOs in helping these people to make their journey back was immense. The NGOs and the volunteers provided food, water, masks, medicine, and other services to facilitate their way back home. The organisation *Janvikas Initiative Institute of Social Studies and Transformation* located in Ahmedabad was running a community kitchen to feed 10,000 migrants. They called it the "dignity kitchen". The same organisation also helped the migrant workers to reach their homes in Shramik trains. The NGO *Jan Sahas* used technology to track 1,22,000 migrant families and distributed ration. They used the longitude migration tracking system. Their intervention was based on an assessment survey of various vulnerable communities, and it was found that the condition of the migrants was the most vulnerable during the COVID situation (Mukherjee, 2020). Organisations like *Aman Biradari Trust* and *Karwan-e-Mohabbat* documented narratives of the migrants and projected the same to mobilise funds (Lounge, 2020). The funds were used to provide food and other essentials to the migrants.

The NGOs, volunteers, and individuals came out in good numbers to help the migrant workers. The digital platforms like WhatsApp, Telegram, and social media were widely used to form a virtual network of volunteers across state borders. The digital media facilitated the formation of the wide network of NGOs and volunteers beyond their respective sectors to work on the issue of migrants. The migrant workers had already started their journey back home amidst lockdown. Negotiation with the state police and supply of daily provisions were required in their journey. NGOs were seen advocating the causes of the migrant population and appealing to provide facilities. Digital media was used to create a pressure group and highlight the woes of the workers. The work of the NGOs in this crisis was upheld by the apex court of India.

Providing Essential Services

During the lockdown, with the loss of livelihoods, many essential services were affected. NGOs across the country have worked tirelessly and innovatively in reaching out to people and delivering services. An organisation named *Utthan* in Gujarat provided daily ration to about 2,500 tribal families from different parts of coastal Gujarat. The food grains were sourced from the community itself, also providing a market to the farmers in the village. *Safa*, a nonprofit organisation based in Hyderabad, focused on generating livelihoods of the youth affected by the pandemic through skill training. It connected to single mothers and daily wage earners in Bengaluru, Karnataka, and Chennai through its network of volunteers and distributed daily essentials (Mazumdar, 2020).

It is important to note that NGOs reached out to the most vulnerable and stigmatised constituencies while delivering and facilitating essential services. In the society, sex workers and transgenders are always in the margins. The sex workers remain in isolated pockets and are often oblivious to prominent welfare agencies. *Citizens for Justice and Peace* and *Jimme Foundation* mobilised funds to address the daily requirements of 200 sex workers families in Kamathipura (Lounge, 2020).

The *Sashakt Foundation* provided meals to the transgenders and the eunuch community in greater Noida. The lockdown had seized all livelihood options available for the community. The members of the community earned on a daily basis. Moreover, the stigma and the taboos associated with the members of the community make them more vulnerable. The NGO and its volunteers provided cooked meals and dry ration throughout the lockdown period (Covid-19 lockdown: Volunteers, NGO help transgenders, 2020).

Addressing Gender-Based Violence

COVID lockdown saw an upsurge in cases related to gender-based violence including cases of domestic violence, sexual crimes, and intimate partner violence. The financial dependency on the abusive partner often becomes the reason of prolong tolerance of intimate partner violence (Evans et al., 2020). The covid lockdown had led to loss of jobs. I would like to highlight the case of a woman who used to work as a domestic help. Her employer refused to pay her during the lockdown citing loss in business and income. She had to depend on her husband for running the household. The husband, who was not used to giving money regularly to his wife for household expenditures, found it frustrating and used to often beat her up. There was no place she could go. The stress of economic instability had led men getting into alcoholism or any other form of substance abuse resulting in more incidents of domestic violence while the women were overburdened with household work and care giving. Existing in close quarters increased friction leading to more violence. Restricted movement, reduced contact with natal family, and unavailability of the formal support system were cited as few of the reasons for the spike in the reported cases of domestic violence (Arora and Jain, 2020).

NGOs have stepped up its work in addressing such concerns. It has come forward with interventions for immediate relief and also strategies to realise the full potential of the issue. For immediate relief, organisations started online counselling and active helplines. An NGO named *Shakti Vahini*, based out of Delhi, reported a reduced number of domestic violence cases. The reason was the lack of space and time to confide. In most cases, the victims were living with the perpetrators, which made it difficult for them to access the services. With the police being engaged in managing the lockdown and COVID protocols, the usual support for rescue was not available. The organisation started a 24-hr helpline to assist the women. However, the number of calls was less owing to the stated given reason (Arora and Jain, 2020) (Jagori, n.d.). The mode of operation for many NGOs had shifted to online counselling through phones.

Work of the NGOs also involved in depth research in different states. Research was mostly in the form of rapid survey remotely carried out to examine the risks of women staying at home. The "risks" refer to domestic abuse, mental and physical. The NGO *Jagori* created a series of infographics named as "At home At risk" based on several such rapid surveys. They have published and made the reports available online. The same organisation also compiled verified support services for women facing violence during lockdown (Jagori, n.d.).

Community Work

The NGOs have a wide network of people at the grassroots. These networks were seen to emerge and take a leading role in carrying forward the work of the NGOs. The lockdown imposed restrictions on mobility for the NGO workers. The organisations made their presence felt through these networks. Village-level institutions were revived and evolved to facilitate community work, which was mostly delivery of dry ration, cooked food, and facilitating primary health care.

Groups and collectives were formed and activated with the sole purpose of making life easy during the COVID lockdown. These groups got engaged in a variety of activities. For instance, in one village, an NGO facilitated a youth group and encouraged them to get constructively engaged in traditional theatre (based on personal interaction with a civil society organisation in Assam). The purpose behind this was to revive an art form among the youth and also to revoke solidarity in the community. The same platform was used to disseminate information about covid protocols and the like.

Advocacy

Under the International Covenant on Economic, Social and Cultural Rights, the signatory governments are obligated to effective steps for the prevention, treatment and control of epidemic, endemic, occupational and other diseases. The pandemic created multiple challenges for citizens to exercise their Right to Health. One cannot deny that the pandemic also pushed the Indian economy to its edge and the health systems were struggling to manage with the limited resources. The NGOs played an important role in advocating for the rights to Health and access to health services.

The NGO CRY has been advocating for the access to better health services to communities and children (Marwaha, 2021). CARE India Team has collaborated with different development partners in advocating for better access to information (Battling COVID 19, n.d.). The Peoples Foundation of India (PFI) is a partner to the Government of India to create digital content to raise awareness on the various health services with special reference to COVID-19. The PFI in collaboration with a renowned theatre and film director Feroz Abbas Khan has created short animation films to demystify and destigmatise the pandemic and the affected ones (Response to Covid 19, n.d.). The PFI also assessed the differential impact of COVID-19 on women and developed a policy recommendation document to ensure that women and girls are central to the COVID recovery efforts (Impact of Covid 19 on Women: Policy Brief, n.d.).

The pandemic and the imposed lockdown posed an impediment to the strategies of advocacy that the NGOs have generally used. There were strict limitations on physically mobilising people for human rights defence across the globe.

In this backdrop, the human rights defenders had to work but without the available resources and people. Due to the lockdown, it was getting difficult to mobilise people to form pressure groups or advocacy groups for various causes. Several organisations working for the protection of human rights changed their strategies of generating public opinion. The digital platform and the print media were popularly used to garner public opinion. The economic anxieties of the people were high and required immediate attention. Audio visual content was created for digital platforms. However, it was also seen that NGOs mostly worked with focus on the economic and social rights of the people and it was also observed that the civil and political rights were given lesser priority owing to the other emergent needs (Seyhan, 2020) (Balaji, 2020).

Education

The education sector came under a huge impact by the lockdown. The classes were curtailed and the shift to online mode of teaching posed several challenges. The children from the underprivileged background did not have the adequate resources to avail the online classes. Many NGOs came forward to help with the crisis. The oracle India Foundation has taken a multipronged approach to address the gaps during online learning. It has collaborated with partner agencies in remote areas to set up child care institutions with Internet facilities and power back up. The children in remote areas are provided with smart phone and other accessories. The organisation is providing skill-building exercises to engage the students constructively during the pandemic. They have reached out to more than 10,000 students across seven states – Maharashtra, Tamil Nadu, Madhya Pradesh, Tripura, Telangana, Karnataka, and Kerala (Chakrabarty, 2020).

The organisation ASHA working in the slums of Delhi has opened its recreational centre called Bal Mandir at the community to engage children in education and recreational activities. The organisation made sure to follow all the COVID protocols. Neighbourhood classes were held with maximum ten children, sticking to the social distancing norms (David, 2020). The organisation PRATHAM has been working with underprivileged children through a new programme called *Karona thodi masti thodi padhai* (Do it: Little Fun and little Study) to aid students to study during the pandemic. It uses multiple aids like radio and WhatsApp to connect with children using new ways. It is also working to make learning resources available to all (COVID 19 Response, n.d.). EKLAVYA, an NGO, has conducted training programmes for parents, siblings, and local youth to teach at spaces with good ventilation and by following the COVID protocols. It also initiated a mobile library system, which rotates between localities and inculcate a reading habit in children.

Mental Health

A study referred to by an English daily stated that over 80 deaths were caused by suicide during the lockdown (PTI, 2020). Several mental health issues have been reported to be associated with the COVID-19 pandemic. A few are anxiety, stress, insomnia, depression, denial, anger, fear, and paranoia (Torales et al., 2020). The lockdown had created a vulnerable situation for all categories of people. The frontline health workers were going through immense stress; the elderly and the children were trying to cope with the new environment; the financial distress was triggering mental health conditions; and the like. A survey conducted by the Indian Psychiatry Society validated a 20% rise in mental health cases after the pandemic broke out (Balaji, 2020).

The NGO *Minds Foundation* has been working in the mental health sector through awareness, education, and care giving. They developed self-care tools and resource material to deal with mental health issues at home during the lockdown period (Balaji, 2020). Another organisation, *The Neptune foundation* launched helpline numbers to assist people facing stress or anxiety (Balaji, 2020). The organisation *Arpan* launched Mental Health Support system through chat-based counselling support via WhatsApp, Facebook, Instagram, and Twitter (Mental Health Support-COVID 19, n.d.). Call-based counselling was also carried out. Organisations conducted several webinars to discuss and talk about different mental health concerns during the lockdown. The White Swan Foundation developed audio visual material to raise awareness on mental health issues specific to the pandemic times (Balaji, 2020). NGOs evolved resource material and used the digital media to disseminate the same among all stakeholders (Balaji, 2020) (PTI, 2020) (Mental Health Support-COVID 19, n.d.) (OUTLOOK The News Scroll, 2020).

Capacity Building

NGOs were seen working towards generating awareness on COVID-19. Awareness drives were organised on the COVID protocols through digital media. As the COVID cases were reported, there was a rise in stigma associated with the disease. People diagnosed with COVID were communally boycotted in neighbourhoods. Though exceptions were also seen, one could not deny the level of ignorance, which eventually had led to the stigma. NGOs worked tirelessly to destigmatise the disease by disseminating information and demystifying the protocols.

The COVID-19 pandemic had created challenging conditions for the animals on the streets and homes. There was a misconception of the virus being spread through animals, due to which many pets were abandoned in the streets. Some NGOs and collectives stepped up to help these animals in distress by feeding, treating, and rehabilitating. *Pawsitive Farm Sanctuary* in Mumbai provided shelter to 114 dogs and cats abandoned by pet owners during the lockdown (OUTLOOK The News Scroll, 2020). The *Anubis Tiger Foundation* is also one such organisation which facilitated the rehabilitation of dogs (Maneckshaw, 2020). The *Just be Friendly* (JBF) organisation, located in Guwahati, fed the street dogs in the city with the help of its wide network of volunteers during the lockdown (based on personal interaction with the NGO personnel). The NGOs thus went beyond the human world to contribute for better lives.

The process of "co production" was witnessed in these covid-created circumstances. Elinor Ostrom defines coproduction as "the process through which inputs used to provide a good or service, are contributed by individuals who are not 'in' the same organization" (Ostrum, 1996). Coproduction refers to the involvement of common man in providing public services, thus creating value for the communities (McGranahan, 2015). Coproduction involves citizens and community groups, who are aware of local conditions and help to assure that interventions reflect specific needs and customs (Verschuere et al., 2012). The NGOs facilitated the coproduction by the "layman" and created various entry points for individual volunteers to come together and contribute in accordance to specific needs and customs.

The "New Normal" for the NGOs

The work of the NGOs has been motivated towards development and welfare. The pandemic did bring a shift in the way organisations functioned. In usual circumstances, NGOs work with an immersive approach, working closely with the stakeholders. The sudden lockdown had limited the mobility of NGO functionaries to carry out the deliverables. The functionaries had to depend upon the local networks for the accomplishment of the tasks in hand. The wide use of digital platforms was seen in the development sector. This allowed the organisations to look beyond their sectoral focus and collaborate across sectors and geographies. NGOs applied innovative methods in research, monitoring, and evaluation. Tools for remote monitoring or data collection were widely used owing to the restricted mobility. As the NGOs shifted to online reporting, remote working has become the new norm. There is a rise in the use of new technology to monitor and validate field-based data flows. While on one hand, the lockdown limited physical movements, it also opened the door to multitude of possibilities through digital platforms.

The Challenges Faced by the NGOs

Though the NGOs went beyond their capacity to work to its full potential in the times of COVID, the challenges were no less. The Centre for Social Impact and Philanthropy at Ashoka University had carried out a research in the months of April and May, 2020 to understand the impact of COVID on the nonprofit organisations. A total of 52 interviews were conducted and the results revealed that one of the crucial challenges that NGOs were facing was the fund crunch. One half of the interviewed NGOs were dependent on the Corporate Social Responsibility (CSR) fund. This fund was being largely diverted to address COVID relief operations including the PM CARES fund. With decreased operations, there is a likelihood of less CSR funding being generated in the near future (Centre for Social Impact and Philantrophy, 2020). International funding agencies were relatively reported to be flexible, and many offered no cost extensions for the projects. However, the recent amendments of the Foreign Contributions (Regulation) Act, 2010 or FCRA created difficult bottle necks for the organisations (Centre for Social Impact and Philantrophy, 2020). This added to the funding woes of the NGOs. There was a rise in crowdfunding platforms and NGOs were seen opting for such during the pandemic. However, for process-oriented work, a consistent flow of funding is necessary, and this was hampered due to the pandemic.

The shift to the digital platforms for daily functioning was a challenge to many NGOs. The organisations located in remote areas were struggling to cope with this shift due to the lack of required skills among the members. Nonetheless, handholding and cooperation among organisations was also witnessed. Community work is a process and a break in the work could be an impediment to the overall progress of the project. The lockdown led to a critical disruption, which had an impact on the stakeholders.

Learnings and the Way Forward

I feel that the "new normal" has brought in a new beginning for the nonprofit sector. Though the lockdown period has posed several crucial challenges for the sector, it has also opened a wide array of opportunities. It has given time and space to examine, rethink, and rediscover nuances of development work. A target-oriented approach within tight time frames laid out by funding agencies compels organisations to focus only on accomplishing the deliverables. In the process, the subtleties of working with communities are often overlooked and long-term impact of tasks is compromised. This creates a dependency of the people on the organisation. Thus, NGOs are often seen as an extension of the populist measures adopted by the state. This phenomenon is not empowering for the people that they work for.

During the lockdown period, NGOs had to widely depend upon the grassroots network. The local institutions were revived, and work was delegated. The participation of people organically evolved in executing the tasks and ownership came along. I want to stress upon the importance of process centric approach of community welfare work to make interventions sustainable. In the future, NGOs must take the lessons forward and negotiate with funding agencies to develop empowering and process-oriented welfare strategies, rather than target-driven activities.

There should also be a preparedness to cope with new technology. The organisations must invest to build the capacities of the members in using updated technology for the operations. The inhibition in using new software tools or reporting applications should be overcome at all levels.

The pandemic gave a new lease of life to collaborative action. NGOs ventured out of their isolated sectoral cocoons and collaborated to work on a common cause, which, in this case, was the pandemic itself. This highlighted the possibilities of collaborative action. Though there is no dearth of consortiums within respective developmental sectors, it is important for actors from diverse fields to come together to bring in holistic and sustainable development in a geography.

References

Arora, K. and Jain, S. K. (2020), "Locked-down: Domestic violence reporting in India during COVID-19", *Oxfam India*, 3 August, www.oxfamindia.org/blog/locked-down-domestic-violence-reporting-india-during-covid-19, accessed 5 January 2021.

Balaji, R. (2020), "These NGOs are helping people deal with mental health issues amid the coronavirus pandemic", *Social Story*, 26 April, https://yourstory.com/socialstory/2020/04/ngos-helping-people-mental-health-coronavirus, accessed 5 January 2021.

Battling COVID 19 (n.d.), "Care India", www.careindia.org/covid-19/, accessed 28 December 2020.

Centre for Social Impact and Philantrophy (2020), 15 June, https://csip.ashoka.edu.in/executive-summary-the-impact-of-covid-19-on-indias-nonprofit-organisations/, accessed 6 January 2021.

Chakrabarty, R. (2020), "How this NGO is helping orphaned underprivileged kids continue their education in Covid-19 lockdown", *India Today*, 3 November, www.indiatoday.in/education-today/featurephilia/story/how-this-ngo-is-helping-orphaned-underprivileged-kids-continue-their-education-in-covid-19-lockdown-1737659-2020-11-03, accessed 6 January 2021.

Covid-19 lockdown: Volunteers, NGO help transgenders (2020), *The Times of India*, 17 April, https://timesofindia.indiatimes.com/city/noida/covid-19-lockdown-volunteers-ngo-help-transgenders-with-food-in-noida/articleshow/75206690.cms, accessed 28 December 2020.

COVID 19 Response (n.d.), "Pratham", www.pratham.org/covid-19-response/, accessed 31 March 2020.

David, S. (2020), *The New Indian Express*, 10 November, www.newindianexpress.com/business, accessed 31 March 2020.

Evans, M. L., Lindauer, M. and Farrell, M. E. (2020), "A pandemic within a pandemic – intimate partner violence during Covid-19", *The New England Journal of Medicine*, May, 2303–2304.

Ghose, T. and Kassam, M. (2012), "Motivations to volunteer among college students in India", *International Society for Third Sector Research*, 2014(25), 28–45.

Human Rights Watch (2021), *Human Rights Watch*, www.hrw.org/world-report/2021/country-chapters/india, accessed 26 December 2020.

Impact of Covid 19 on Women: Policy Brief (n.d.), "Population foundation", https://populationfoundation.in/impact-covid-19-women-brief/, accessed 29 March 2021.

Jagori (n.d.), *Jagori*, www.jagori.org/covid-19, accessed 26 December 2020.

Kaur, P. (2020), "How volunteer groups are helping municipalities across the country with COVID-19 funerals", *The Wire*, 14 August, https://thewire.in/rights/india-covid-19-deaths-burials-volunteers-municipal-authorities-help, accessed 29 March 2021.

Lounge, T. (2020), *Livemint*, 31 March, www.livemint.com/mint-lounge/features/how-to-help-the-most-vulnerable-during-the-covid-19-lockdown-11585631303316.html, accessed 28 December 2020.

Maneckshaw, F. (2020), "First, the pandemic made Indians abandon pets, then they rushed to adopt them", *The Print*, 2 August, https://theprint.in/opinion/first-the-pandemic-made-indians-abandon-pets-then-they-rushed-to-adopt-them/472539/, accessed 28 December 2020.

Marwaha, P. (2021), "Celebrating the role of Indian NGOs in combating the COVID-19 pandemic", *Down to Earth*, 27 February, www.downtoearth.org.in/blog/governance/celebrating-the-role-of-indian-ngos-in-combating-the-covid-19-pandemic-75697, accessed 28 December 2020.

Mazumdar, M. (2020), "Coronavirus: These NGO's are working around lockdown restrictions to feed the needy", *The Hindu*, 30 March, www.thehindu.com/news/cities/chennai/these-ngos-are-working-around-coronavirus-lockdown-restrictions-to-feed-the-needy/article31192583.ece, accessed 7 April 2021.

McGranahan, G. (2015), "Realizing the right to sanitation in deprived urban communities: Meeting the challenges of collective action, coproduction, affordability, and housing tenure", *World Development*, 68, 242–253.

Mental Health Support-COVID 19 (n.d.), "Arpan", www.arpan.org.in/mental-health-support-covid-19/, accessed 7 January 2020.

Mukherjee, R. (2020), "From food grains to PPE kits, this NGO leaves no stones unturned to help migrant workers tide over COVID-19 crisis", *The Logical Indian*, 24 May, https://thelogicalindian.com/campaign/ngo-provides-food-clothing-and-protection-amid-covid-19-crisis-21274.4, accessed 25 December 2020.

Ostrum, E. (1996), "Crossing the great divide: Coproduction, synergy, and development", *World Development*, 24(6), 1073–1087.

OUTLOOK The News Scroll (2020), *Outlook India*, 29 June, www.outlookindia.com/newsscroll/pawsitive-farm-sanctuary-a-haven-for-the-covid-abandoned/1880296, accessed 26 December 2020.

PTI (2020), "NGOs deserve all appreciation for helping migrants during COVID-19 pandemic: SC", *The Hindu*, 9 June, www.thehindu.com/news/national/ngos-deserves-all-appreciation-for-helping-migrants-during-covid-19-pandemic-sc/article31786947.ece, accessed 28 December 2020.

PTI (2020), "Suicide leading cause for over 300 lockdown deaths in India", *The Economic Times*, 5 May, https://economictimes.indiatimes.com/news/politics-and-nation/suicide-leading-cause-for-over-300-lockdown-deaths-in-india-says-study/articleshow/75519279.cms?from=mdr, accessed 28 December 2020.

Qing, M., Schwarz, S. and Schwarz, G. (2021), "Responding to COVID-19: Community volunteerism and coproduction in China", *World Development*, August, 137. Doi: 10.1016/j.worlddev.2020.105128.

Response to Covid 19 (n.d.), "Population foundation", https://populationfoundation.in/pfis-response-to-covid-19/, accessed 7 January, 2021.

Seyhan, E. (2020), "Pandemic powers: Why human rights organizations should not lose focus on civil and political rights", *Public Health Emergency Collection*, 31 August, 268–275. https://doi.org/10.1093/jhuman/huaa035.

Shanker, K. S. (2020), "Ost recovery, NGO volunteers turn guides at govt. hospitals", *The Hindu*, 20 July, www.thehindu.com/news/cities/Hyderabad/post-recovery-ngo-volunteers-turn-guides-at-govt-hospitals/article32132629.ece, accessed 7 January, 2021.

Torales, J., O'Higgins, M., Castaldelli-Maia, J. and Ventriglio, A. (2020), "The outbreak of COVID-19 coronavirus and its impact on global mental health", *International Journal of Social Psychiatry*, 66(4), 317–320.

Verschuere, B., Brandsen, T. and Pestoff, V. (2012), "Co-production: The state of the art in research and the future agenda", *Voluntas: International Journal of Voluntary and Nonprofit Organizations*, 23(4), 1083–1101.

Part III

On the Periphery

8 Home, Violence, and the Pandemic

Sociological Discourses and Re-imagination in India

Rukmini Sen

Introduction

All over the world, several countries (Vatican News, 2020) had taken cognisance of the undeniable spike in the cases of domestic violence against women and raised concerns through public addresses and advisories and support extended. The "shadow pandemic" (UN Women, 2020), as the UN Women termed it, has been witnessed in countries such as Argentina, Germany, the United States, China, France, Spain, the United Kingdom, and India. Several women's rights activists and civil society partners have flagged the rise in the number of cases of domestic violence during the crisis. In India, we have received a number of advisories but none on the increase in domestic violence due to lockdown or advisory on mental health of abused women and children at home facing violence.

Both the WHO and the Ministry of Health and Family Welfare (MoHFW), which issued several important advisories everyday relating to COVID-19 virus, the lockdown and its effects on people, identified home as the safety net from the virus with their slogan "stay home stay safe". However, not all homes are safe and neither all people have the luxury of home, nor have the means to maintain social distance in a small room occupied by many members in the household. This chapter will engage with the many ways that domestic violence increased during the pandemic in India – mapping reasons for those and recommending certain policy measures that could have far reaching implications applicable even for non-crisis times. Through this analysis, this chapter will also propose a re-imagination of the home or domestic. The pandemic gave an important opportunity for sociologists to conceptualise the home, as distinct from the family.

Stay Home, Stay (Un)Safe

Countless women, including trans and queer women, have faced the immediate gendered impact of the mandatory lockdown – domestic violence. The lockdown has made it difficult to respond to domestic violence cases with the police (Harsh, 2020).[1] While India was getting ready to prepare for a

DOI: 10.4324/9781003282815-12

lockdown, the MoHFW initiated advisories, which indicated that all members of the household were to remain inside their respective homes for the duration of the lockdown, and practice what was termed as social distancing, together with work from home.

However, in all challenges posed by the lockdown, the National Commission for Women[2] reported that the number of reported cases of violence was increasing. As a response, the Commission announced a WhatsApp number for women to register complaints. As per NCW, between the beginning of March and 5 April 2020, the NCW received 310 grievances of domestic violence and 885 complaints for other forms of violence against women, many of which were domestic in nature – such as bigamy, polygamy, dowry deaths, and harassment for dowry (Sen, 2020). This was two and a half times more than the number of the global figure of domestic violence, which had also increased with the United Nations expressing alarm at a horrifying global surge on domestic violence (New York Times, 2020).

The UN Secretary General appealed to put women's safety first to world leaders as they fought the pandemic. The WHO in 2021 indicated that globally about one in three (30%) of women worldwide have been subjected to either physical and/or sexual intimate partner violence or non-partner sexual violence in their lifetime. While we acknowledge that domestic violence increased during the pandemic, it is important to understand the intersectional nature of this violence and that specific categories of women have faced different kinds of violence in relation to the domestic sphere, some of which may not even in non-pandemic times be recorded as domestic violence. Women living with disabilities, Muslim women, LGBTQ+ individuals, women living with HIV-AIDS, or sex workers have already been drastically impacted in terms of access to basic amenities and health care (The Week, 2020) and have experienced specific forms of violence.

In a report released by Rising Flame and Sightsavers titled "Neglected and Forgotten: Women with Disabilities during the COVID crisis in India" on 14 July 2020, a total of 82 women with disabilities and 12 experts across 19 states and nine self-identified disability groups participated in a survey on women with disabilities. In India, the "Comprehensive Disability Inclusive Guidelines for Protection and Safety of Persons with Disabilities for COVID-19 response" by the Department of Empowerment of Persons with Disabilities does not mention gender inclusive response. The "shadow pandemic" was a reality for women and girls with disabilities. Participants who worked in disability persons organisations and were helping women with disabilities through these issues reported a lack of privacy and accessibility for women with disabilities to seek peer support or redressal. Independent and assisted community living, which enables better mental health for people with disabilities, was disrupted by the lengthy lockdown. This resulted in women having to relocate to live with their family – who might have an abusive relationship with them. While there are some helplines, how can d/Deaf or deafblind women "call" to seek help? Besides the barriers, there is not much clarity in intervention strategy in domestic violence cases especially with regard to availability of care alternatives for women with disabilities facing violence from caregivers. One of the recommendations made in this report was helplines should also be available at the local levels to ensure that information is available in local languages and in the regional sign language.

Another infographics report titled "At Home at Risk" (Jagori et al., 2020) clearly interrogating the Stay Home Stay Safe advisory, was based on a Rapid Survey Series for seven days in seven states on the DV redressal ecosystem in COVID-19 pandemic released by eight women's rights, queer rights organisations in India (Jagori et al., 2020). While the space of the home became violent, the shelter homes in various states also refused shelter to women. As per an April 2020 Supreme Court directive, women's shelters were asked to avoid overcrowding and prevent the spread of COVID-19 (PTI, 2020).

Nearly all shelter homes spoken to, as per the findings of this report, refused to admit survivors of domestic violence, unless they were forced to or felt compelled. The reasons were fear of COVID-19, lack of space, and no quarantine facility. Except shelters in Assam, those in the other six states either had no knowledge of SOPs or had not received any. Most scrambled for information about safety measures or received virtual instructions without monetary or PPE assistance. A queer feminist resource group, part of this survey, described

> We received calls from many queer and transpersons during the lockdown, asking for shelter or safe spaces. Some could not leave home because of the lockdown; those who could leave had no safe spaces to go to. Our calls went up from 1 (on an average) call per week to 7 (on an average) calls every week during the lockdown. Most callers from across the country reported emotional and mental violence by the natal family.

There is nothing in the Indian laws to consider violence faced by sex workers as domestic violence – since there is no concept of a shared household or domestic relationship as the Protection of Women from Domestic Violence Act 2005 needs to prove domestic violence. Three kinds of information related to sex workers have been reported: (a) The president of the All India Network of Sex Workers (AINSW) on its 17 May 2020 news report said that over 60% of the sex workers in Delhi left for their home states – around 3,000 sex workers out of registered 5,000 (PTI, 2020). Shalini, one such worker, as mentioned in the report, moved back to her village in Uttar Pradesh after living for eight years in Delhi. "I ran away from my abusive home in UP at the age of 18. I wanted to be an actress but got into prostitution to survive in this city", 26-year-old Shalini told. She further said, "After getting into this business (sex trade), at least I was not struggling for food,

I was not on streets. But ever since the Coronavirus outbreak and the lockdown, I have zero customers and money is drying up". Many had to go back to abusive familial relationship, giving up on source of individual income. The president said that they feel that all the work which they did in the past years for HIV and other diseases would be of no use (The Hindu, 2020 (a)).

Many of them who escaped abusive homes can again become victims of domestic violence. (b) A second situation was experienced through another sex worker Rashmi (annonymised) who resumed work after lockdown restrictions were eased, and lives in fear of contracting COVID-19. Geeta, coordinator, Sadhana Mahila Sangha, working for the rights and welfare of street-based sex workers, in Bengaluru, said that while the state government had announced assistance to various professionals like drivers and barbers, it had failed to even acknowledge sex workers. "The pandemic has completely snatched their livelihood. Yet, the government has not come to their aid" [The Hindu, 2020 (b)]. (c) Thirdly, there are reports which say that sex workers are getting back to business through technology – phone sex, video shoots, using FB messenger or WhatsApp, etc. and payment through Google Pay [Live Mint, 2020 (a)].

There were a number of ways through which the courts intervened to address domestic violence during the pandemic. The courts took suo moto cognisance in case of the Jammu and Kashmir High Court (The Leaflet, 2020), which on 18 April 2020 offered interim directions to include creation of special funds. They designated informal spaces for women such as grocery stores and pharmacies where women could report abuse without alerting the perpetrator. Other safe spaces like empty hotels/education institutions could also be as shelters for women. The Karnataka High Court too asked the state government about the condition of helplines and report the necessary measures and action taken on domestic violence complaints (Livelaw, 2020).

The state in its reply reported that helplines, counsellors, shelter homes, and protection officers are working round the clock to help victims of violence in Karnataka [The New Indian Express, 2020 (a)]. In Tamil Nadu, protection officers appointed under the Domestic Violence Act 2005 were allowed to move during the lockdown and *Anganwadi* workers were placed as coordinators to receive and escalate calls of domestic abuse to their immediate superior officials. They were also provided with smart phones [ibid. 2020] in Uttar Pradesh; the state government initiated a special helpline for victims of domestic abuse under the title "Suppress Corona not your voice" with the state police asking women to call a helpline number and assured them that women police officers will visit them in the event of a complaint as part of an enhanced response to cases of violence against women.

Although various measures of tackling pandemic-induced domestic violence was being raised in India, there has been little or no systemic measure proposed by the state to deal with the issue at a comprehensive policy level. In fact, in Delhi when the All India Council of Human Rights, Liberties and Social Justice petitioned the courts, some courts issued directions to the state to provide protection to women and children. The Delhi High Court directed the centre and the AAP government to hold top-level meetings to deliberate on measures to curb domestic violence and protect the victims during the Coronavirus lockdown [The Economic Times, 2020]. The court heard the matter via video conferencing on 18 April 2020 and issued notice to the centre, the Delhi government, the National and Delhi Women Commissions, seeking their stand on the petition. The state in its reply said that it had put a protocol in place where a survivor if once called the helpline would have the telecaller take the complaint who in turn will forward it to the counsellor who will then establish a phone communication with the survivor during the lockdown. The court disposed of the petition after the status report was filed by the government.

We understand from the earlier reports released by civil society organisations and in newspapers as well as the court interventions that the impact of the pandemic has been felt by women both generally and specifically. Increase in domestic violence, loss of livelihood, returning back to abusive homes, being abused by the caregiver, and absence of adequate shelter homes all have been experienced due to the pandemic. It is important at this juncture, in the wake of a public health crisis, to recognise various experiences as violation to human dignity happening as a result of being in a home – dominant imagination of which is heterosexual, monogamous, and with biological reproduction.

Government Advisories and Home/Housing

While the Stay Home Stay Safe guideline meant the commonsensical popular imagination of the family, it reinforced heterosexual and elite stereotypes that there is an enclosed property that most Indians have which they call the "home" within which dwells a genealogical family who will remain "safe" if they stay with each other. That home has for long been associated with situations/emotions like "caged" or "trapped" especially in feminist writings (Naaz, 2017). The increase in domestic violence during the pandemic only reinforced the ongoing crisis inside the homes. This section does a survey of the government advisories around specific settlements – either slums or gated complexes, which find separate mention and specific COVID protocols, which indicated class-caste biases in these advisories.

The MoHFW broadly identified two kinds of housing arrangements through its advisories published on their website for issuing guidelines for the public. The two guidelines in question here are the guidelines on "Advisory for Gated Residential Complexes with regard to COVID-19 (17 July 2020)"[3] and "Preparedness and response to COVID-19 in Urban Settlements[4] (16 May 2020)". The former delineates provisions for ensuring protection from COVID-19 by suggesting measures such as thermal screening of "visitors/staff at entry points such as vendors, household helps, car cleaners, delivery personnel etc." to undergo such screening daily. Additionally the guidelines emphasise the importance of maintaining physical distance "in all common areas, inclusive of parks, corridors, lift lobbies, gyms, clubs". There is little or no discussion on surveillance unless a residential colony was declared as a containment zone, which would render local health authorities to "ensure that all houses are covered under daily surveillance" (MoHFW 17.07.20).

The Ministry, on the other hand, describes urban settlements as

> informal settlements within cities that may have mushroomed due to migration with inadequate housing and poor living conditions. These settlements are affordable and accessible to the poor in the cities. The main reason for the proliferation of these settlements is the rapid and non-inclusive patterns of urbanisation catalysed by increasing rural migration to urban areas.

The guidelines outlined overcrowding as a key vulnerability to the virus and affirmed that these spaces are "characterised by poor structural quality of housing, inadequate access to safe water, poor sanitation and insecure residential status and gaps in health and healthcare services" (MoHFW 16.05.20).

These guidelines also emphasised on the importance of strengthening surveillance system especially for such informal settlements for contact tracing mechanism, which would entail identification of the health workers in the health posts/dispensaries, Auxiliary Nurse-Midwife (ANM), Accredited Social Health Activist (ASHA), *Anganwadi* Workers, municipal health staff, sanitation staff, community health volunteers, and other volunteers. This trained manpower was expected to be contacted for deployment at short notice as per the advisory (MoHFW 16.05.20).

Another advisory issued on 14 April 2020 on "Enabling Delivery of Essential Health Services during the COVID 19 Outbreak"[5] highlighted the role of home visits by ASHAs in the aforementioned informal urban settlements, especially for high-risk pregnant women or newborn, elderly, and disabled individuals. The advisory mentions, if "during home visits, ASHAs should be alert to the possibility of increased gender based violence, inform the Medical Officer[6] and support the victim to access appropriate health and social services". It also mentions services to victims of "sexual and physical violence should be ensured as per protocols wherein the information about support services under social welfare department, NGOs, one stop crisis centres and helplines would be provided to the victim" (MoHFW 14.04.20).

However, these measures are evidently not sufficient since the home and the living arrangements are diverse and lie outside the binary of residential and informal settlements arrangements. Moreover, providing financial help and legal help to those facing domestic violence was also a challenge that remained along with the problem of accessing institutional support at a time when office, transport, and courts were closed. The need for a more inclusive approach in responding to distress calls and creating more awareness and accessibility was felt. Issuing advisories was not enough with the burden of domestic violence still left on the survivors with the para-medical staff on the ground exposed to similar violence and the threat of infection.

Additionally, there were different categories of people identified through these advisories which also reveal the popular imagination of family and home. The MoHFW identified certain categories of people dwelling inside the homes since it issued specific advisories addressing the mental and physical well-being of individuals. These advisories ranged from "Taking care of mental health of elderly during COVID-19" or "COVID-19: Pregnancy and Labour Management" for pregnant women at home; or tips on "Taking care of mental health of children during COVID-19" or releasing a video carrying "Tips for parents and students coping with anxiety and stress during the lockdown". Another video titled "For parents to learn 'Connecting with little ones during the COVID19 Lockdown" suggested that "this is the time to re-bond and to create a family time together to deal with anxieties". This was proposed as a way to tackle mental health issues and anxiety related to the lockdown.

While these advisories were important and indicated that the government was attaching importance to different categories of people – pregnant women, children [their parent(s)], elderly (grandparents), as well as recognising mental health awareness as necessary during the pandemic, yet the heteronormative imagination represented through these guidelines and visuals prepared for circulation cannot be missed. The homeless somehow did not find any space in these advisories. Also those who were separated from their "families" due to sudden declaration of the lockdown, without adequate time and planning, were missing. As a result, we saw a huge exodus of people walking back, crowding railway platforms, bus stands to return back to their hometowns from where they migrate to cities (seasonally or for longer durations), either as individuals or with their kins in search of jobs.

What we understand from the above set of advisories and guidelines is that home was a pre-given entity and it was pre-given as to who would reside within it – young children with parents while elderly parents by themselves. There was clearly no concept of either single-person households or domestic spaces which are shared by friends or flat mates. Neither was there a thought on hostels (not only those attached to colleges and universities, since they were directed to be vacated), paying guest accommodations – all of which are so much a part of urban realities. The class-based approaches to the ways of ensuring COVID protocols in gated communities and urban settlements are indicative in the advisories – the approaches and concerns are different based on what classes of people live where.

Home: Encountered and Re-imagined

All kinds of public health crisis or natural disasters have seen gendered impacts – increase in domestic violence, increase in child marriages and trafficking, increase in dropout rates among girls from schools, healthcare workers being infected more, sometimes even mortality rates being higher among women due to infections. The Spanish Flu, Ebola crisis, Tsunami disaster, or the Bhuj earthquake all had witnessed some or all of these. This pandemic, due to its insistence on social distancing norms and nationwide lockdown, brought into public discourse a continuous imagery of the home. Home was encountered and experienced – it was constructed and preserved. It is necessary for a sociological re-imagination of this home. There were contestations around five meanings around home, as emerging in this crisis all of which have gender-based implications and consequences.

Firstly, *Stay at home* to reduce the spread of the virus. In India, the first advisory came on March 16 (Ministry of Health and Family Welfare, 2020) directing regulations on mass gathering, closure of schools, ensuring physical distancing of minimum one metre between tables in restaurants, postponement of examinations, avoidance of non-essential travel. It was only a matter of time before we understood that the implications of stay at home in conjunction with work from home were going to be serious for gender-based household work. Secondly, *work from home* for most of the urban upper middle-class women in India has meant disproportionate increase in domestic labour. Finding the work – life balance became difficult if not impossible [The Indian Express, 2020 (a)] primarily because the increase in care work in addition to the professional work from the confines of home, without assistance from paid domestic helps for at least the first two months (varied depending upon when a household would feel comfortable letting the "outsider" in) of the lockdown impacted women's lives in manifold ways. It is valuable for us to note that traveling to the workplace is an important liberating journey for most women, which is also true for college going women students.

Thirdly, *violence inside the home*, or domestic violence. Fourthly *migrants walking back home* – a bulk of whom were women with children, family migrants sometimes with their non-human companion, walking or cycling unimaginable distances, travelling by bus, tempos wherever possible due to the sudden announcement of nation-wide lockdown. What this clearly demonstrated is that big cities do not become homes for migrant labourers; they come there to work seasonally, mostly as construction workers and short-term migrant workers experiencing a complete sense of precarity if there is no daily work in the city [Live Mint, 2020 (b)]. Thus the need to go back to the village or the town from where they had come from, where maybe the assurance of food remained even though it could mean absence of livelihood.

Fifthly, the anxiety and hope of *home coming* for many students who stay in halls of residence away from their parents, or in rented apartments in cities where they work, within or outside the country, away from their original usually natal homes [The Indian Express, 2020 (b)] Travelling back home for a certain class of people, take a flight or an AC train to "come" home or the country of original residence had been disrupted and shaken up in ways that have never happened in the recent past. It is important to recognise the class difference between the precarity of walking back home and the anxiety around flights getting discontinued and home coming getting delayed. While these were the different metaphors of home encountered during the pandemic, the chapter will conclude with a discussion on the need to reimagine the home in the context of increased violence inside the home.

The UN Women September 2020 report suggests that measures to protect women from violence must be a standard part of government responses to the pandemic, as well as long-term recovery packages. Safe access to support services and emergency measures, including legal assistance and judicial remedies, is urgently needed. In countries like India, it is important to emphasise on increasing government budgets for providing shelter homes, hostels for working women and other housing schemes so that women do not need to remain inside abusive homes. There are three routes through which the need for accessible, affordable home and housing can be traced – firstly through policy initiatives that Housing and Land Rights Network (HRLN) or National Forum for Housing Rights have articulated over the years – "homes for all" in India mainly in the context of the urban poor, eviction, and displacement. As per 2012 records, India has a shortage of 18.78 million houses in urban areas, according to the housing and urban poverty alleviation ministry [Live Mint, 2012 (c)]

A second route to take is through *Pinjra Tod* – a campaign by women students in Delhi against hostel rules and regulations. They raised voices against curfew timings, library timings, for more affordable accommodation, and regularisation of rents in private accommodation which abound the Delhi University area. All of these signalled an emphasis on women's autonomy, collectivisation, and the ability for them to take control of their lives and for collective bargaining with patriarchal structures in built in an institution (Anveshi, 2018).

Affordable hostels for all came to be discussed in the context of higher education post the tragic death of Rohith Vemula as well as through this campaign. It created a vocabulary about the importance of secure yet non-judgemental places of habitation, away from family homes. A third route that can be taken is the need to talk about housing rights as concomitant to ethical and just cities. In a recent piece Sushmita Pati asks, "given how diversified the landscape of housing is, there is a need to make housing a political question" (The Wire, 2020). In a Muslim family, single women find it extremely hard to find a place to rent across cities. Older, Brahmin-dominated localities in Bangalore and Chennai have consistently refused to let out to "non-vegetarians", who are more often than not, non-Brahmins (ibid. 2020). Housing is clearly not an individualised problem and the pandemic has brought out the universal necessity of affordable housing in big cities and demonstrated that it is a social issue.

From understanding the multiple meanings attached to the home to articulating the need for affordable collective housing, the pandemic gives us an opportunity to situate the experience of domestic violence in a much broader sociological assessment. This coupled with policy-level changes like placing women and girls at the centre of preparedness, response, and recovery in any situation of crisis is absolutely vital. The need and importance of improved gender data collection and expanded research on the gendered impacts of COVID-19, particularly on those most marginalised is tremendous. This chapter, by discussing specific situations of women with disability or sex workers, has demonstrated this need for gender-segregated data on domestic violence. While a crisis situation enables critical public discussion on immediate issues emanating, what is important is to continue to engage with these and transform the contours and conceptualisation of some of these discourses – like violence and home as this chapter shows.

Notes

1 Harsh (2020), Stories Asia, 25 April, www.storiesasia.org/2020/04/25/covid-19-lockdown-india-is-failing-domestic-violence-victims/,

2 The National Commission of Women, a government body which receives complaints of domestic violence from all parts of the country, recorded more than twofold rise in gender-based violence during the lockdown, which led to NCW to launch a WhatsApp number (7217735372) for distress calls. The NCW Chairperson Rekha Sharma revealed that "most of the complaints were received via email as people are scared of going to the police".

3 www.mohfw.gov.in/pdf/AdvisoryforRWAsonCOVID19.pdf,17.07.2020.

4 www.mohfw.gov.in/pdf/PreparednessandresponsetoCOVID19inUrbansettlements.pdf, 16.05.2020.

5 www.mohfw.gov.in/pdf/EssentialservicesduringCOVID19updated0411201.pdf

6 Medical Officer acts as primary administrator responsible for implementing all activities grouped under Health and Family Welfare delivery system in Public Health Centre's area.

References

Anveshi Research Centre for Women's Studies (2018), "Breaking the Chains: Understanding the 'Pinjra Tod' campaign", email interview by Rani Mohini Raman w.anveshi.org.in/broadsheet-on-contemporary-politics/broadsheet-on-contemporary-politics-no-14/breaking-the-chains-understanding-the-pinjra-tod-campaign/, accessed 7 March 2021.

The Economic Times (2020), "Implement steps to curb domestic violence during COVID-19 lockdown: High court to Centre, Delhi government", *The Economic Times*, 20 April, https://economictimes.indiatimes.com/news/politics-and-nation/implement-steps-to-curb-domestic-violence-during-covid-19-lockdown-high-court-to-centre-delhi-govt/articleshow/75249397.cms?from=mdr, accessed 10 March 2021.

Francesca Merlo (2020), "Global rise in domestic violence cases since coronavirus lockdown", *Vatican News*, 1 April, www.vaticannews.va/en/world/news/2020-04/increase-in-number-of-domestic-violence-cases-since-lockdown.html, accessed 27 February 2021.

The Hindu (a) (2020), "Lockdown: Over 60% sex workers in Delhi return to their homes", *The Hindu*, 17 May, www.thehindu.com/news/cities/Delhi/lockdown-over-60-of-sex-workers-in-delhi-return-to-their-home-states/article31606490.ece, accessed 27 February 2021.

The Hindu (b) (2020), "Desperation forces sex workers to risk COVID-19", *The Hindu, 16 July* www.thehindu.com/news/cities/bangalore/desperation-forces-sex-workers-to-risk-covid-19/article32105196.ece, accessed 28 February 2021.

The Indian Express (a) (2020), "The struggle of urban working women to strike a balance at home and work during the pandemic", 22 September, https://indianexpress.com/article/express-sunday-eye/why-women-are-struggling-to-balance-home-and-work-during-the-pandemic-6565804/, accessed 8 March 2021.

The Indian Express (b) (2020), "Homecoming will never be the same again', https://indianexpress.com/article/express-sunday-eye/homecoming-will-never-mean-the-same-again-diwali-6996980/, accessed 25 February 2021.

Jagori, Ekta, Action India, Nazariya, Visthar, Vimochana, NEN, Sangama (2020), *At Home at Risk: A Rapid Survey Series Across 7 States on the Domestic Violence Redressal Ecosystem during COVID-19 Outbreak.*

Leaflet (2020), "COVID-19: J&K HC takes suo moto cognizance of increase in domestic violence cases amidst Lockdown", *The Leaflet*, 18 April, https://theleaflet.in/covid-19-jk-hc-takes-suo-moto-cognizance-of-increase-in-domestic-violence-cases-amidst-lockdown/#, accessed 10 March 2021.

Livelaw Plumber, M. (2020), "Karnataka HC asks state about action taken on increasing complaints of domestic violence during lockdown [read order]", *Live Law*, 22 April, www.livelaw.in/news-updates/hc-asks-state-about-action-taken-on-increasing-complaints-of-dv-during-lockdown-155639, accessed 27 February 2021.

Live Mint (a) (2020), "How sex workers are using technology to service clients during lock down", *Live Mint*, 22 May, www.livemint.com/mint-lounge/features/how-sex-workers-are-using-technology-to-service-clients-during-the-lockdown-11590152476385.html, accessed 7 March 2021.

Live Mint (b) (2020), "Why India's 'migrants' walked back home?" www.livemint.com/news/india/why-india-migrants-walked-back-home-11590564390171.html, accessed 27 February 2021.

Live Mint (c) (2012), "Forum to persuade government to provide home to all", www.livemint.com/Politics/b6rCP5AL2XbZbmKqCQspLM/housing-rights.html, accessed 10 March 2021.

Ministry of Health and Family Welfare (2020), Advisory on Social Distancing Measure in view of spread of COVID-19 disease March 16, 2020, *The Government of India*, www.mohfw.gov.in/pdf/SocialDistancingAdvisorybyMOHFW.pdf, accessed 7 March 2021.

Ministry of Health and Family Welfare (2020), "Taking care of mental health of elderly during COVID -19", April 1, *The Government of India*, www.mohfw.gov.in/pdf/mentalhealthelderly.pdf, accessed 10 March 2021.

Ministry of Health and Family Welfare (2020), "Taking care of mental health of children during COVID – 19", April 1, *The Government of India*, www.mohfw.gov.in/pdf/mentalhealthchildrean.pdf, accessed 7 March 2021.
Ministry of Health and Family Welfare (2020), Tips for parents and students coping with anxiety and stress during the lockdown, April 5, *The Government of India*, www.youtube.com/watch?v=lELlhPGm2Nk, accessed 7 March 2021.
Ministry of Health and Family Welfare (2020), "COVID-19 (Pregnancy & labour management), Webinar by AIIMS, New Delhi", April 7, *The Government of India*, www.mohfw.gov.in/pdf/COVID19PregnancyAIIMSWebinar.pdf, accessed 7 March 2021.
Ministry of Health and Family Welfare (2020), "Enabling delivery of essential health services during the COVID 19 Outbreak: Guidance note", April 14, *The Government of India*, www.mohfw.gov.in/pdf/EssentialservicesduringCOVID19updated0411201.pdf, accessed 10 March 2021.
Ministry of Health and Family Welfare (2020), "Preparedness and response to COVID-19 in urban settlements", May 16, *The Government of India*, Directorate General of Health Services. Emergency Medical Relief Division, www.mohfw.gov.in/pdf/PreparednessandresponsetoCOVID19inUrbansettlements.pdf, accessed 10 March 2021.
Ministry of Health and Family Welfare (2020), "Advisory for Gated Residential Complexes with regards to COVID-19", July 17, *The Government of India*, Directorate General of Health Services (EMR Division), www.mohfw.gov.in/pdf/AdvisoryforRWAsonCOVID19.pdf, accessed 10 March 2021.
Ministry of Health and Family Welfare (2020), "27.03.2020 Dr. Shekhar P. Seshadri on 'Connecting with little ones during the COVID19 lockdown- English", March 27, *The Government of India*, www.youtube.com/watch?v=OYD9bogtJlU&feature=youtu.be, accessed 10 March 2021.
Naaz, Hira (2017), "The caged bird who sang: The life and writing of Rashsundari Devi", https://feminisminindia.com/2017/03/23/rassundari-devi-essay/, 23 March, accessed 25 February 2021.
National Commission for Women, Helplines for women in distress, www.ncw.nic.in/helplines, accessed 27 February 2021.
The New Indian Express (a) (2020), "Officials providing help, relief to domestic violence victims: State to HC", *The New Indian Express*, 26 April, www.newindianexpress.com/cities/bengaluru/2020/apr/26/officials-providing-help-relief-to-domestic-violence-victims-state-to-hc-2135401.html, accessed 27 February 2021.
The New Indian Express (b) (2020), "Effective steps taken to curb domestic violence during lockdown, TN tells Madras HC", *The New Indian Express*, 25 April, www.newindianexpress.com/states/tamil-nadu/2020/apr/25/effective-steps-taken-to-curb-domestic-violence-during-lockdown-tn-tells-madras-hc-2135296.html, accessed 27 February 2021.
The New York Times (2020), "The new COVID-19 crisis: Domestic abuse rises worldwide", *The New York Times*, 6 April, www.nytimes.com/2020/04/06/world/coronavirus-domestic-violence.html, accessed 7 March 2021.
Ngcka (2020), "Violence against women and girls: The shadow pandemic: Statement by Phumzile Mlambo-Ngcuka, executive director of UN Women", *UN Women*, 6 April, www.unwomen.org/en/news/stories/2020/4/statement-ed-phumzile-violence-against-women-during-pandemic, accessed 27 February 2021.

PTI (2020), "SC extends preventive guidelines to include women shelter homes", *PTI*, 21 April, www.thehindu.com/news/national/coronavirus-sc-extends-preventive-guidelines-to-include-women-shelter-homes/article31396433.ece, accessed 26 February 2021.

Rising Flame and Sightsavers (2020), *Neglected and Forgotten: Women with Disabilities during the COVID Crisis in India.*

Sen, Rukmini (2020), "Stay home, stay safe: Interrogating violence in the domestic sphere", *Economic and Political Weekly*, 20 June, 55(25), www.epw.in/engage/article/stay-home-stay-safe-interrogating-violence, accessed 7 March 2021.

The Week (2020), "The gendered impact of COVID-19 in India", *The Week*, 9 April, www.theweek.in/news/india/2020/04/09/opinion-the-gendered-impact-of-covid-19-in-india.html, accessed 28 February 2021.

The Wire (2020), "Pati, Sushmita the right to speak of housing rights in India is right now", https://thewire.in/urban/housing-rights-covid-19-city-space-delhi-mumbai, accessed 7 March 2021.

UN Women (2020), "The Shadow Pandemic: violence against women during COVID-19", https://www.unwomen.org/en/news/in-focus/in-focus-gender-equality-in-covid-19-response/violence-against-women-during-covid-19, accessed 20 February 2021.

9 The Unwanted Citizen

Dalit Precarity and the Pandemic in India

N. Sukumar and Shailaja Menon

Introduction

Wars and revolutions alter the cartographies of states and continents. Similarly, epidemics and pestilences too can amend the global order. The Black Death bacterium caused plague from the sixth to the eighth century AD and killed more than 100 million people. Some have linked plague to one of the first known examples of biological warfare when the Mongols catapulted plague victims into cities. Before Rome, we know also of the plague in Athens in the second year of the Peloponnesian war. It continued for four years (430–426 BC) and claimed 100,000 lives including those of Xanthippus and Pericles. But, more importantly Thucydides, who survived the war and gave detailed description of the epidemic, wrote how fear and self-interest to which people submitted, guided not just their actions, but affected the fate of the nation as well. Thucydides talks of the practical and moral weaknesses, which had a disastrous impact. Athens lost the war, which continued for a long period, but, as historians noted, it led to the decline of the Athenian democracy. The Black Death in England in 1348 led to far-reaching changes in the agrarian structure (Samaddar, 2020). In the last decade of the twentieth century, pneumonic plague broke out in the city of Surat in Gujarat in 1994 leading to fear and anxiety but the situation was rapidly brought under control and the transmission of the disease was checked (Pallipparambil, 2021)

The Body, Disease, and Its Cultural Milieu in India

In the Indian context, it is impossible to view any "body", human or animal, divorced from its caste-based cultural milieu. They embody a specific semiotics in the cosmology of the everyday social relations of production. Some bodies, whether human or animal, enjoy a privileged status with greater access to resources, whereas an untouchable body is cordoned off from any routine communication through religious diktats which are discriminatory. Such practices continue to prevail in both rural and urban spaces with the

DOI: 10.4324/9781003282815-13

lower castes entering the privileged domain for only menial tasks, considered unclean by their social superiors. As Gopal Guru succinctly argues

> [T]he discourse on untouchability is built up around the idea of touch. Unlike other societies, socially dominant groups within India have developed a distinct understanding of touch. The idea is embedded in their minds with enormous power to fragment, discipline, segregate and quarantine large chunks of humanity. What is so distinct about touch is its moral 'economy', which achieves this fragmentation with no investment of power; that is to say, it is withdrawal from, rather than engagement with, bodies that creates the other-the untouchable. Thus, touch is powerful because it privileges some bodies through insulation rather than assimilation.
>
> (Guru, 2006)

Untouchability as a negative value gets ontologically linked to the corporal body, which remains the same in all the spheres of life. That is to say, the body as the recipient of repulsion is denied a generic advantage. The reverse of this mediating ideology reproduces a logical counterpart, that is, the profane or the ritually defiling body. Ideological mediation assigns a repulsive meaning even to the corporal body, reducing the latter to the level of the "walking Carrion", as Barrington Moor Jr. would describe it (Guru, 2006).

When colonial rule gradually ensconced itself in the sub-continent, they encountered strange climates and diseases. In an attempt to protect the white bodies from being infected by the bizarre miasma and odours prevalent in the hostile environment, the colonial medical practitioners devised novel systems of health and hygiene vis-à-vis the native population as described by the British. Western medicine gradually worked as a cultural agency of colonial ideological domination. The epitome of such policies was witnessed when plague broke out in the Bombay Presidency in 1897 and the Epidemic Diseases Act was passed, which authorised the colonial state to enforce draconian measures to contain the disease.

While introducing the Epidemic Diseases Bill in the Council of the Governor-General of India in Calcutta for "better prevention of the spread of dangerous epidemic diseases", John Woodburn, the council member who introduced it, himself considered the powers mentioned in it as "extraordinary" but "necessary". Woodburn emphasised that people must "trust the discretion of the executive in grave and critical circumstances". This act empowered the colonial authorities to detain the plague suspects, destroy or demolish infected property and dwellings, prohibit fairs and pilgrimages, and examine the passengers at will. In this regard, particularly emotive was the issue of the "check-up" of Indian women at railway stations and public places. It was soon translated by the Hindu and the Muslim elites alike as colonial interference in the "private sphere" and an attempt to "dishonour"

Indian women. In fact, the Plague Riot of Kanpur in April 1900 was fuelled largely by the rhetoric around the issue of women's "honour". It appeared as if the anti-plague campaign "was directed more against the natives than the plague bacillus"(Woodburn as stated in Rai, 2020).

David Arnold in his study of medicine in colonial India has noted that people resisted the intrusion of their body during the plague epidemic by medical practitioners by concealing their symptoms or evading surveillance by the state. Such incidents were triggered by the belief among Indians that epidemics signified the Divine's way of punishing rampant sin among the people. Orthodox Muslims feared that "surrendering" to anti-epidemic measures was against the principle of *taqdeer* (predestination); Brahmans feared for their caste; Rajputs and Muslims could not let their women be seen without *pardah*; Jains, with their utmost belief in *ahimsa*, loathed the idea of killing rats during Bubonic plagues (Lone, 2020). Hence, it can be argued that Indian society was no stranger to the norms of social distancing as it was embedded in the habitus of everyday life. The COVID-19 pandemic exposed the physical, social, economic, and cultural distancing practiced by the socially dominant communities, in both the rural and urban spaces.

The Dalit Body and Its Precarity

In a meeting with Gandhi on 14 August 1931, Ambedkar declared, "Gandhiji, I have no homeland" (Patel, 2000). After almost nine decades, Dalits are forced to recall this prophetic statement when their survival is threatened by multiple agents: the apathetic ruling class, an "uncivil society", and a pandemic. The pandemic can be construed as a natural phenomena, but the former is a deliberate act to deprive the most marginalised sections of our society the nominal protection of citizenship. The Dalit migrant cannot wish away the curse of caste even in times of extreme precarity. Ambedkar's brief exposition of his experiences, his daily encounters with the caste ridden Hindu society and his observation "that the untouchables regard the village in every way as their home – and yet never touch or be touched by any one belonging to the village".

Ambedkar in his "Waiting for a Visa" speaks eloquently of his vulnerability. He felt exclusion deeply all along in his life: whether it was while travelling in bullock cart or when searching for water to quench his thirst; whether it was when he looked for living quarters or his stint in the Baroda State services post his education in Columbia; the sense of being an "outsider" prevailed. Ultimately, Ambedkar was forced to lie in order to get shelter, silently bear the humiliation of his fellow colleagues in the office, and suppress his anger. Ambedkar learnt a very valuable lesson: that a caste Hindu person can be a menial but has a dignity by which he can look upon himself as a person who is superior to any untouchable, even though the latter might be a barrister-at-law (Ambedkar, 2013). Surely, these experiences are also reflected in the city spaces even after almost nine decades of independence.

The coronavirus originated in foreign shores and was brought into India by those who travelled by air. Paradoxically, the price of living and surviving this disease was paid by the commoners who were struggling to lead a fairly decent life. It took a couple of months for countries to cobble together a response to avert the spread of the virus and by then scores of people across the globe had been infected and thousands succumbed to the disease. In a bid to contain the virus, the Indian state imposed a strict lockdown on the entire country under the colonial era Epidemic Diseases Act 1897.

Needless to mention, such stringent measures generated panic and gave rise to rumours. There were incidents of people from the North East of India being subjected to racist attacks and being pejoratively linked to the virus (Taskin, 2020). Similarly, there were reports of "corona jihad" trending on social media as a gathering of the Tablighi Jamat in Delhi was accused of spreading the virus (AP News, 2020). David Arnold has shared analogous incidents during the plague in Bombay. In October 1896, the infectious diseases hospital at Arthur Road in Bombay (today the Kasturba Hospital) was mobbed by hundreds of mill workers when a local woman was forcibly taken there. The workers believed that "there was 'something diabolical' about a hospital 'which claimed so many victims'". Patients, it was said, were "bled to death through the soles of their feet" (Kumbhar, 2020).

The state and medical personnel emphasised social distancing amidst the lockdown and gradually, a "new normal" came into existence. For the well-fed and well-housed citizen, the state arranged the re-runs of Ramayana and Mahabharata. For further entertainment, one could binge-watch digital platforms or even videos of celebrities doing their "bartan, jhadoo pocha". There were pronouncements by the political class that we should be generous and neighbourly with our fellow beings (Menon and Sukumar, 2020). Social media was awash with images of men who took pride in the fact that they were also performing the domestic chores. Majority of the people were assuaged that lighting lamps and beating utensils would defeat the virus and things will slide back to the old routine.

The Mordant Theatre of Politics

During the months of April and May 2020, Ambedkar's prescient observations were validated by scenes reminiscent of partition, which were witnessed in most of our cities – men, women, and children clutching their meagre possessions, desperate to avail any means of transport and reach home. A tribal girl, Jamlo Makdam (Outlook, 2020), died on the arduous trek from Telangana to her village in Chattisgarh. The Child Protection Council apparently never investigated as to why she was forced to work in the chilly fields instead of being in school. The mangled bodies of migrant labourers and chapattis strewn on the railway tracks bear silent testimony to the unfolding tragedy (The Hindu, 2020). The bodies of migrant workers who were killed in Uttar Pradesh's Auraiya road accident were stuffed in a truck with other workers and sent to West Bengal and Jharkhand (Hindustan

Times, 2020). During the first two months of the lockdown, 139 migrants lost their lives in various accidents in a bid to reach their homes (Indian Express, 2020). Their fate is to die unwept, unhonoured, and unsung. They were considered as collateral damage by a society, which constructed a new "lakshman rekha" to sanitise itself from the disease. The state, the media, and even the medical profession emphasised social distancing to contain the virus. In a caste-ridden society, this form of segregation is however socially sanctioned and easily normalised. (Social distance is used to maintain purity in a caste-based society. It is in this context that the term is used as caste is a form of exclusion.)

For thousands of migrants, surviving hunger was a major challenge compared to the pandemic. The lockdown cut off their source of income without which it was difficult to survive. A few samaritans did help out but it was too little too late. Their fate also testified to the lopsided development of the country and the neglect of socio-economic conditions, health, and education of the Dalits and tribals. For several years after independence, Mumbai, Kolkata, and Delhi were considered hotspots for employment. Gradually, the southern states of India rapidly developed due to better investment in quality education, infrastructure, health, industrial growth, and eventually the IT sector. Among the six largest metropolitan cities, Hyderabad saw the biggest inflow of migrants in the 2001–11 period, followed by Chennai and Bengaluru (Devulapalli, 2019).

The special trains overflowing with migrant labour desperate to reach back to their local/home villages in North India speak volumes about the uneven development that leads to poverty and unemployment and eventually migration. During the present crisis, the Kerala government was compelled to set up call centres to communicate with the migrants in their local languages. Those manning the lines could speak five languages – Hindi, Bengali, Odia, Assamese, and Garwahli. Kerala had the highest number of state-run relief camps for migrant workers. The state had 18,912 camps that housed over three lakh migrant workers. Uttar Pradesh was a distant second with 2,230 government-run camps while Maharashtra was third with 1,135 relief centres, according to data submitted by the Home Ministry to the Supreme Court on 8 April 2020 (Arnimesh, 2020).

The Hindi belt is the main source of migrant labour. Nearly 70 to 80% of labour who left Dharavi (Mumbai), a sprawling slum of about 8.5 lakh people packed into a geographical area of 2.4 square kilometre, were single men of all ages, with impoverished families in Bihar, Uttar Pradesh, and Jharkhand (Iyer and Modak, 2020). According to the 2011 census, four states – Uttar Pradesh, Bihar, Rajasthan, and Madhya Pradesh accounted for 50% of India's total inter-state migrants. On the other side, Maharashtra, Delhi, Gujarat, Uttar Pradesh, and Haryana housed 50% of the country's inter-state migrants. These shares are much higher than the share of these states in India's total population (Jha and Kawoosa, 2019).

If we take away the mask and remove the shroud of anonymity, majority of the migrant labour comprises the Dalit-bahujans, women, Muslims, and tribals who exist on the peripheries of society. Poverty and lack of opportunity in their hometowns drove 93 million Indians from disadvantaged castes and tribes in 2011 to migrate to other areas within their states in the hope of securing education or employment. The total number of internal migrants in India, as per the 2011 census, was 45.36 crore or 37% of the country's population. The annual net flows amount to about 1% of the working age population. As per census 2011, the size of the workforce was 48.2 crore people. This figure is estimated to have exceeded 50 crore in 2016, the Economic Survey pegged the size of the migrant workforce at roughly 20% or over ten crore in 2016 (Singh and Magazine, 2020).

But these migrants are plagued by social segregation and unequal access to the labour market which adversely impacts their life chances. Internal migration, both within a state and across states in India, improved households' socioeconomic status, and benefited both the region that people migrate to and where they migrate from, as reported by India Spend in August 2019 (Singh and Rawat, 2020). Remittances can help reduce poverty in the migrants' places of origin. But scheduled castes (SC) – castes considered "lower" in the social hierarchy – and scheduled tribes (ST) – Indigenous tribal populations – benefited less from migration as social discrimination continued to impact them in the places they migrated to (Singh and Rawat, 2020). *(SC/ST are official terms which have been used in the* chapter. *The term "Dalit" is not part of the official discourse.)*

In a study of slum dwellers in four Indian cities to investigate the correlation between caste and job market participation, it was found that those from higher caste groups seem to have better endowments required for absorption in the urban labour market. Also, the costs of migration are possibly easy for them to bear compared to those from disadvantaged castes. From the occupational choice model, it is again evident that migrants from lower castes (SCs) and the non-migrants across different social categories have a lower probability of joining the relatively better jobs, indicating that migrants from higher castes are better off in the urban job market. Though the results are based on slum survey, comprising mostly the low-income households, the findings confirm that among them, those who belong to higher castes are economically better off. The disadvantaged castes are not even in a position to take the benefits of migration as they are either unable to bear the cost of migration or unlikely to get absorbed in the urban labour market in relatively better jobs. This reflects the importance of special programmes, which can help reduce the vulnerability of the disadvantaged castes by providing improved access to livelihood opportunities (Chandrasekhar and Mitra, 2018).

About 16% of the total intra-state migrants in India belong to the SCs and 8% to the STs, almost equal to their share in the total population, as per the census 2011 data. This proportion has remained constant since 2001, when SCs made up 15.7% and STs 8% of intra-state migrants. Inadequate government policies often push migrants, from all social groups, to the fringes of cities that have limited civic infrastructure and municipal facilities, which in turn makes migrants prone to poor health and living conditions, as reported by India Spend in October 2019. The impact of such policies on migrants from the SCs and STs is greater, as these migrants comprise some of the poorest in the country as reflected by the government's National Sample Survey on expenditure in 2011–12 (Thorat and Ahmad, 2015). Thus, the 2011–12 data indicates that the Muslims and the Buddhists (most of whom belong to the SC) are the poorest in comparison to other religious groups including the Hindus, Sikhs, and Christians. Both the Muslims and the Buddhists suffer from multidimensional poverty and thus remained the most backward and poorest religious communities in the country (Thorat and Ahmad, 2015).

For the migrants, their misery is compounded as they cannot access state-specific schemes like the public distribution schemes. Those belonging to the SC and tribes cannot avail of any reservation benefits like seeking government jobs or getting enrolled in state-run educational institutions, when they migrate from one state to another and their caste is not notified there, according to a Supreme Court judgment (The Hindu, 2020) in 2018. This makes it difficult for migrants from historically marginalised communities to seek state support to better their lives.

Over 45.58 crore Indians were found to be "migrants" for various reasons during the enumeration exercises of census 2011. The previous census (2001) had recorded the number of migrants at 31.45 crore – more than 30% lower than the 2011 figure. According to the website of the Registrar General & Census Commissioner, India, "When a person is enumerated in Census at a different place than his/her place of birth, she/he is considered a 'migrant' ". Migration data began to be collected with the census of 1872, but was not very detailed until 1961. Changes introduced in 1961 continued until 2001; in the census of 2011, a more detailed format for collecting information on migrants was adopted (Yadav, 2019). The SC figures for intrastate migration increased from 42 million in 2001 to 62 million in 2011. Similarly, the ST migrants increased from 21 million in 2001 to 31 million in 2011 (Singh and Rawat, 2020).

While there is no official data for the inter-state migrants in the country, estimates for 2020 have been made by Amitabh Kundu of Research and Information System for Developing Countries. His estimates, which are based on the 2011 census, NSSO surveys, and economic survey, show that there are a total of about 65 million inter-state migrants, and 33% of these migrants are workers. By conservative estimates, 30% of them are casual workers and another 30% work on regular basis but in the informal sector. If one adds street vendors, another vulnerable community, which is not captured by the worker data, that would mean that there are 12 million to 18 million people who are residing in states other than that of their origin and have been placed at a risk of losing their income. A study by the Centre for the Study of Developing Societies (CSDS) and Azim Premji University in 2019 estimates that 29% of the population in India's big cities is of daily wagers (Singh and Magazine, 2020) (Amitabh Kundu as cited in the report by Singh and Magazine, 2020).

Women Seeking Work

The migrants from the dominant communities are equipped with more socio-cultural and educational capital to negotiate for better paying jobs in the urban areas. In the case of women, social location and access to resources play a decisive role in the nature of migration. Dwindling forest resources are a major reason for many tribal women who migrate to seek work. Interesting insights into the social implications of different types of migration are revealed when the distribution of the relative shares of the various types of migration among female migrants is analysed by social group/caste categories. It is noticeable that for upper caste women, the share of long- and medium-term migration is predominant with 75% of them concentrated in long- and medium-term migration. In contrast, short-term and circulatory migration accounted for 59% of migrant women workers from ST and 41% of SC women migrants. The concentration of SC and ST in this mass of general labour that circulates at the lower end of the productive economy, in which casual labour in agriculture, construction, and brick making figure prominently, draws attention to the limitations of the migration enterprise as conditioned by the prevailing economic system, in effecting transformation of degrading feudal hierarchies. At the same time, it is noticeable that among upper caste women, irregular short-term migration is more significant than for all other caste categories. This is possibly because responses to pauperisation may be differentiated along the status grades established by the caste system (Agnihotri et al., 2011).

Types of migration are very closely correlated with sectors and occupations. The diversified service occupations, for example, are more linked with long-term and medium-term migration. Hard manual labour-based occupations, generally attached to degraded conditions of work, are on the other hand more closely correlated with short-term and circular migration. When examining the more detailed data on individual migrant workers, the earlier mentioned study (Agnihotri et al.) found that 66% of upper caste female migrant workers were in the fairly diversified service sectors such as professional technical and related workers, call centre, sale workers, nursing, and other white-collared services.

As one proceeded further down the caste hierarchy, there was progressive concentrations in bhatta (brick making), seasonal agriculture, and paid domestic work. Migrant women workers from other backward castes (OBC) were also relatively more concentrated in paid domestic and agricultural seasonal work although 36% of them were distributed across a wide ranging white-collared services. SC women appeared to be more concentrated in bhatta labour, while ST migrant women were more concentrated in construction. More than 22% of SC women migrants were in brick making while 28% ST women migrants were construction workers. The corollary of such concentrations of SC and ST women in hard labour-based manual occupations of a casual nature was their low proportions in white-collar services. White-collar services accounted for 19% of SC and 18% of ST women migrants (ibid.).

In contrast to these extremes separating workers across caste categories, paid domestic work occupied a significant place in the occupational profiles of all caste categories while textile-based manufacturing was significant in all categories other than among ST migrant women workers. As such, the indications are that concentration in migrant manual labour in agriculture, construction, and brickmaking at one end, and more diversified and relatively more settled forms of employment for migrants at the other end, are more determined by initial location in caste hierarchies. On the other hand, gender that is not so differentiated along caste lines is the primary axis that determines migration for paid domestic work. The migrant female workforce in production work in modern textiles also appeared to have less of a caste bias, although our data indicates that ST workers had almost no entry into such work (Agnihotri et al., 2011).

In a similar research study of tribal women's migration seeking remunerative work, from the states of Orissa, Chattisgarh, Jharkhand, and Madhya Pradesh, it was observed that about 60% of the migrant women were working as domestic help followed by wage labour (34%). More than three fourths of Chhattisgarh, Jharkhand and Orissa states find tribal women working as domestic servant maids, whereas within the state of Madhya Pradesh, tribal women are engaged in wage employment. Some women are also reported in the professions of private job (2%) and very few are seen in government jobs, in shops/hotels, students and in other miscellaneous occupations (3%) (Planning Commission, 2010). Unemployment, poverty, and lack of basic facilities of education, health, and hygiene are still a major problem in the tribal areas forcing them towards out-migration to various towns and cities. The migrant tribal women and girls in cities suffer from poor housing conditions. Most of them have their houses in slum areas surrounded by unhealthy environment. In addition, more than 50% of the migrant tribal women and girls are living in rented houses. The average monthly income of migrant tribal women and girls is observed to be very low. This is because of the fact that a large number of them are employed as domestic servants where Minimum Wages Act is not applicable. It is also not effectively implemented in construction industry, factories, and other organisations where these migrant tribal women and girls are employed (Planning Commission, 2010).

The extreme precarity of the migrant labour is reflected in their earnings. According to the "Politics and Society Between Elections Survey" from 2017–2019 conducted by CSDS (Centre for the Study of Developing Societies, Delhi), the monthly household income of 22% of daily and weekly wagers is up to Rs. 2,000; 32%, earn between Rs. 2,000 and 5,000; 25%, between 5,000 and 10,000; 13%, between Rs. 10,000 and 20,000; and 8% get more than Rs. 20,000. A CSDS survey during the recent Delhi Assembly elections also found that 20% of respondents reported their monthly household income to be less than Rs. 10,000. Among migrants from Bihar and UP, this was even higher at 33% and 27%, respectively (Singh and Magazine, 2020).

The Long Trek Home

On 24 March 2020, a nationwide lockdown was imposed with a notice of four hours, catching everyone by surprise. Initially, it was announced for three weeks anticipating that the virus will somehow disappear. However, the latter seemed to further entrench itself and the lockdown kept stretching. After the first couple of days when the material resources gradually started depleting, the workers became restive. There was no work, no pay, and no source of any support from the state. They were left at the mercy of kind-hearted citizens. The choice was stark: either stay put and battle hunger and the virus or trek home by any means possible and hope for succour from the family. For the elites, "work from home" turned into a viable option ensconced in the comfort of their homes. Therefore, "work from home" was not a mere act of social distancing to avoid the disease, but it also turned out to be a potent middle-class privilege; the middle-class luxury that comes along with paid holidays and job security. It is a hierarchical professional segregation reflecting a new form of untouchability: the essential service providers must remain functional to serve and protect the life requirements of the middle-class elites, even in the most contaminated environment (Wankhede, 2020).

For the political class and the privileged classes, the image that emerges of the worker is hazy, faceless lacking any human semiotics. "Home" exists for the tax payers. The wretched of the earth have no claims to a "home". How can a *kaamwali bai* or a casual labour assert his or her agency and say that "we need to go home for our families are there". A stage show unfolded in Karnataka with the workers being prevented from leaving as the real estate sector required their labour (The Wire, 2020). The trains from Bengaluru were cancelled only to resume after a public protest. It seems that the state is battling more for the capitalist class. The Vande Bharat Mission is for the rich and the middle-class NRIs, rather than for the poor with the former apparently supporting the current political dispensation more. Many of them comprise techies from premier institutes who seem to work well under the guidance of multinationals. Where does a poor migrant, who gains importance only during elections, stand amidst such glorious statistics? (Menon and Sukumar, 2020)

There were widespread protests by migrant workers in various states. In Gujarat, police had to lob tear gas to control agitated workers in Surat. A group of 50 migrant workers in Surat tonsured their heads in protest against the delay in sending them back home, pointing out that many of them had sold their watches and mobile phones to pay the Gujarat government for the bus fare. Migrant workers protested on the streets of Rajkot, too. Hundreds came out on the road in the Shapar-Veraval industrial area on the city outskirts, demanding that they be sent back home (The Telegraph, 2020). Many states were reluctant to accommodate their returning migrant labour and failed to make adequate provisions for their travel. In many places, there were horrifying accounts of workers being sprayed by sanitisers. As a resident pointed out in Darbhanga in Bihar, "During the lockdown, Nitish first did not let migrants return, and then sprayed them with sanitizers like animals" (The Indian Express, 2020).

The plight of the migrant labourers during the COVID-19 pandemic testifies to their precarity as observed by Guy Standing. They are being habituated to a life of unstable, insecure labour, lacking an occupational identity or narrative to give meaning to their lives. They must do much work for labour, not counted in official statistics or political rhetoric, but which if not done can be costly, such as retraining, networking, refining résumés, filling forms, and waiting around for jobs. Despite their labour, they are not counted in official statistics. Often, they obtain jobs below their education or qualifications, and have low upward mobility. The precariat is losing citizenship rights, often not realising until they need them. This is cruelly affecting the growing number of migrants and other deprived groups as they tend to lose their cultural, civil, social, economic, and political rights. They feel excluded from communities that would give identity and solidarity; they cannot obtain due process if officials deny them benefits, they cannot practice what they are qualified to do, and do not see in the political spectrum leaders who represent their interests and needs (Standing, 2018).

The pandemic forced the state and civil society to acknowledge the marginality which envelops the lives of the migrant labour. The state has failed to collect any concrete data on the deaths of migrant workers during the pandemic (Rhea Binoy, 2021) Similarly, there is no data on the number of Dalit and tribal children who cannot access education and other amenities. Evidence from the nationally representative CMIE-CPHS survey as well as from some of the purposive sample surveys shows that Dalits, and to some extent Adivasis, were relatively more affected among workers broadly categorised into four caste groups – SC, ST, OBCs, and the general category. Fifty-one per cent of Dalit workers lost their jobs during the months of the strict lockdown, while at the other end, relatively far fewer upper-caste workers lost their jobs. "The relatively less drastic impact for Adivasis (out of all the non-upper caste categories) could be partly explained by higher dependence on agriculture, which was least impacted in terms of employment loss" (Azim Premji University, 2021). Only through proper documentation and policy measures the state can ensure social security benefits to these workers so that they may enjoy their constitutional entitlements as citizens.

References

Agnihotri, Indu, Mazumdar, Indrani and N. Neetha (2011), *Gender and Migration: Negotiating Rights, a Women's Movement Perspective*, New Delhi: Centre for Women's Development Studies, p. 49.

Ambedkar, B. R. (2013), *Waiting for a Visa, Writings and Speeches*, (eds) Vsant Moon, B. R. Ambedkar, Vol. 12, New Delhi, Ambedkar Foundation, pp. 663–671.

Arnimesh, Shankar (2020), "Rotis, mobile recharges, carrom boards – how Kerala fixed its migrant worker anger", *The Print*, 18 April, https://theprint.in/, accessed 15 May 2020.

AP News (2020), "As Muslims face stigma and blame for surge in infections, India's coronavirus fight weakens", *News 18*, 25 April, accessed 20 April 2020.

Azim Premji University, State of Working India (2021), *One year of Covid-19. Centre for Sustainable Employment,* Azim Premji University, Bengaluru, 5 May.

Bannerjee, Shoumojit and Mahale, Ajit (2020), *The Hindu*, 8 May, www.thehindu.com/news/national/other-states/16-migrant-workers-run-over-by-goods-train-near-aurangabad-in-maharashtra/article31531352.ece, accessed 30 May 2020. www.youtube.com/watch?v=PAECxmYwx1Q, Shimla (Himachal Pradesh), Apr 26 (ANI): Prime Minister Narendra Modi on Thursday said that the government is committed to provide poor people an easy and economical way of travelling. PM Modi said that his government is working to develop 25 to 30 airports for commercial purposes.

Bihar outside Bihar: Kept out in lockdown, 'sprayed like animals', Dehradun workers seek change (2020), *The Indian Express*, 5 November, https://indianexpress.com/.

Binoy, Rhea, Centre Still Collecting Data on the Death of Migrant Workers During Lockdown, (2021), *The Leaflet*, 12 February, www.theleaflet.in/, accessed 10 March 2021.

Chandrasekhar, S. and Mitra, Arup (2018), *Migration, Caste and Livelihood: Evidence From Indian City-Slums, Urban Research & Practice*, London: Routledge, pp. 11–12.

Coronavirus lockdown: So far, over 130 migrants killed in accidents en route to their home states (2020), *Indian Express*, https://indianexpress.com/article/india/coronavirus-lockdown-count-of-migrants-killed-in-accidents-enroute-their-home-states-6412475 / Also the Hindu, May 20, 2020, accessed 25 May 2020.

Devulapalli, Sriharsha (2019), "Howindialives.com, Migrant flows to Delhi, Mumbai ebbing", *Livemint*, 20 September, www.livemint.com/news/india/migrant-flows-to-delhi-mumbai-ebbing-1568981492505.html, accessed 25 September 2020.

Guru, Gopal (2006), "Power of touch", *Frontline*, 29 December.

HT Correspondent (2020), "Migrant workers travel with dead bodies of those killed in UP's Auraiya", *Hindustan Times*, 18 May, www.hindustantimes.com/india-news/migrant-workers-travel-with-dead-bodies-of-those-killed-in-up-s-auraiya/story-kFlKkHm7yrdiYWL2vsTdrN.html, accessed 5 January 2021.

Iyer, Kavitha and Modak, Sadaf (2020), "In Mumbai slums, signs of exodus: Locked doors, empty lanes", *The Indian Express*, 19 May.

Jha, Abhishek and Kawoosa, Vijdan Mohammad (2019), "What the 2011 census data on migration tells us", *Hindustan Times*, 26 July, www.hindustantimes.com/delhi-news/migration-from-up-bihar-disproportionately-high/story-K3WAio8TrrvBhd22VbAPLN.html, accessed 15 December 2020.

Kumbhar, Kiran (2020), "India's tumultuous history of epidemics, religion and public health policy", *The Wire*, 8 April.
Lone, Suhail-ul-Rehman (2020), "What epidemics from the colonial era can teach us about society's response", *The Wire*, 8 April.
Menon, Shailaja and Sukumar, N. (2020), "Who will mourn the walking dead? A requiem for Jamlo Makdam", 21 May, http://roundtableindia.co.in/index.php?option=com_content&view=article&id=9914:who-will-mourn-the-walking-dead-a-requiem-for-jamlo-makdam&catid=119:feature&Itemid=132.
Migration of Tribal Women: Its Socioeconomic Effects – An In-depth Study of Chhatisgarh, Jharkhand, M.P. and Orissa (2010), *Planning Commission*, Government of India, Society for Regional Research and Analysis, October, pp. 41–42.
Pallipparambil, Godshen Robert (2021), "The Surat plague and its aftermath, insects, disease and history, Montana state university", 20 January, www.montana.edu/historybug/yersiniaessays/godshen.html.
Patel, Jabbar, Dr. Babasaheb Ambedkar, (Film) 2000, Produced by National Film Development Corporation.
PTI (2020), "Migrant workers erupt in protest in Surat", *The Telegraph*, 4 May, accessed 5 January 2021.
PTI (2020), *Outlook*, 21 April, www.outlookindia.com/website/story/india-news-lockdown-12-year-old-girl-who-left-for-home-on-foot-dies-after-150-km/351151, accessed 27 April 2020.
Rai, Saurav Kumar (2020), "How the epidemic diseases act of 1897 came to be", *The Wire*, 2 April.
Samaddar, Ranabir (2020), *Borders of an Epidemic, Covid 19 and Migrant Workers*, Kolkata: Calcutta Research Group, pp. 1–2.
SC/ST members from one State can't claim quota in another, rules apex court (2018), *The Hindu Business Line*, 30 August, accessed 30 January 2021.
Singh, Priyansha and Rawat, Chitra (2020), "How caste impacts migration and its benefits", *IndiaSpend*, 16 January, www.indiaspend.com/how-caste-impacts-migration-and-its-benefits/, accessed 30 January 2021.
Singh, Sushant and Magazine, Aanchal (2020), "Explained: Indian Migrants, across India", *The Indian Express*, New Delhi, 6 April.
Standing, Guy (2018), "Who are 'the precariat' and why do they threaten our society?" *Euronews*, 2 May, | www.euronews.com/2018/05/01/who-are-the-precariat-and-why-they-threaten-our-society-view, accessed 10 February 2021.
Taskin, Bismee (2020), " 'Corona' is not just a virus. Indians are using it as a slur against people from northeast", *The Print*, 26 March. Also see Kimi Colney, Indians from the northeast face intensified racism as coronavirus fears grow", *The Caravan*, 3 April 2020.
Thorat, Sukhadeo and Ahmad, Mashkoor (2015), "Minorities and poverty: Why some minorities are more poor than others?" *Journal of Social Inclusion Studies*, Sage, 126–142.
To Appease Builders' Lobby, Karnataka Cancels Trains for Migrant Workers (2020), *The Wire*, 6 May, https://thewire.in/government/karnataka-trains-migrant-workers.
Wankhede, Harish (2020), "The virus and class divide", *The Wire*, 6 April.
Yadav, Shyamlal (2019), "India on the move: What data from Census 2011 show on migrations", *The Indian Express*, 26 July.

10 COVID-19 and Queer Community in India

Transgender Precarity Versus Homovivah

Pushpesh Kumar and Vallala Sravya

Introduction

This chapter tries to understand class stratification within the queer community which revealed itself more prominently during the COVID-19 pandemic. Visuals of the middle and affluent classes enthusiastically beating thalis and lighting lamps upon the prime minister's call to acknowledge frontline workers gave these occasions an aura of mass festive rituals. Parallel to this, the precarity of daily wage earners continued to multiply and escalate, and domestic workers and people in low-paid jobs bore the brunt of the lockdown and other regulatory measures enforced by the authorities.

Though lives turned difficult for many, the most visible impact of the pandemic was witnessed in the lives of transgender communities. Transgender persons inside and outside the community struggled for food, medicine, transitioning, and therapy along with loss of sources of income and livelihood with very minimal state support. They mostly survived through community support, NGOs, and voluntary organisations. The mainstream media barely captured their plight. Amnesty International surmised it thus: "As the World comes together, India's transgender community fights COVID alone" (Trivedi, 2020). Posters were stuck in Hyderabad city, for example, warning people not to talk to transgender persons to avoid contracting the Coronavirus, leading to housing complexes asking transgender persons to vacate their rented accommodation (ibid.).

Against the plight of transgender communities on the verge of multiple precarities triggered by the pandemic and its several lockdown phases, how does one understand the filing of petitions for marriage rights/equality in the Delhi High Court by certain gay and lesbian persons during the pandemic?[1] From "marriage rights" to the loss of livelihood and precarity, it is pertinent to explore the priorities of these divided queer groups during the pandemic. It is equally important to ask whether the privileged queer filing cases in the Delhi High Court for marriage equality have expressed any concern towards the transgender persons' vulnerabilities. We turn to Twitter and converse with a few transgender intellectuals and activists to understand who celebrates same-sex marriage (SSM), who disapproves of

DOI: 10.4324/9781003282815-14

marriage equality, who are indifferent, and who are sceptical in these times. With hindsight, we submit that SSM is more desirable for the financially independent, individualistic, affluent queer persons who, through their class position and financial security, can undermine and transcend community, caste, ethnic, racial, and even national boundaries.

We begin this chapter by outlining some of the polarised debates on gay marriage in the western context, mainly the assimilationist and equality perspective versus the critical queer perspective. Following this, we engage with the class and cultural privileges of those who filed cases for same-sex marriage rights in the Delhi High Court, contrasting them with precarious majority among the transgender communities. While the pandemic has been an existential battle for the latter, for the former, civil rights ensuring conjugality, inheritance, property rights, and insurance nomination as available to heterosexual citizens (read middle class) emerged as issues. Then, we examine the Twitterstorm of #Homovivah to understand the priorities of the culturally privileged classes of queer persons and their global supporters. We end with the concerns, anxieties, and alternative imaginations of some transgender intellectuals and activists and their reactions to legalising SSM.

Gay Marriage: Assimilationist Versus Equality Perspective

Although a wide spectrum of sexual ideologies exists in the US LGBT communities, some fairly discernible ideological types can be identified, an important one being the assimilationist view versus the radical view on the debate around SSM (Yep et al., 2003). The contention between the two groups relates to the desirability and/or pitfalls and troubles with marriage equality for queer liberationist politics. The assimilationists have sought SSM rights as the true and unmistakable sign that gays and lesbians have "arrived" in terms of being treated equally (ibid.). Andrew Sullivan, the anti-left face of the gay movement in the United States, urges the LGBT communities to move in the direction of homogeneity and become more mainstreamed (Sullivan, 2009). Sullivan claims that in the past years, it was important for gays to rebel, but now "gay marriage" also presses more responsibilities upon the gays: gay relationships are not better or worse than straight relationships and legalising gay marriage would offer homosexuals the same deal society now offers to the heterosexuals (ibid.:169). Another related argument is that SSM – like the major functions of heterosexual marriages – would allow for raising children in a stable, socially sanctioned, highly functional, and economically viable setting (Yep et al., 2003). If one takes this position, then single mothers, female-headed households, and single queer and transgender persons might become disqualified for rearing and raising children.

The opposing position on SSM emphasises that entering a monogamous marriage would amount to participation in a patriarchal, oppressive, and state-governed institution of marriage, create new hierarchies within queer communities, further marginalise those who choose alternative relationships, and trivialise non-monogamous relations through a hostile and restrictive version of morality (ibid.: 170–171). Queer studies scholars have also pointed out that the demand for marriage equality mostly emerges from the privileged queers than those whose lives are entangled in precarity due to class and racial disadvantages (Duggan, 2003).

Arlene Stein's (2013) comparative study of the suburbs of Maplewood, New Jersey, and Newark clearly illustrates that queer people of colour are, for a variety of reasons including the lack of access to capital, greater embeddedness in non-nuclear familial networks, feelings of loyalty to and belonging to racial and ethnic minority groups, the fear of stigma, and higher religiosity, among others, less likely than their white middle-class counterparts to make sexuality a primary identity. Maplewood's affluent middle-class gays and lesbians, a fair chunk of whom have got into civil unions, want their neighbours to recognise them as not only different but also similar (as members of the family-oriented middle class); they want the state to grant them the legal rights and economic benefits enjoyed by their heterosexual neighbours (ibid.). In contrast, in the poverty-stricken Newark, queer persons of colour consider marriage as a luxury and consider a safe street, descent jobs, and access to quality health as priorities (ibid.).

Lissa Duggan (quoted in Stein, 2013) raises concerns about the long-term implications of SSM on the LGBT movement itself. Duggan argues that marriage is a strategy for privatising gay politics and culture for the neoliberal world order (ibid.). The privileged advocates of marriage equality with heterosexuals do not contest dominant heteronormative assumptions and institutions, but uphold and sustain them while promising the possibility of a demobilised gay constituency and a privatised, depoliticised gay culture anchored in domesticity and consumption (ibid.). The question arises here: "can the poverty, inequality, stigma and vulnerabilities of transgender communities in India, intensifying in the context of the pandemic, allow them the luxury of domesticity and consumption"? Certainly not. In such a situation, the transgender communities cannot prioritise marriage rights; rather, they raise fundamental questions of livelihood, employment, financial and other support, health care, affirmative policies, and safety.

Demand for Marriage Rights Versus Precarious Transgender Subjects

Elopements and (un) successful attempts at marrying and/or escaping the tyranny of family and kinship by queer persons did exist in post-colonial India (Vanita, 2005), and photos of a few pompous and affluent gay weddings[2] emerged at times in glossy magazines and webzines for an exclusive class of readership. However, in the post-377[3] India, there is a renewed emphasis on legalisation and marriage equality, equivalent to the heterosexually married majority. It is in examining the backgrounds of those who are fighting and demanding for marriage equality that one can observe the stratifications within the LGBTQI+ community falsely assumed to be a homogeneous group. In further sections, we elaborate the concerns of these two groups during the pandemic that we, for the sake of simplifying the argument, placed on two extreme ends of privilege. The right to marriage is a civil right outside the state's financial and infrastructural commitments. In contrast, the right to food, medicine, livelihood, access to gender-affirming needs, and HIV/AIDS treatment would require allocating and distributing resources to the underclass. The specific temporality of the Corona pandemic revealed the differing priorities of the two different classes of queer – one seeking the legality of marriage parallel to heterosexual couples, while the more subaltern transgender persons struggling to get a fair share of necessary resources from the state. The latter want their daily meals and an institutional mechanism to safeguard their emergency and gender-affirming health needs, which is not so much of a priority for the former. There has not been significant interlocutory moment and dialogue between these two groups when they together constitute the collective, LGBTQIA+, or the "sexual minority". In annual pride marches across cities, media reports erase differences and reinforce this collective identity: similar to the popular opinions about other minority groups identified through a singular fixed marker like religion or ethnicity, society and media homogenise and minoritise all within gender and sexual non-conforming groups on the basis of an alternative sexuality. An overemphasis on sexuality erases other intersecting inequalities emphasised by the more marginalised within the group. Therefore, it seems pertinent to reflect on the class position of the petitioners for SSM equality and the basis of their justification for the latter. Following this, we contrast the same with the situations of transgender persons during the pandemic lockdowns.

Towards Unbreakable Bonds: Privileged Queer and Marriage Rights

Given the predominance of heteropatriarchy, there is no denying that the privileged classes of queer do have issues and problems that compel them to petition the High Court for marriage legalisation. Among the three petitions filed, Kavita Arora and Ankita Khanna, two mental health professionals, who have been living together for the past eight years as partners saw that the lack of legal rights put them in a certain precarity disallowing them to take medical decisions on behalf of each other and pass on their property and responsibilities to the other person in the event of sudden demise (Kripal, 2020). They filed a petition in the Delhi High Court in October 2020 highlighting their difficulties in opening a joint bank account as a couple, in nominating a same-sex partner in their insurance policy, gratuity, and pension, and applying for a passport, citing the constitutional provisions of justice and non-discrimination. They invoked their right to marry through the Special Marriage Act (SMA).

Jain and Mehta filed their petition for legal recognition under the Foreign Marriage Act, 1969, in the Delhi High Court after the Indian Consulate denied recognition of their marriage registration in New York. The couple's 2019 wedding in Texas, resembling any "mainstream" caste Hindu wedding amidst family and kin, had gone viral in Indian media. The act allows Indian citizens abroad to certify their marriage by a consular officer so that their spouse can legally participate in health directives, inheritances, and similar matters (Sorabhji, 2021), including travelling home during an emergency.

Both these petitions were filed by Arundhati Katju and Surbhi Dhar and argued in court by Menaka Guruswamy (Kirpal, 2020). Guruswamy and Katju, who filed and represented the case of Kavita and Ankita, speak of their marriage rights advocacy mission as a "marriage project", citing this as central to the Indian society,[4] implying that marriage is the most crucial gateway for LGBT acceptance in Indian society. Guruswamy proclaims in the Oxford Unity Society's invited speech – "we (the Indians) are a marriage society", where there is a complete erasure of feminist and queer critics on marriage being discussed and debated in India. Marriage *inter alia* is associated with dowry, domestic violence, unequal work burden, restrictions on women's mobility, and endogamy, which reproduces the exploitative caste structure in India. Katju and Guruswamy underplay these concerns in their formal speech. But the question is, who can afford this "depoliticized", "privatized" (homo) normative life (Duggan, 2003) and articulate a habitus that is almost similar to the elite and consumptive middle classes (Sender, 2001)?

It is here that it becomes important to examine the privileges and social positions of the petitioners and the lawyers representing them. The petitioners come from affluent families and had the privilege of coming out and being accepted by their families. Their generational capital in the form of wealth, caste, urban location, education, and the resulting career and income have all contributed towards making such a rare luxury possible for them. They also enjoy cis privileges, which allow them to access to the capital passed on to them generationally. Hence, the couples can be thought of as the most privileged among the LGBTQI+ community, which is plagued with struggles for survival such as basic needs of food and livelihood, employment, housing, safety in public spaces, and public health services, which are commonplace concerns for working-class queer and transgender persons. A majority of transgender persons are disowned by their families and have no choice in coming out. The issue of withdrawal of familial support is also faced by most queer youth in India, which leads to their discontinuation of education and exposure to violence and abuse. Given the low acceptance rate, working-class queers are forced to marry heterosexually, and "coming out" would sound alien to them.

While the rights to joint bank accounts and nominations and co-owning apartments are serious concerns, it is important to critically ask if marriage and conjugality should be considered as the only basis to claim them legally.

While projecting homosexual couples as victims of a discriminatory law, the parties involved tacitly reinscribe these relationships as superior to other intimacies and partnerships. Halberstam (2020) associates queer existence with wilderness, theorising the wild as an unbounded and unpredictable space that offers sources of opposition to modernity's orderly impulses (ibid.). While the unpredictability of life during the pandemic compels privileged same-sex couples to think of civil entitlements, what remains in the background are monogamy, bounded love, and, of course, entitlements parallel to that of heterosexual couples. When an imitation of the heteronormative middle class is the prime aspiration, the poor material conditions of fellow queer and the subversive politics of queer movement disappear from the agenda. The wilderness of queer bodies and uncertainties of queer existence, as articulated by Halberstam (2020), are overshadowed. From the amount of media attention, both news coverage and social media traction, given to issues of privileged queers, it is evident that their issues are considered more important than that of the lower rungs.

Preceding Kavita and Ankita's case, on 8 September 2020, a petition was filed in the Delhi High Court to legalise SSM within the purview of the Hindu Marriage Act (HMA) of 1955 by Mitra, Madurai, Thadani, and Oorvashi. The majority of these petitioners are again from a privileged class background. Seeking SSM legalisation within the HMA excludes the personal laws of minority communities in India, including that of transgender persons who mostly cannot afford to file such petitions to legalise their marriages, normativising and Hinduising the legal reform.

Despite the Indian illegality of SSM, the super acceptance of family and kin and other privileges disable elite queers such as the petitioners, from seeing and fighting against the troubles and traumas of being transgender in the street (Edelman, 2015), unable to earn their livelihood during a pandemic. This can be seen as a validation of Duggan's fear that marriage rights depoliticise queers as they allow them to participate in middle-class consumptive culture staying within the comforts of home, marriage, and domesticity. In that, solidarity towards community, which is assumed among sexual minorities, is complicated. For this reason, the poor transgender persons may connect to the politics of other marginalised communities along with their sexual and gender marginalities (Kumar, 2017, 2020) in contrast to the privileged classes of petitioners who enjoy cis-normative privileges, even attaining a celebrity status, representing what Sender (2001) refers to as an elite gay habitus.

Count Us as Humans: Transgender Communities and the Pandemic

We now turn to the plight of transgender communities during the pandemic lockdown. Amit Sharma's short film *Hamari Bhi Kar Lo Insano Mein*

Ginati (count us as humans) attempts to start the dialogue on the transgender community's experiences amidst the unprecedented lockdown in India (Ganguli and Singh, 2021). According to one study, more than 87% of transgender persons are dependent on traditional forms of livelihood like "badhai" – earning money by giving blessings during celebrations – begging and sex work; all this came to a stop during lockdowns (Ratnam, 2020). A National Human Rights Commission 2017, survey revealed that 98% of the transgender community do not own any property, and over 50% of bank account holders among them have less than 2,000 rupees in savings (Maji, 2021). It was a massive challenge for many to afford food and medicine (Sebastian, 2020) with little savings and social security benefits during the initial 21 days of complete lockdown in India.

During the same lockdown phase, a transwoman posted in social media that there was no food for her to eat; another transwoman mentioned that she had resorted to "sex work" to raise money for food (Tankha, 2020). Some of them are HIV+ and require medicines daily, but no help seemed to be arriving on that account (ibid.). Those who had undergone sex-reassignment surgery had to be under oestrogen hormones costing around Rs. 1,200, but many had no money to cater to this gender-affirming need (ibid.). As mentioned earlier, more than 2,000 transgender persons wrote to the union ministries of home, finance, and social justice seeking a special package for the community, which had no permanent sources of income and were as vulnerable as daily wagers amid the lockdown (The Indian Express, 4 July 2020).[5] They requested the government to provide an assured subsistence of at least Rs. 3,000 per month to every transgender person until the situation returned to normalcy (ibid.). "This is necessary because most trans persons do not have ration cards, no pension is provided in most states, and many transgender persons live in rented accommodations", their letter to the ministries said (ibid.). They also urged the government to universalise the Public Distribution System to ensure food security for all needy citizens, including transgender persons (ibid.). The letter requested the government to issue a mandate that no transgender person shall be forced to pay rent or face eviction by their house owners for non-payment of rent during the lockdown (ibid.).

Transmasculine persons were subjected to gender dysphoria as lockdowns did not allow them to access gender-affirming hormones and therapy. It became equally difficult for many intersex persons who might need therapy to procure support from formal and informal sources (see Mukherjee and Kumar, 2021). In recent years, there have been many litigations by the transgender communities demanding affirmative action in employment and education, and health benefits under certain schemes, but the state is yet to accommodate and act on these demands. The above instances suggest a world of difference between the precarious existence of the majority vis-a-vis the elite existence of a few within the transgender community.

The Twitterstorm #Homovivah: Class Aesthetics and Marriage Equality

This section constitutes a reflection on the Twitterstorm #Homovivah to understand some of the supporters of SSM, their aesthetic sensibilities, and the ideas and beliefs underpinning their support. On 14 October 2020, the Delhi High Court held the hearing on a petition for the legal recognition of SSM. Following that, there was an explosion of tweets using the hashtag YesHomoVivah sending outpouring support to the move on legalisation.

A significant part of the supporting voices came from the GenZ BTS ARMY in Twitter. BTS is a boyband from South Korea who, although are not vocally queer, do play it "unsafe" sometimes and reveal their queerness in their performances. The BTS band, therefore, is considered as queer icons. One of the interesting tweets says, "I checked the news channel but they are showing political news, and not even one line dedicated to decisions about homovivah", while their bio also says "keep politics away from me". The battle for SSM, hence, presents itself more as a cultural aspiration inspired by pop culture icons. The ARMY also gave calls to trend the hashtag YesHomoVivah since they believed it would make a difference in the decision of the court. The ARMY also called for non-desi moots to trend the hashtag YesHomoVivah in order to drown out the hashtag NoHomoVivah and then to post queer content using the same.

Another major trend also involved sharing pictures of viral, lavish, and large-scale[6] queer weddings. The viral weddings of Bianca Maileli and Saima Ahmad, Sufi Malik and Anjali Chakra, and Amit Shah and Aditya Madiraju, many of whom are social media influencers, were reported in Indian mainstream news outlets.[7] The couples are based abroad and are significantly rich.[8] Maileli and Ahmad are from India and Pakistan, respectively. The tweets claimed their identities as a Hindu-Muslim marriage, even though, in reality, it was a marriage between a Christian and a Muslim.[9]

The critical voices here are few. One user called for the Transgender Act of 2019 to be discussed, highlighting that there are different punishments for the rape of a transwoman and a ciswoman, that is an imprisonment for a maximum of 2 years and 7 years, respectively, and emphasising that homovivah will not solve any problems. Another post said "marriages aren't the solution, they are a candy given to you to look away from the violence that is normalised against queer community inside out; #homovivah is transphobic". A queer vegan of colour and a lecturer at the University of Paris asked if gay marriage will be interfaith or inter-caste or if it is just for the dominant Hindus. Another account also pointed out that HomoVivah is not the right word since it has exclusionary implications. Marriages outside of marriage rituals based on religion should also be accommodated. One of the well-known queer activists and a research student said: "strange times to have agreements over popular opinions. Systems of marriage have to be destroyed not entered into. Queers against patriarchal marriage system; #nohomovivah".

There is recognition of differential privileges within the queer community as well as the problematisation of the marriage system in India along with its inherent class and caste interests. At the same time, there are also voices that feel marriage is redeemable only if it is rid of its class, caste, and religious interests. The transgender communities who use Twitter for political issues were indifferent and unenthusiastic about the issue altogether as they were worried about the issues of livelihood, health, safety, security, starvation, and many other uncertainties in these times hit by the pandemic.

Same-sex Marriage, Pandemic, and Transgender Concerns

Here, we offer the views of a few representatives from the transgender and gender non-binary communities to reflect on marriage legalisation. Most of our interlocutors are English-speaking and have had access to higher education; most of them feel alienated from their natal families and prefer staying away from close kin. A few of them are transitioning, while others were forced to go back to their natal families during the pandemic and are experiencing dissonance, dysphoria, and depression. Their English-speaking status has not enabled them to articulate proximity to a heteronormative middle-classness. The transness of bodies and cross-gender identities disentitle members of transgender communities from taking up jobs, staying in a "respectable" heteronormative middle-class neighbourhood, and sustaining corporate jobs. Hence, those with transgender and non-binary identities are more likely to experience phobia and overt and covert discrimination vis-à-vis the cis-normative gay and lesbian persons. Belonging to affluent classes adds further privileges and entitlements for the latter group.

Our interlocutors, who were interviewed in March 2021, seemed to be least concerned about marriage rights/equality petitions in the Delhi High Court. They talked about more fundamental rights for the transgender communities, including employment, livelihood, affirmative action, the discriminatory Transgender Act of 2019, safe street, access to gender affirmative, and general health needs. Many transgender activists were busy filing petitions in the court for access to rations and financial help, mobilising support for the community through fundraising and approaching NGOs and civil society organisations. A non-binary transgender interlocutor, A, submits: "When people (transgender persons) are on the verge of starvation and precarity; marriage seems rather frivolous". A few of them surmised "people who have the privilege and money to approach the court and hire high-profile lawyers for advocating their case of SSM are yet to mount a challenge against the blatantly unconstitutional Transgender Act (of 2019)". "The celebratory lawyer couple (referring to Guruswamy and Katju) are tight-lipped on the Transgender Bill, which amounts to a criminal silence". C, another gender non-binary transgender person pursuing doctoral research, refers to Keshav Suri, the wealthy (gay) hotelier and one of the petitioners against Section 377 of the Indian Penal code, and remarks that he would not file a petition for transgender women's fundamental rights. A further shares: "many transitioning trans-persons had to go back to their natal families on account of the loss of jobs or the closure of public places and institutions where they were studying. For several of them, staying with natal families meant painful de-transitioning (assuming their assigned gender at birth) under familial pressure". While responding to the question whether marriage would pave the way for availing certain benefits available to the heterosexually married couples, most of our interlocutors were sceptical, asking "why should a state-recognized dominant patriarchal institution like marriage be the only way to access such entitlements"? The state needs to authenticate other ways of organising personal and intimate lives to democratise inheritance, care, and various kinds of insurances. Civil partnerships and intimate partners beyond marriage need to be recognised for such entitlements.

To A, marriage restricts the number of people who can gain by such entitlements and benefits. Emphasising the alternative life world of the Hijra community, A cites the mentor (guru)/disciple (chela) relationship through which kinship ties are forged. If a chela or a guru has no visitation rights during hospitalisation and a medical emergency, marriage equality will not help either. Reacting to #Homovivah, many interlocutors resented and labelled Vivah as Brahmanical, Hindu, and North Indian, implying that a Sanskritised caste and dominant religion are reinforced through the Twitterstorm. R, a self-identified transgender woman, iterated the mental distress of transgender women arising from the loss of livelihood and the absence of counselling services for them during the pandemic. She further adds how the lockdowns hindered Hijra and transgender women from meeting their general health needs, apart from accessing Anti-Retroviral Treatment (ART), shooting viral loads for those infected with HIV/AIDS.

Many in rural and remote areas could not travel to urban centres for ART, and those in urban areas witnessed the conversion of ART centres into COVID centres, creating confusion and uncertainty. R further points out that for transgender communities and others in alternative family and kinship arrangements, the demand should be for the legal recognition of consensual living relationships and community bonds. C claims that it is possible for two individuals to open a joint bank account without being married, and for passing on property, one can simply write a will. For C, fundamental rights are more important than these civil rights, which are unavailable to most transgender persons. They end by saying that entitlements to food, shelter, education, and reservations in jobs are more needed than insurance and inheritance for transgender persons.

Conclusion

SSM is perceived by many of the privileged class queer as a crucial right. The argument supporting SSM is based on the access to the legal equality and civil rights as within heterosexual conjugality. Critiques in both the western and non-western contexts have pointed at the depoliticisation of queer through marriage equality and their participation in a heteronormative world view.

Contradictions and differences within the queer community appeared more sharply during the pandemic. Caste and class and the lack of cisnormative privileges render the majority of transgender women vulnerable. Whereas the corporate and the privileged queer began demanding for marriage equality, transgender persons were fighting for their fundamental rights, such as food, shelter, safety, gender affirmative needs, employment, and acceptance into public spaces. One can see the disconnect between these two classes of queer – the former is silent about transgender existential struggles during the pandemic, while the latter expressed ignorance, indifference, or scepticism to marriage equality and hold marriage as a state-recognised patriarchal institution. The differences in priorities among these groups, which are on extreme ends of the spectrum, warrant us to critically look at LGBTQI+ community as complex and internally stratified. It also points towards the difficulty in building solidarities in the community. It is important to build such solidarities reflecting the tensions in queer politics.

Notes

1 In one of the petitions filed in the Delhi High Court to legitimise gay marriage under HMA, two transgender persons also figure in. One of them belongs to a privileged class and cannot be regarded as the representative of the majority of marginalised, transgender persons.
2 See (124) Pinterest.
3 Post-377 indicates the reading down of Section 377 of the Indian Penal Code which criminalised homosexuality since 1861 in September 2018 by the Supreme Court of India.
4 See Menaka Guruswamy and Arundhati Katju | Full Address and Q&A | Oxford Union – Bing video.
5 Transgender community demands special package amid COVID-19 lockdown | India News, The Indian Express.
6 "5 Times Indian LGBT Couples Set Serious Wedding Fashion Goals". *ETimes*. Entertainment Times, 16 January 2020. https://timesofindia.indiatimes.com/life-style/fashion/buzz/5-times-indian-lgbt-couples-set-serious-wedding-fashion-goals/photostory/73296517.cms.
7 Kumari, Pradamini. "18 Couples Who Rewrote Society's Rules on How Weddings & Marriages Should Be." *ScoopWhoop*, 19 October 2020.; www.scoopwhoop.com/culture/couples-who-rewrote-indian-society-wedding-rules/.; Sonoma, Serena.
8 Anjali, Sufi and *Taking My Girlfriend on Vacation w My Mom + Sis: Hawai'i Vlog*. *YouTube*. YouTube, 2020. www.youtube.com/watch?v=v_BBGuBSCq8.
9 Sonoma, Serena. "This Indian-Pakistani Lesbian Marriage Gave Us All the Feels". *Out Magazine*, 2 September 2019. www.out.com/lesbian/2019/9/02/indian-pakistani-lesbian-marriage-gave-us-all-feels.

References

Duggan, Lissa (2003), *The Twilights of Equality? Neoliberalism, Cultural Politics and Attack on Democracy*, Boston: Beacon Press.

Edelman, Elijah Adiv (2015), "Walking while transgendered: Necropolitical regulations of transfeminine bodies of colour in the US national capital", in J. Haritaworn, A. Kuntsman and S. Posocco (eds), *Queer Necropolitics*, New York: Routledge.

Ganguly, Debapriya and Singh, Rajni (2021), "*Hum Bhi Hain Insaan*: The transgender humanitarian crisis during Covid-19 Pandemic in India", in *Intersections: Gender and Sexuality in Asia and Pacific*, Intersections: Hum Bhi Hai Insaan': The Transgender Humanitarian Crisis during the Covid-19 Pandemic in India (anu.edu.au).

Halberstam, Jack (2020), *The Disorder of Desire*, Durham: Duke University Press.

Kirpal, Saurabh (2020), "Why its time to consider same sex marriage", Why It's Time to Consider Same Sex Marriage – Article 14 (article-14.com).

Kumar, Pushpesh (2017), "Radicalizing community development: Changing face of queer movement in the Hyderabad City", *Community Development Journal*, 52(3), 470–487.

Kumar, Pushpesh (2020), "Mapping queer celebratory moment in India: Necropolitics or substantive democracy?" *Community Development Journal*, 55(1), 159–176.

Maji, Sucharita (2021), "There are some less cared for", There are some less cared for (dailypioneer.com), accessed 23 June 2021.

Mukherjee, D. and Kumar, P. (2021), "Subordinate and marginalised masculinities and the COVID-19 Pandemic", *Economic and Political Weekly*, 56(11), 2349–8846. https://doi.org/ISSN (Online).

PTI (2020, April 28), "Transgender community demands special package amid Covid-19 lockdown", *India Express*, https://indianexpress.com/article/india/transgender-community-demands-special-package-amid-covid-19-lockdown-6383015/, accessed 25 July 25, 2021.

Ratnam, Dhamini (2020), "Covid 19 lockdowns put transcommunity in a spot", Covid-19 lockdown puts trans community in a spot | Latest News India – Hindustan Times.

Sebastien, Swan (2020), "Covid 19: What about transgender community?" COVID-19: What about the transgender community? (downtoearth.org.in).

Sender, Katherine (2001), "Gay readers, consumers, and a dominant gay habitus: 25 Years of advocate magazine", *Journal of Communication*, 52(1), 73–99.

Sohrabji, Sunita (2021), "Indian American couple files precedent-setting petition in Delhi high court, urging India to recognize same-sex marriages", Indian American Couple Files Precedent-Setting Petition in Delhi High Court, Urging India to Recognize Same-Sex Marriages | Global Indian | indiawest.com, accessed 25 June 2021.

Stein, Arlane (2013), "What's matter with Newark? Race, class, marriage. Politics and limits of queer liberalism", in M. Bernstein and V. Taylor (eds), *The Marrying Kind: Debating Same Sex Marriage Within Gay and Lesbian Movement*, Minneapolis: University of Minnesota Press, pp. 39–66.

Sullivan, Andrew (2009), *Same Sex Marriage: Pro and Con*, New York: Vintage.

Tankha, Rajkumari Sharma (2020), "Transgender plight during coronavirus pandemic", Transgender's plight during coronavirus pandemic. *The New Indian Express*.

Trivedi, Divya (2020), "Covid 19 and plights of transgender community", COVID-19 and the plight of the transgender community – Frontline (thehindu.com).

Vanita, Ruth (2005), *Same Sex Marriage in India and the West*, New Delhi: Palgrave Macmillan.

Yep et al. (2003), "A critical appraisal of assimilationist and radical ideologies underlaying same sex marriages in LGBT communities in the United States", *Journal of Homosexuality*, 45(1), 45–63.

11 Life of the Marginalised and the Pandemic

The Case of Tribes in India

Jagannath Ambagudia and Virginius Xaxa

Introduction

Human society has been confronted with numerous unprecedented challenges over time. Some have been short-lived, while others were *long duree* and with implications on communities. Some of the challenges have been severe while others were moderate. The most critical challenges are generally visible in the sphere of the health of groups and communities on the margin of the society. Of such groups, Indigenous/tribal people have been the worst sufferers across the globe. India is no exception. However, although some sporadic attempts have been made to address the overall health issues of tribal communities in India (Pati, 1998; Hardiman, 2007, 2008; Mishra and Sarma, 2011), the existing social science scholarship has not given due attention to tribal health in the context of calamities such as the present case of the COVID-19.

Tribal communities are marked by various issues, concerns, and challenges of different magnitudes and forms. They have low socio-economic, educational, political, and health indicators compared to non-tribal communities. Due to these, they are more prone to multiple risks. Low health status, among others, has exposed the communities to more significant health risks. However, such a phenomenon among them is not a recent phenomenon. It has been there with them for centuries. Historically, critical health risks, such as the impact of the pandemic, have been a significant problem for tribal communities resulting in a larger number of pandemic deaths. Against this backdrop, this chapter looks at the ramifications of COVID-19 on tribal communities in India. While doing so, it briefly looks at the phenomenon in historical contexts as tribes were exposed to a similar phenomenon in the past as well. It then moves to address what Coronavirus meant for the tribal communities of India. It also critically examines the role of the state in addressing the problems posed by the COVID-19 to tribal communities in India.

Tribes, Well-being, and Calamities in History

COVID-19 affects everyone, but it does not impact all populations evenly. It is likely to affect those communities the most who live with vulnerabilities.

DOI: 10.4324/9781003282815-15

Tribal people in India are one such community with distinct and specific vulnerabilities; thus, they are likely to be the most adversely affected. The development indicators of tribal communities are the poorest of all social categories in India (Government of India, 2014). Poverty, low literacy, unsafe drinking water, deteriorating environment, and poor essential health services are widespread problems in the tribal region. These have had an adverse bearing on their present health status that may expose them to the infection, resulting in high mortality. Indeed, contagious diseases and Indigenous peoples have a long and painful history. Hence, it would not be out of place to briefly spell out their economic, educational, and health status.

A low standard of living may have characterised tribal society in India, but poverty in the form of hunger death had generally been marked by absence. If there was starvation and hunger death at all, it was more based on natural calamities such as famine, cholera, malaria, and infectious diseases due to contact with the outside world. In such a case, the community as a whole suffered, and not some particular individuals and families. The Andaman and Nicobar Islands illustrate it best. In 1858, when the penal settlement started, the population of the Andamanese tribes was almost 4,800. However, they declined to 625 by 1901, to 90 by 1930, and 28 by 1988. The declining of Andamanese tribal population was perhaps due to the warfare with the colonisers at the initial period. However, diseases, such as pneumonia, measles, and syphilis, also contributed to their declining number at a later period. The disease infected the Onges, resulting in a decline in their numbers from 670 in 1901 to 250 in 1930. Their number had further declined to about 100 in 2006 (Minority Rights Group International, 2008). Even in mainland India, tribes as a whole suffered a substantial decline in their absolute number during 1891–1901, 1911–1921, 1921–1931 due to famine or epidemics (Maharatna, 2005).

In settings other than famine and epidemics, an increase in number has not been a problem. The proportion of tribal population ranged from 2.26 to 3.26% during 1881–1941, whereas the Hindu proportion steadily declined from 75.1% to 69.5% during this period. In *The Population of India and Pakistan* (1951), Kingsley Davis explains the reasons for such differences attributed to the high fertility of the tribal population compared to the Hindu population (cited in Maharatna, 2000: 3039). This meant that the nutritional status of tribes was positive. Tribes, in fact, had subsisted for generations with a reasonable standard of health because forests provided them food, such as fruits, leafy vegetables, honey, and juice. The caloric intake of many of the traditionally food-gathering tribes is entirely from collections made by them from the forest. Even many settled agriculturist tribes derive substantial nutrition from forest products. Medicinal plants, which they have been using to treat diseases and maintain health, are today a source of modern medicine.

The existing data suggests that tribal communities in India suffer a high incidence of poverty than other social groups. Though there is a slight decline in the poverty ratio among the tribal communities, the figures still indicate a higher level. For instance, the tribal population living below the poverty line (BPL) has declined from 47.4% in 2009–2010 to 45.3% in 2011–2012 in rural areas. Similarly, the poverty ratio of tribal communities in urban areas has declined from 30.4% in 2009–2010 to 24.1% in 2011–2012 (Government of India, 2021a: 41). However, the overall poverty ratio of tribal communities stands at 40.6% compared to 20.5% among the non-tribal communities (Government of India, 2018: 17). As per the 2011 census, the tribal literacy rate was just 59% compared to 73% for the country. However, the dropout rate in school education among tribal students is still alarming. For instance, the dropout rate was 8.54, 9.58, 8.88, 26.96, and 8.40 in primary, upper primary, elementary, secondary, and grade XI-XII in 2016–2017 (Government of India, 2021a: 36).

The government-appointed Committee on Tribal Health indicates the sorry state of tribal health in India (Government of India, 2018). About 65.1% of tribal women in the age group of 15–49 suffer from anaemia. The tribal population constituted 50% of the total deaths due to malaria. About 75% of pregnant and lactating women and about 68–71% of tribal children had inadequate intakes of protein and calories. In 2014, the infant mortality rate was 44.4 per 1,000 live births for the tribal population than 32.1 for others, that is, non-SC, non-ST, and non-OBC populations. The child mortality rate among the tribal communities was 13.4 per 1,000 live births against 6.6 for others. Similarly, the figure for under-five mortality, the great pointer of malnourishment, was 95.7 per 1,000 live births against 38.5 for others (Government of India, 2018: 27). This is the national scenario. However, if one were to situate them in the regional context, the problems are even more revealing.

The Expert Committee on Health showed that the tribal population bears a disproportionate burden of communicable diseases like malaria, tuberculosis, skin infection, sexually transmitted diseases, HIV, typhoid, viral fever, and cholera (Government of India, 2018). Such being the situation and context of the Indigenous/tribal people worldwide, most international agencies such as the United Nations Organization bodies, International Labour Organization, and International Fund for Agricultural Development have shown concern and advised the national governments for effective measures to address their problems arising from the pandemic. For instance, Anne Nuorgam, Chair of the United Nations Permanent Forum on Indigenous Issues, urged the member states and international community to "include the specific needs and priorities of indigenous peoples in addressing the global outbreak of COVID 19" (United Nations, 2020).

COVID-19 and Plight of Tribal Communities

COVID-19 has disproportionally impacted various communities in India, and it has caused multiple disruptions to tribal communities. Some of the critical areas, such as health, livelihood, migration, and education, where the pandemic has profoundly impacted the tribal communities, are discussed later.

Health Situation of Tribes

COVID-19 has exposed the fragile health system present in rural areas in general and tribal areas in particular. The tribal areas lack health infrastructure and human resources. The MoTA provides statistical evidence of the shortage of health infrastructure in tribal areas. The all-India-level aggregate data indicates that as of 31 March 2019, the tribal areas experienced a shortage of 7,054, 1,204, and 326, constituting 21.74, 24.80, and 27.12% of the required sub-centres, primary health centres, and community health centres based on population norms, respectively (Government of India, 2021a: 151). The statistics also indicate growing state-wise disparities in health infrastructure and human resources in the tribal areas (Government of India, 2021a: 151–156).

Tribal communities are most vulnerable to nutritional deficiency. The existing data demonstrates a considerable difference in nutritional status between the tribal and the non-tribal communities in India (International Institute for Population Sciences, 2017: 305–342). ST women are more prone to nutritional deficiency and chronic energy deficiency, raising serious concerns about the nutrition status among the STs in India (Government of India, 2013: 38). Tribal children are nutritionally deficient (Government of India, 2013: 38). The National Family Health Survey (NFHS-4) indicates that 42% of tribal children are underweight, 1.5 times higher than non-tribal children (Government of India, 2018). The NFHS-4 indicates that only 30.8% of tribal households are covered by a health scheme or health insurance (International Institute for Population Sciences, 2017: 372). Situating COVID-19 in tribal public health indicates that the vulnerable tribal communities are more prone to communicable diseases such as the Coronavirus. Though tribal areas seem to have been less affected by the deadly impact of COVID-19, at least at the initial stage of spreading, shortage of healthcare facilities would undoubtedly test the state of tribal public health. However, unlike the first stage of transmission of Coronavirus, the rural areas are no longer exceptional to the clutch of the virus. The number of COVID-19 positive cases gradually increased in tribal areas too.

It may be unrealistic to argue that the state of tribal health has been exposed to significant risk at a time of Coronavirus. Such a scenario was always there much before the pandemic hit the world. Nevertheless, the pandemic has made the already vulnerable tribal communities more vulnerable in the health sector. The ethnic communities experience the health risks unequally and differently. The global slogan of "social distancing" that has now literally converted into "physical distancing" to contain the further spread of the disease has become unrealistic in tribal India and has posed a more significant challenge for the implementing authorities as tribal communities continue to struggle for basic facilities.

The tribal communities lag behind other social groups regarding basic amenities like housing, drinking water, and sanitation (Government of India, 2013: 68). The requirements of home quarantine for the returned tribal migrants became another burden due to the insufficient number of rooms to accommodate people. In the absence of reliable sources of water facilities and acute water shortage, tribal households (especially in remote tribal areas) have to travel miles to collect drinking water. Therefore, the recommended 20 or 30 seconds hand wash has become a distant dream for tribal India. Meanwhile, lack of or low awareness about the dynamics of the pandemic, at least at the initial stage, also had critical implications for tribal communities, especially when there was a need to adhere to the dos and don'ts while fighting the COVID. Tribal communities encounter this unprecedented health crisis mediated by profound inequalities in power, resources, and visibility (Meade, 2020: 379).

Issues of Migration

Broadly, migration occurs in two forms in tribal areas: inward migration and outward migration. Inward migration facilitates the migration of non-tribes into tribal areas. This dimension of migration suggests that the tribal areas are recipients of large chunks of outsiders in tribal areas. The non-tribals have facilitated this process at their level. At the same time, more often, the state also takes the responsibility of converting tribal areas into the hotbed of migrant rehabilitation. Ambagudia (2019), Bhaumik (2009), and Singh (2010) deal with the processes of state-initiated migration to tribal areas and explore the relationship between the tribal and non-tribal communities. These studies show that the migration of non-tribal communities has put considerable pressure on locally available opportunities, infrastructural facilities, and other civic amenities.

The inward migration has also resulted in the alienation of tribal land and substantially reduced the tribal communities' possession of resources. The dispossession of resources also affects marginal, small, semi-medium, medium, and large-scale operational landholdings. Over the years, there has been a gradual decline in the number and area of operational holdings of tribal communities in India. For instance, there is a decline from 56,000 in 2005–2006 to 52,000 in 2010–2011 concerning the number of operational landholdings. This further declined to 48,000 in 2015–2016. The area operated by the tribal communities has declined by 2.4% from 18.22 million hectares in 2010–2011 to 17.78 million hectares in 2015–2016. The average operated area of tribal communities has declined from 1.76 hectares in 2000–2001 to 1.64 hectares in 2005–2006, which has further declined to 1.52 hectares in 2010–2011, and 1.40 hectares in 2015–2016 (Government of India, 2012: 42–44; Government of India, 2015: 55–60; Government of

India, 2020a: 48–53). Such statistics indicate the gradual decline of land possession among the tribal communities in India.

Migration has also led to the scarcity of resources in tribal areas, which has, in turn, led to community conflicts over resources between the tribals and the non-tribals (Ambagudia, 2019; Singh, 2010). The dispossession of resources has substantially reduced the capabilities of tribal communities in fighting against the pandemic. Meanwhile, non-tribal communities were also recruited as school teachers and were posted in schools located in tribal areas. When physical classroom teaching was suspended, and schools were temporarily closed during the pandemic, school teachers from coastal areas preferred to return to their native places. However, opening the schools in the middle of the pandemic compelled them to return to the tribal areas, which increased the possibility of infection in the tribal areas.

The outward migration from tribal areas occurs when the tribal people move out of their native place to seek better livelihood on both a short-term and long-term basis. Tribal people moved to the urban areas, near and far-away cities and towns, to work in brick kilns, construction areas, agriculture fields, and the service sector. However, the COVID imposed lockdown and suspension of manufacturing, and social sector activities resulted in job losses for tribes. Consequently, they were compelled to return to their native places. During the initial stage of the pandemic, the spread of the virus in tribal areas was accounted for by the reverse migration of tribal communities, thereby raising concerns. The need for a dedicated community targeted policy framework was felt as there was also news of returned tribal migrants getting emotionally hurt as they were asked to go into quarantine in schools located outside the villages, which led to suicide (Hindustan Times, 2020).

Issues of Livelihood

COVID-19 has disrupted the strategies and means of tribal livelihood. Minor forest produce (MFP) has been an essential means of tribal livelihood, contributing to about 20–40% of the annual income of tribal communities in India (Behera and Dassani, 2021: 19). Due to COVID-imposed social distancing and lockdown of local markets, collection and selling of the MFP have become challenging. While focusing on the strategies to negotiate livelihood, Haokip et al. (2020) discussed the impact of the pandemic on the livelihood of urban tribal women vendors in Manipur. These tribal women experienced the loss of income and difficulty in rent payment (as they migrated from the hill districts of Manipur and lived in rented houses) and their struggle to pay for children's education. They highlighted the inability of tribal women to cope with the challenges posed by the pandemic. Similarly, Wakharde (2021) underlined that COVID-19 led to food insecurity and loss of home and livelihood means for tribal women of the Nanded district of Maharashtra, thereby mounting their struggle for emergency services for livelihood and survival. Consequently, the pandemic contributed to the further vulnerability of tribal communities in India.

Tribal Education

COVID-19 also has had critical ramifications over the educational sphere. The closing down of schools, colleges, and universities due to COVID-imposed lockdown compelled the authorities to introduce the online teaching-learning process in India. The educational crisis due to the pandemic has exposed the digital divide between rural and urban India (around 90% of tribal communities live in rural India). Digital access has exposed the poor network in tribal areas and created divisions between different social groups, with tribal communities remaining at the margins of society with poor accessibility to digital facilities. Such a scenario has critical implications for tribal students' access to online classes via different gadgets, preferably mobile phones and laptops. Tribal communities are more prone to digital infrastructural vulnerabilities as far as the possession of mobile phones is considered.

The MoTA acknowledged that most tribal students did not have access to smartphones/tablets for accessing online resources (Government of India, 2021a: 74). The available statistics indicate that 57.39% of rural tribal households do not possess any phones, and only 41.37% of rural tribal households own mobile phones (Government of India, 2017: 31). It indicates the difficulties that tribal students have had to endure in attending online classes during this new normal created by the pandemic. Kasi and Saha (2021) discuss the impact of the pandemic on tribal youth, where educational vulnerabilities are widely visible during the pandemic time.

The COVID-imposed lockdown has completely disrupted the education of tribal students in India. They have their own testimony regarding the accessibility of online education during the pandemic. The tribal students of Malkangiri and Keonjhar districts of Odisha expressed their inability to afford smartphones for attending online classes (Odishatv Bureau, 2020). On the contrary, those who have access to smartphones also have to travel to the hilltop to detect the network. The District Welfare Officer of Malkangiri admitted that only 10% of the students in the district could successfully attend online classes, and the tribal students were the worst victims of the virtual mode of teaching (Sahu, 2020). The digital divide in accessing virtual classes even has compelled tribal students to migrate to earn money for purchasing a smartphone for online classes. It was reported that a tribal student from the Malkangiri district of Odisha was rescued from migrating to the neighbouring state to buy a smartphone for online classes (Barik, 2020). Such has been the story of tribal India.

Role of the State

The Indian state has taken various steps to address the pandemic crisis. Anticipating the difficulties that various categories would encounter due to the lockdown, the Government of India announced Rs. 1.70 lakh crore relief package under the Pradhan Mantri Garib Kalyan Yojana to help the poor sections of society. The announcement included health workers, women, senior citizens, poor widows, and the poor disabled. It did not categorically mention the vulnerable tribal communities of India (Government of India, 2020b). However, the tribal communities appear to have been included when it was announced to financially assist the poor workers and farmers under the Mahatma Gandhi National Rural Employment Guarantee Act, where tribal communities form a substantial part of the composition.

Meanwhile, when six members from the particularly vulnerable tribal groups (PVTGs) of Odisha tested COVID positive in the last week of August 2020, the National Commission for Scheduled Tribes considered this a "matter of grave concern" due to the poor health status of these communities (Mohanty, 2020). The MoTA also issued a press release indicating its steps to assist the tribal communities during the pandemic. The steps included the preparation of a roadmap for restoring economic growth in the post-COVID situation, relaxation of COVID guidelines concerning the collection, harvesting, and processing of MFP, revision of minimum support price (MSP) for MFP, the addition of 23 new items under the MSP for MFP, provision for utilising funds from the tribal sub-plan towards providing financial assistance to tribal communities, preparation of Tribal Health Action Plan, developing Swasthya Portal for addressing health infrastructure and manpower shortage in 177 tribal districts among others (Government of India, 2020c). It also launched the GOAL (Going Online As Leaders) programme in collaboration with Facebook to enhance the digital skill of tribal youth to facilitate their learning of a new way of doing business and get connected with markets at different levels (Government of India, 2021b).

In addressing the problems of the pandemic vis-a-vis the tribes, the focus generally has been on the rural setting, as tribes are predominantly dependent on agriculture and forests for their livelihood and hence inhabit the villages. This is also reflected in MoTA's response towards tribes. The response has been aimed at minimising the effect of COVID-19 on tribal health and livelihood. To this end, the State Nodal Departments were expected to prepare plans for mitigating the challenges of COVID-19. Consequently, based on the proposals of various state governments, the MoTA provided funds to the states for undertaking wide range of livelihood activities ranging from farm-based activities, such as agriculture, horticulture, animal husbandry, and fisheries, to various non-farm-based livelihood activities (Government of India, 2021b).

The Tribal Co-operative Marketing Federation of India (TRIFED), which claims to transform the lives of tribal communities in India under the MoTA, has also taken several initiatives to address the plight of tribal communities. The TRIFED has launched an e-market portal (www.tribesindia.com) and partnered with other e-commercial portals such as Amazon, Snapdeal, Flipkart, Paytm, and GeM to facilitate the selling of tribal products online. As of 31 October 2020, 3,093 artisans had enrolled, and 12,760 products had been uploaded on the online commercial platform (Government of India, 2021a: 102).

However, the state's pandemic measures and subsequent engagement with tribal communities and tribal areas have raised many issues and concerns that require broader deliberations. The consequences of the outbreak of COVID-19 in tribal regions, as elsewhere in the country, have been economic distress, especially during the lockdown. This was addressed by distributing free ration and providing employment through NREGSA and MSP for MFP schemes. In this context, on 4 May 2020, a group of civil society organisations, activists, researchers, and experts working with tribals and forest-dwelling communities submitted a preliminary assessment report to the MoTA. The report highlighted the socio-economic distress situation in tribal areas during the pandemic period and urged the government to take urgent steps to ensure support for the tribal communities.

The group demanded urgent action by MoTA to ensure adequate awareness and healthcare and protect the rights and livelihoods of the tribal communities. The report was based on preliminary information collected from civil society organisations working with tribals and forest dwellers and secondary information from media reports. The main findings of the report delved into health, livelihood, severe distress on the PVTGs, specific problems of the pastoral and nomadic communities, tenurial insecurity arising from non-recording of forest rights, restriction on movement to national parks and wildlife sanctuaries, forest land diversion, environmental impact assessment, and compensatory afforestation (Ground Xero Report, 2020).

While there have been initiatives to address immediate problems arising from the pandemic, the central government has also been simultaneously taking measures that would strengthen and expedite the process of its control over tribal land: through land acquisition on the one hand, and through tightening its control over forests at the cost of the violation of the Forest Rights Act (FRA) on the other hand. The state has taken such initiatives bypassing orders which have relaxed land acquisition rules and diverted forest land for mineral exploitation and other government projects. For instance, the Forest Advisory Committee, in its meeting on 30 March 2020, via video conferencing, recommended the diversion of forest land for mining purposes in the Keonjhar district of Odisha and automatic extension of forest clearance to five National Mineral Development Corporation mines in Chhattisgarh (Nandi, 2020). This was evident in the lack of due recording of existing forest rights of tribes and forest dwellers exposed to tenurial insecurity and increased vulnerability. Having titles to land that was their right would have spared them from adverse impact (on livelihood and food security) in the period of lockdown and later.

Somewhat of similar bearing was the advisory instruction of the Ministry of Environment, Forest and Climate Change (MoEFCC) issued on 6 April 2020, instructing all states and union territories to reduce the human-wildlife interface by restricting people's movement to national parks/

sanctuaries/tiger reserves. This advisory immediately impacted about three million to four million people living in and around protected areas, predominantly tribal communities, including PVTGs, nomadic, and pastoralist communities. They are most dependent on the natural resources within and around the protected areas for their livelihoods. The danger of this advisory is that it may be misunderstood and misused to alienate the tribes further and restrict their access to natural resources (Ground Xero Report, 2020). The preliminary report of the group of civil society organisations, activists, researchers, and experts working with tribals and forest-dwelling communities further maintained that the diversion of forests continues to happen during the pandemic even without securing the consent of the Gram Sabha and thereby violating the provisions of the FRA (Ground Xero Report, 2020).

The Forest Conservation Act Rules amended in 2014 eased the process of conservation by making the provision that the certificate from the Gram Sabha is no longer required under the FRA, and only the certificate of the District Collector would suffice to diversion of land (Bijoy, 2020). Such ease in the diversion of land has continued to guide the government even during the pandemic period. In a series of meetings during the lockdown, both the Expert Appraisal Committee (coal, hydro and river valley, thermal and non-coal mining, infrastructure, coastal regulation zone (CRZ, industrial) and the Forest Advisory Committee recommended approximately 120 projects, deferred 90 projects, returned 30 projects, and rejected two projects. It has been observed that a quarter of recommended projects fall in tribal areas (Pinto, 2020). The clearance of projects falling in schedule areas requires the consent of the Gram Sabha. However, the clearance of the projects via video conferencing seems to have not obtained the consent of Gram Sabha.

Further, on 28 March 2020, the MoEFCC amended the rules for Environment Impact Assessment (EIA), 2006. The amendment exempted several projects from the requirement of environment clearance without considering the short- and long-term impacts of such decisions on the livelihood security of tribal and forest-dwelling communities. The EIA amendment has also diluted the provision to obtain written consent of the Gram Sabha under FRA. Moreover, attempts at pushing for post facto environment clearance for projects that have already started defying environmental norms are also being made during the pandemic period (Ground Xero Report, 2020).

The central government auctioned 41 coal blocks for commercial mining covering the states of Jharkhand, Chhattisgarh, Madhya Pradesh, Odisha, and Maharashtra at a time when all people were under strict lockdown and subjected to physical and social distancing (International Work Group for Indigenous Affairs, 2020: 7–8). Of the 41 blocks, 11 blocks of mines are from Madhya Pradesh, nine each from Chhattisgarh, Jharkhand, and Odisha, and three from Maharashtra. The majority of districts where these mines are located are predominantly tribal areas. These areas fall under the Fifth Schedule to the Indian Constitution, which provides constitutional and administrative safeguards to tribal communities in India. In short, it seems that the state has strategically exploited the crisis, which has far-reaching implications for the dispossession, deprivation, and marginalisation of tribal communities in India.

Conclusion

Indigenous/tribal people are among the poorest, most excluded, and most marginalised sections of the world's population. They not only suffer disproportionately from the loss of their traditional and customary resource base but also are disproportionately represented among those who are illiterate with poor health status and facilities. Hence, it is not surprising that the United Nations Organization/Department of Economic and Social Affairs has urged the member states and international community to include the specific needs and priorities of Indigenous/tribal people in addressing the global outbreak of COVID-19.

Due to the aforementioned characteristics, Indigenous/tribal communities are more prone to multiple risks. Poor health indicators, among others, have exposed the communities to a greater health risk. Catastrophic loss of livelihood is not just the outcome of the pandemic but results from how societies are organised around exploitation, inequalities, and neo-liberal ideology (Kenny, 2020: 4). The Indian state has taken some steps to address the impact of the pandemic on tribal communities. However, at the same time, it has also initiated some interventionist measures, which are detrimental to tribal communities in contemporary India. Today, tribal communities are in a situation where their access to natural resources is closed, and landholding has become small, leading to their increased vulnerability and precarity. Such a scenario in tribal India has reduced the capability of tribal communities to fight against the deadly Coronavirus.

References

Ambagudia, Jagannath (2019), *Adivasis, Migrants and the State in India*, London and New York: Routledge.

Barik, Satyasundar (2020), "Odisha tribal student migration to earn a smartphone for online schooling rescued", *The Hindu*, 22 October, www.thehindu.com/news/national/other-states/odisha-tribal-student-migrating-to-earn-a-smartphone-for-online-schooling-rescued/article32918165.ece, accessed 4 April 2021.

Behera, Minaketan and Dassani, Preksha (2021), "Livelihood vulnerabilities of tribals during Covid-19: Challenges and policy measures", *Economic and Political Weekly*, 56(11), 19–22.

Bhaumik, Subir (2009), "Just development: A strategy for ethnic reconciliation in Tripura", in Sanjib Baruah (ed), *Beyond Counter-Insurgency: Breaking the Impasse in Northeast India*, New Delhi: Oxford University Press, pp. 293–307.

Bijoy, C. R. (2020), "Repeated amendments to land diversion laws threatening forest, people", *Business Standard*, 28 September, www.business-standard.com/

article/current-affairs/repeated-amendments-to-land-diversion-laws-threatening-forests-dwellers-120092800967_1.html, accessed 22 April 2021.

Davis, K. (1951). *The Population of India and Pakistan*, Princeton: Princeton University Press.

Government of India (2012), *All India Report on Agriculture Census 2005–06*, New Delhi: Department of Agriculture & Cooperation, Ministry of Agriculture.

Government of India (2013), *Statistical Profile of Scheduled Tribes in India, 2013*, New Delhi: Ministry of Tribal Affairs.

Government of India (2014), *Report of the Socio-Economic, Educational and Health Status of Tribal Communities in India*, New Delhi: Ministry of Tribal Affairs.

Government of India (2015), *All India Report on Agriculture Census 2010–11*, New Delhi: Department of Agriculture, Cooperation, & Farmers Welfare, Ministry of Agriculture & Farmers Welfare.

Government of India (2017), *Annual Report 2016–17*, New Delhi: Ministry of Tribal Affairs.

Government of India (2018), *Report of the Expert Committee on Tribal Health in India: Bridging the Gap and Roadmap for the Future*, New Delhi: Ministry of Health and Family Welfare and Ministry of Tribal Affairs.

Government of India (2020a), *All India Report on Agriculture Census 2015–16*, New Delhi: Department of Agriculture, Cooperation, & Farmers Welfare, Ministry of Agriculture & Farmers Welfare.

Government of India (2020b), *Finance Minister Announces Rs 1.70 Lakh Crore Relief Package Under Pradhan Mantri Garib Kalyan Yojana for the Poor to Help Them Fight the Battle against Corona Virus*, New Delhi: Ministry of Finance, https://pib.gov.in/PressReleaseIframePage.aspx?PRID=1608345, accessed 26 February 2021.

Government of India (2020c), *Steps Taken by Government to Support Tribal Communities During Covid Pandemic*, New Delhi: Ministry of Tribal Affairs, https://pib.gov.in/PressReleasePage.aspx?PRID=1655632, accessed 27 February 2021.

Government of India (2021a), *Annual Report 2020–21*, New Delhi: Ministry of Tribal Affairs.

Government of India (2021b), *Year End Review-2020-Ministry of Tribal Affairs*, New Delhi: Ministry of Tribal Affairs, https://pib.gov.in/PressReleaseIframePage.aspx?PRID=1685572, accessed 5 April 2021.

Ground Xero Report (2020), "A report on the covid lockdown impact on tribal communities in India", 7 May, www.groundxero.in/2020/05/07/a-report-on-the-covid-lockdown-impact-on-tribal-communities-in-india/, accessed 25 March 2021.

Haokip, Hoipi, Haokip, Arfina and Gangte, Tingneichong (2020), "Negotiating livelihood during Covid-19: Urban tribal women vendors of Manipur", *Economic and Political Weekly*, 55(46), 19–22.

Hardiman, David (2007), "Healing medical power and the poor: Contests in tribal India", *Economic and Political Weekly*, 42(16), 1404–1408.

Hardiman, David (2008), "Practices of healing in tribal Gujarat", *Economic and Political Weekly*, 43(9), 43–50.

Hindustan Times (2020), "Tribal labourer about to be quarantined commits suicide", *Hindustan Times*, 24 April, www.hindustantimes.com/bhopal/tribal-labourer-about-to-be-quarantined-commits-suicide/story-drPKMueqJfrsYa9nYwqXcK.html, accessed 22 December 2020.

International Institute for Population Sciences (2017), *National Family Health Survey (NFHS-4), 2015–16: India*, Mumbai: International Institute for Population Sciences.

International Work Group for Indigenous Affairs (2020), *Bearing the Brunt: The Impact of Government Responses to Covid-19 on Indigenous Peoples in India*, Copenhagen: The International Work Group for Indigenous Affairs.

Kasi, Eswarappa and Saha, Atrayee (2021), "Pushed to the margins: The crisis among tribal youth in India during Covid-19", *Critical Sociology*. Doi.org/10.1177/0896920521994195.

Kenny, Sue (2020), "Covid-19 and community development", *Community Development Journal*, 55(4), 699–703.

Maharatna, Arup (2000), "Tribal fertility in India: Socio-cultural influences on demographic behaviour", *Economic and Political Weekly*, 35(34), 3037–3047.

Maharatna, Arup (2005), *Demographic Perspectives on India's Tribes*, New Delhi: Oxford University Press.

Meade, Rosie R. (2020), "CDJ editorial-what is this Covid-19 crisis?" *Community Development Journal*, 55(3), 379–381.

Minority Rights Group International (2008), "World directory of minorities and Indigenous Peoples-India: Andaman Islanders", www.refworld.org/docid/49749d133c.html, accessed 2 April 2021.

Mishra, Arima and Sarma, Sumita (2011), "Understanding health and illness among tribal communities in Orissa", *Indian Anthropologist*, 41(1), 1–16.

Mohanty, Aishwarya (2020), "Covid-19 reaches remote tribes of Odisha: Why is it a matter of concern?" *The Indian Express*, 23 September, https://indianexpress.com/article/explained/explained-the-remote-tribes-of-odisha-covid-19-has-reached-6605476/, accessed 25 January 2021.

Nandi, Jayashree (2020), "Covid-19: Environment ministry panel for automatic extension of forest clearance", *Hindustan Times*, 5 April, www.hindustantimes.com/india-news/covid-19-env-min-panel-for-automatic-extension-of-forest-clearance/story-e6W7xbhu5b16xidB855rHK.html, accessed 22 April 2021.

Odishatv Bureau (2020), "Online classes remain 'out of bound' for students in rural Odisha", *Odisha TV*, 4 October, https://odishatv.in/odisha-news/online-classes-remain-out-of-bounds-for-students-in-rural-odisha-480890, accessed 4 April 2021.

Pati, Biswamoy (1998), "Siting the body: Perspectives on health and medicine in colonial Orissa", *Social Scientist*, 26(11/12), 3–26.

Pinto, Aditi (2020), "How the government diluted forest rights of Adivasis during lockdown", *BehanBox*, 19 July, https://behanbox.com/2020/07/19/how-the-government-of-india-used-the-lockdown-to-dilute-the-forest-rights-of-communities-voices-of-the-people-affected-by-hydro-electric-projects/, accessed 22 April 2021.

Sahu, Diana (2020), "Great digital divide: Here's how online education poses massive challenges in rural Odisha", *The New Indian Express*, 9 August, www.newindianexpress.com/states/odisha/2020/aug/09/great-digital-divide-heres-how-online-education-poses-massive-challenges-in-rural-odisha-2181055.html, accessed 4 April 2021.

Singh, Deepak K. (2010), *Statelessness in South Asia: The Chakmas Between Bangladesh and India*, New Delhi: Sage Publications.

United Nations (2020), *Covid-19 and Indigenous Peoples*, New York: Department of Economic and Social Affairs, www.un.org/development/desa/indigenouspeoples/covid-19.html, accessed 5 April 2021.

Wakharde, Sonali Baliram (2021), "COVID-19 pandemic and tribal women in Nanded District of Maharashtra", *Economic and Political Weekly*, 56(11), www.epw.in/engage/article/covid-19-pandemic-and-tribal-women-nanded-district, accessed 11 April 2022.

12 Tracing Challenges, Coping, and Resilience Among Older Persons Amidst Corona Pandemic

A Case of Urban India

Archana Kaushik

Introduction

Coronavirus (COVID-19) has posed unprecedented challenges, globally threatening the health and life of humans and impacting almost every aspect of our lives. The elderly, due to their health concerns, have emerged as one of the most vulnerable social groups during the pandemic. The sudden announcement of lockdown and related measures prescribed to curtail the spread of COVID-19 added to the woes, vulnerabilities, problems, and challenges among the older persons, severely impacting their well-being and social support.

Deterioration in health and strength of the body is a characteristic feature of old age and Corona infection along with pre-existing co-morbidities like respiratory ailments, diabetes, heart disease, and cancer may have deleterious effects on the aged population, notes the World Health Organization (2020). Daoust (2020) collating data from 27 countries covering Vietnam, the United States of America, the United Kingdom, the United Arab Emirates, Thailand, Taiwan, Sweden, Spain, South Korea, Singapore, Saudi Arabia, Philippines, Norway, the Netherlands, Mexico, Malaysia, Japan, Italy, Germany, France, Finland, Hong Kong, Canada, Brazil, Australia, and Denmark confirms that the elderly are the most vulnerable population group amidst COVID-19 pandemic across these nations.

The United Nations (2020) calculates that nearly 50% of COVID-19 deaths occurred among older persons with chronic ailments, and mortality rates for octogenarians and older are five times higher than the global average. Similar trends are observed in the United States (Novel, 2020) and China (Liu et al., 2020), indicating higher fatality rates among the elderly, which increase with age and intensity of co-morbidities. With India being no exception to it, the Ministry of Health and Family Welfare (2020) assesses that the elderly population is experiencing the worse outcomes of COVID-19 in contrast to the general population with about 63% deaths being reported among older people due to Corona infection. Reportedly, the infected older patients have increased hospitalisation, intensified symptoms,

DOI: 10.4324/9781003282815-16

greater discomfort, faster disease progression, delayed recovery, and almost double the time of their need of mechanical ventilation and oxygen therapy (Liu et al., 2020; Shahid et al., 2020). Three-fourth of the elderly, in a survey by Agewell Foundation (2020), admitted encountering health complications due to the inability to visit doctors for regular check-ups and accessing healthcare services for their ailments. Ample cases of medical triaging are reported where lowest priority is given for life-saving treatment among older persons in Italy (Rosenbaum, 2020), China, and the United States (Arya et al., 2020; Xie et al., 2020).

The mental health consequences of the pandemic on the elderly are equally worse. Banerjee (2020) shows that the imposed lockdown and social distancing norms have resulted in increased instances of elder neglect, abuse, isolation, anxiety, and depression. Institutionalised elderly faced accentuated deprivations and reported higher mental ailments. Even good-intentioned initiatives like maintaining social distance to protect older citizens from COVID infection resulted in social isolation, detachment, and loneliness among them (Van Orden et al., 2020), especially those in assisted living (Brooke and Jackson, 2020). Research studies have proved that loneliness and isolation (which has increased among the elderly during COVID pandemic) have high propensity of outcomes like anxiety, depression, negative coping like alcoholism and smoking, re-hospitalisation, and even increase in mortality (Kuiper et al., 2015; Hwang et al., 2020).

On similar lines, Agewell Foundation (2020) brings out that nearly 54% aged respondents (out of the sample of 5,000) claimed that their quality of life was hampered due to COVID-19 lockdown restrictions. Some of the instances given in the study are – fear of infection even while interacting with their family members coming from outside is paramount among the elderly; more than one-third reported anxiety, lack of appetite, sleeplessness, hopelessness, death anxiety, and depressive moods; about 55% admitted that their intergenerational relations have become bitter and nearly 20% reported rise in abuse by their younger relatives. Likewise, Aylaz and others (2020) find that cases of loneliness, anxiety, depression, and post-traumatic stress disorders have increased among the elderly due to the quarantine protocols. They also have exhibited the guilt of being the carriers of Corona. Armitage and Nellums (2020) show higher rates of suicidal ideations and attempts among the aged people amidst the COVID-19 pandemic. While there is a sharp rise in the intensity and instances of mental health problems among the elderly, reporting and access to services and support structures have reduced intensely.

Senior citizens living alone were among the worst affected as during the lockdown, they faced problems in meeting their basic needs with domestic help not available and their inability to access medical services and other civic amenities (Aylaz et al., 2020). The United Nations (2020) has highlighted that the elderly, especially in the less developed nations, have highly restricted access to digital technologies along with lack of skills, which might impact receiving and comprehending information related to prevention and precautions vis-à-vis COVID-19 pandemic. In the United States Monahan et al. (2020) observe that stay at home and social distancing orders have posed serious constraints among older workers to pursue their jobs, impacting their economic stability. Several other studies (Agarwal, 2020; Grills and Goli, 2020, *Times of India*, 11 May 2020; United Nations, 2020) also bring out the heightened economic vulnerability among the elderly due to the pandemic leading to poverty, hunger, and starvation coupled with ageism.

In this backdrop, this chapter focuses on the coping and resilience among the senior citizens in urban areas as they adapt and bounce back to successfully and effectively deal with the crisis. It attempts to locate factors influencing positive coping and resilience among the elderly in an Indian context. While doing this, it seeks to trace the life of urban elderly during the lockdown period; understand the challenges faced by the older persons and document the coping and resilience exhibited by them amidst the pandemic; examine the factors influencing their resilience; and gain insight into the role and scope of human service professionals in enhancing resilience among the senior citizens and ensuring their well-being and empowerment.

Method of Data Collection

The nature of the research is qualitative in the framework of descriptive research design. Sample unit was a person aged 60 years or more living either alone or with his/her family in an urban setting. Sample area is a group housing society in the National Capital Territory of Delhi. Data was collected from 50 elderly persons through participant observation and multiple sessions of interviews. Their interviews were sometimes quick and occasionally in-depth, through telephone, WhatsApp video calls, and even online meetings. Purposive and convenience sampling was employed.

The site of research is a residential complex that has 120 apartments. The residents are mainly retired employees from a nationalised bank and their spouses. To meet the research objectives, it was necessary that the respondents freely shared their feelings and emotions. A bit of prior acquaintance and familiarity of the researcher with the elderly living there was quite helpful. The researcher's parents live in the vicinity and her dad has been a retired bank employee. This made it easier for the researcher to form a rapport with the people she was interacting with.

The period of study included the months of March (last week), April, and May 2020. During data collection, the focus was not only on seeking information on the problems and challenges that the elderly were facing during the lockdown but also on the coping, adaptation, and resilience displayed by the respondents.

Certain ethical guidelines were adhered to along with the strict abiding of the protocols issued to prevent and curb Corona infection. Prior consent and permission were sought and interviews, largely conducted telephonically, were scheduled as per the convenience of the respondents. Interviews were rescheduled whenever the researcher realised that the respondents are not comfortable to talk at the scheduled time. Their choice to decline at any moment to participate in the study was clearly informed prior to interviews and respected throughout the data collection period. Confidentiality was maintained and pseudo-names are used in the case studies to protect the identities of the respondents.

The researcher ensured that no intentional or unintentional harm was incurred to the respondents during the study. Rather, the elderly respondents claimed that they got an opportunity to connect and share their problems and fears, to shed away their loneliness and depressive feelings by interacting with the researcher, especially amidst the lockdown. During the process of data collection, the researcher was able to link the older persons with certain services such as provision of medicines and grocery at their doorstep. A compassionate ear was provided to the elderly respondents during the interviews, which, as reported by several, was therapeutic, especially for those living alone.

While the study provides empirical evidences of vulnerabilities, coping and resilience among the older individuals during the COVID-19 pandemic, certain limitations of the study may be spelled out. The research was restricted to the urban senior citizens from the middle income group. Due to the qualitative nature of the study and the small sample size, findings may not be generalised.

Key Findings

In the study, 27 elderly women and 23 aged men participated. Their age range was from 63 to 92 years. The respondents exhibited a high degree of homogeneity with regard to variables such as educational attainments, socio-economic status, occupational patterns, and income levels. Among the senior citizens living in the sampled area, most males were retired employees of a nationalised bank while females have been mostly housewives. Out of the 50 sampled elderly, six women and one man were living alone and 11 elderly couples were staying alone while the rest of them were living with their married children.

On 24 March 2020, the prime minister announced for the complete nationwide lockdown initially for 21 days to curb the spread of COVID-19. This step has severely affected the elderly in several ways accentuating their problems and vulnerabilities. Some of the excerpts from the interviews of the older respondents are as follows:

R32 (68-year-old widower): "I was able to keep my diabetes under control by maintaining a strict routine of morning and evening walks for two hours alone with diet management. Now, I am afraid that my sugar levels are going to shoot up. I have become very anxious of my health".

R09 (72-year-old widow living alone): "My domestic help is not able to come due to lockdown, she used to cook and do all the household chores including buying grocery and medicines from the market. All alone, I feel bewildered, panicky and utterly disoriented, even having proper meals is jeopardised. I get up in the midnight perplexed fearing that I am dying and nobody will even come to know about it, my body is unattended and decomposed for weeks together".

R19 (67-year-old lady): "My daughter-in-law and grandchildren have gone to their maternal home, they are caught up there only due to lockdown; I had stopped cooking, even preparing tea for years together as my daughter-in-law efficiently takes care of everything. Now I feel jittery and clueless . . . I even don't know where pulses and spices are kept in the kitchen".

R22 (60-year-old lady): "I am facing mobility issues due to osteoarthritis and was to be operated upon for knee replacement soon. The lockdown has not only postponed the surgery for indefinite period but also added to my woes. My husband is totally bed-ridden and I am unable to do household work as domestic help is not there".

R15 (87-year-old gentleman): "I received the news of the death of my younger brother and his wife in a road accident and the lockdown happened at the same time. I can't explain in words how painful the situation is for me . . . I can't even visit my nephews and nieces to console them and worse is that I couldn't see my brother one last time, he was cremated and none of us could go. . ".

There was disruption in the routine life of the elderly due to the abrupt imposition of the lockdown. Following are the main challenges and problems faced by the elderly respondents in this study:

i. Before the lockdown, domestic helps had been playing a pivotal role in the everyday life of most of the elderly, facilitating them in household management, shopping of daily need items, cooking, assisting in Activities of Daily Living (ADL), to mention some. As domestic help stopped coming, the aged respondents encountered numerous problems. Those living alone were most affected with challenges in having proper meals. Two elderly with disabilities were almost bedridden.
ii. Apart from domestic workers, electricians and plumbers, would extend help to the elderly residents in procuring grocery from the nearby market. The usual services of hawkers selling vegetables and fruits just outside the gate of the residential complex were stopped. The aged were deprived of this support system too.
iii. Many senior citizens faced problems in procurement of their regular medicines of blood pressure control and diabetes as their existing stocks were exhausted.
iv. The senior residents preferred payment of bills of public utility services, mobile recharge by physically going to the respective offices and shops, which became a constraint after the lockdown.

v. Planned surgeries were postponed indefinitely causing discomfort and anxiety among the senior citizens.
vi. Routine health check-ups, pathological screenings, and consultations with their doctors for their chronic ailments used to provide a sense of relief and comfort among the elderly. Lockdown jeopardised this aspect too.
vii. The mornings and especially evenings used to be lively and vibrant in the residential complex – the site of the study – with children playing in the park, elderly taking walks, doing yoga, and sitting and chatting with friends. Lockdown snatched away the vivacity disrupting not only the health maintenance behaviours of the elderly but also severely curtailing their social life.
viii. In few cases, health emergencies like food poisoning, vomiting, and injuries due to fall could not be addressed properly on time. Likewise, many elderly requiring physiotherapy sessions and post-operative care neither could visit the hospital nor avail these services at home due to strict lockdown protocols.
ix. Some respondents faced peculiar challenges such as the indefinite postponement of the marriage of their granddaughter and stoppage of renovation work of the household; in two families, middle-aged children lost their jobs and in three similar cases, the family business was almost shut down due to the pandemic.
x. The retired people used to go to their bank on monthly or bi-monthly basis to fetch their pensions. When lockdown period increased and advisories from the government were out asking elderly people to be strictly homebound, there was anxiety over getting pension and having cash in hand to meet daily expenses.
xi. Reportedly, elderly living alone felt lonely, depressed, and experienced heightened death fear, as they were cut off from the active social life which they had carved out for themselves as a positive coping. They used to engage in society's office work, *satsang* [a spiritual discourse or a sacred gathering] and other activities of the Resident Welfare Association (RWA). Sudden lockdown not only stopped their social interactions but also put them in anxiety and turmoil.
xii. Some respondents experienced elder abuse, largely verbal in nature. They shared that they couldn't comprehend when they became "a source of COVID-19 infection" from being a "vulnerable social group". They started receiving comments from their children like "don't go out, you will bring home Corona and infect us" and "please don't stand in the balcony, if you get infected, we all will". A few respondents admitted that they desired to talk to the researcher freely and share their grief, agony, and pain but with family members being around, they could not; their daughters-in-law and sons kept an eye on them. In two cases, abuse was intense and the aged respondents asked the researcher to provide them addresses of old age homes.

xiii. Most of the respondents were not techno-savvy and for them digital disconnect became a social disconnect too. While the younger generation resorted to social media platforms to reactivate their social life, the elderly were left isolated. Some respondents shared that their children staying abroad tried connecting through WhatsApp and online meeting platforms but they remained clueless. The COVID pandemic changed the normative funeral practices with recommendation of minimal assembling of relatives. This made the elderly feel jittery and depressed for not being able to fulfil the last rites properly, which, as per their notion, hampers the soul of the deceased to achieve peace.

Coping and Resilience

Adapting oneself to the surrounding conditions is one of the characteristic features of living organisms. Human species is known for its exemplary dexterity in adaptation, coping, and resilience. Most of the work on resilience has been done with regard to natural calamities and disasters, with scanty literature available specific to the elderly people. Klasa et al. (2021) applied National Academy of Science Disaster Resilience Model to gerontology, in which resilience is taken as the ability of older persons to plan and prepare for, recover from and thereby adapt to the adverse events, here the corona pandemic. The model emphasises on the incorporation of extrinsic structural factors to equip the elderly with the adverse implications of the crises. They visualised resilience as the decline and recovery of critical functions after the adverse events.

In the study, it was noticed that as days passed by, the aged respondents started adapting to the new situation; major ones are mentioned later:

As depicted in the findings, the lives of the elderly were severely impacted during the lockdown. Keeping in view the fact that a significant proportion of the residents were older persons, special measures were taken by the RWA to prevent the COVID-19 infections. Thermal screening was done at the gate and no-touch hand sanitisation equipment was kept at the entrance points of elevators. The RWA management, which comprised the retired residents, was sensitive and empathetic towards the apprehensions, fears, needs, and challenges of their fellow beings. These measures gave respite and confidence to the senior residents of the society.

The security guards of the residential colony went out of the way to extend help to the senior residents. They started delivery of milk and daily essentials at their doorsteps. Whenever needed, they would go to the chemist shop and buy medicines for the elderly. A plumber working in the society for many years became the "man Friday" for most senior citizens – from buying grocery, medicines, paying bills, to withdrawing money from the banks and ATMs, he was available 24×7.

For the aged respondents suffering from certain life-style diseases, maintaining daily routine of exercise was crucial in health management and restoring confidence. Losing the sense of control over one's body is quite a shattering experience for the ageing individuals. Daily exercise like morning and evening walks, and light yoga is of significance and a vital step towards positive coping and resilience. It was noted that many of the elderly "adapted" to the new situation and started their walk or yoga within the household, with some rearrangement of the furniture. The aged respondents reorganised themselves to revert back to their exercise regime, definitely by remaining indoors.

It was quite heartening to note that the senior citizens reached out to their peers and neighbours through phone calls. On a daily basis, they would call up their ailing and vulnerable friends, checking up on their health. For those living alone, these calls of their friends provided the vital psychological boost and courage to deal with loneliness, death anxiety, and depression.

It was noted that the immediate neighbours of the elderly living alone and their friends in the vicinity would keep cooked and packed meals at their doorstep, ring the bell, and leave. This not only took care of the nutrition needs of senior citizens who were staying alone and did not feel like cooking for themselves but also provided a sense of being cared for and fulfilment. The younger residents too offered help to the senior citizens in bringing items of daily needs from the market, making online payments of bills, especially for the aged couples or single elderly.

Reportedly, barring a few cases, within the joint family system, the lockdown period paved way for intergenerational amicability in familial relations after initial hiccups. Some respondents initially expressed that their presence was not liked by the younger members, and they were being ignored or avoided, if not overtly abused. With all the members staying all the time in the household, space constraints and privacy issues cropped up with the elderly being the weaker and powerless group, facing the heat. However, after some days, things started to improve. As elderly ladies provided help in cooking and household work and aged men played with their grandchildren (indoor games), the youngsters realised their importance in the family. There was a positive shift in the behaviour of younger family members as they began to involve their elderly in day-to-day discussions and household chores.

There used to be regular *satsang* (spiritual discourses) and *kirtan* (devotional singing often accompanied with playing of musical instruments) by a group of elderly ladies on every Tuesday apart from festivals and special occasions. All members would gather in one lady's house for three to four hours for *kirtan*, which was a major source of recreation, catharsis, and social connection for the senior women. Two weeks after the lockdown, the *kirtan* group rebooted itself through WhatsApp conference call, with the members again connecting and singing songs collectively. This initiative acted as an antidote for most of the elderly women suffering from loneliness, alienation, and isolation. It pepped up every member putting a smile on their face.

A positive and heartening change is observed in the contents of the WhatsApp messages circulated by the elderly among their peers and relatives. In the initial days of the lockdown, the messages were having contours of fear, gloom, and heightened susceptibility of Corona infection but subsequently and gradually, the contents reflected a positive mind-set with success stories of older individuals surviving COVID infections being shared.

It was observed that various agencies in the service delivery system took certain initiatives to reach out to the elderly and create an enabling environment for them. Since mid-April 2020, the bank transferred the pension of the retired people to their nearest bank branches, waiving off the need to physically come to sign papers in the office. Similarly, medicines were couriered at their doorsteps after receiving e-mails from the beneficiaries. These steps eased off many troubles faced by the elderly.

A philanthropic organisation, Sai Charitable Trust, offered free packed lunch at the doorstep for the needy elderly and those staying alone (The Times of India, 31 October 2020). These services were available on a phone call. HelpAge India widely publicised their helpline numbers to provide services of volunteers in making available items of daily needs and medicines to the elderly. It also provided digital literacy sessions for the senior citizens where technical know-how of conference calls, video calls, online consultation with the doctor, online banking, paying bills, and such other features were taught (HelpAge India, 2020).

Further, many senior citizens contributed money for meeting the survival needs of the stranded migrants and poor families staying in the neighbourhood. They claimed that this little act of donation filled them with peace and satisfaction.

Some excerpts from the conversations with the elderly respondents are as follows:

R03 (82-year-old widower living alone): "Sudden lockdown has posed big problems for me and others like me living alone. The biggest anxiety was to have food. . . . I can't cook proper meals, the cook was not coming and on the fourth day of the lockdown, I was thinking that now I will have to starve . . . and then the doorbell rang, I was about to open the door when I received a phone call from my neighbor . . . saying that he had sent *idli-sambhar* for my breakfast and some items for lunch . . . I was speechless . . . overjoyed, deeply touched with his gesture . . .".

R23 (62-year-old widow): "In the initial time of the lockdown, I could feel that my *bahu* (daughter-in-law) and grandchildren were not happy with my staying with them, they would ignore and overlook me . . . definitely it feels bad . . . earlier the interaction time was very limited as the children would go to school and *bahu* to her office, now 24x7 we were at home. Gradually, with patience and little efforts, I could win their hearts again. I had taken over the responsibility of cooking daily and I even made sweets for them . . . now, I have become the favourite granny of my grandchildren and developed amicable relations with my *bahu* too".

R49 (68-year-old lady): "Weekly gatherings in *kirtans* used to be a great opportunity for us – the aged ladies, we would casually chat, discuss society's matters, share household problems with our friends and feel lighter and energized. Lockdown stopped all that. One day, I was feeling very low and lonely, missing my *kirtan* group, and suddenly my phone rang, it was a conference call . . . many of my age-mates were on the call and they were singing devotional songs . . . I was astonished, overjoyed . . . so elated that I started crying . . . see, we made Corona lose the battle . . .".

R21 (75-year-old gentleman): "On 12th April 2020, it was the silver jubilee of my wedding anniversary and our children had planned for a big celebration for it, but lockdown washed away the opportunity to even meet our children and grandchildren and me and my wife were a bit depressed . . . none of our relatives and friends even called to wish us since morning. Hardly could we know that my daughter has planned a surprise for us. At 4:00 pm, she called me to click some link on my WhatsApp . . . and here I was seeing all my relatives and friends from India and abroad, on the screen wishing us and celebrating our anniversary, she even played a small video capturing moments of our 25 years of togetherness. There were tears of joy in our eyes. We sang songs, revisited memories of our marriage, cracked jokes, and laughed a lot. I don't think that the actual celebration of that day could have been better than this virtual celebration . . .".

R06 (70-year-old lady): "My husband has been suffering from acute respiratory disorder and his condition is deteriorating with age. One month before the lockdown, our son got transferred and moved with his family to Hyderabad. On 24th April 2020, he experienced breathlessness and chest congestion and fainted. I panicked and called one of his friends. He immediately came and arranged for his hospitalisation. Daughter-in-law of my friend who knew driving came and within ten minutes we were in the hospital. My daughter staying in another city could come only the next day. After eight days of hospitalisation, he was relieved and now he is better. People here are so helpful and amazing, they actually saved his life. I could not have done anything without their support".

R05 (68-year-old lady): "I could see so many positive aspects of this lockdown . . . it gave us a chance to be with our family members, share those little joys of togetherness which we had somehow lost over these years . . .".

R40 (70-year-old gentleman): "This Corona pandemic is God's way to teach us that life is to be lived in the present moment, don't run after money and success, be grateful for what you have and the most important – learn to differentiate between what is essential and what is non-essential in life. Now even with minimal we all are happily living . . . that is to be appreciated"

R20 (89-year-old lady): "I have lived a fulfilled life, I would not mind dying even now . . . Humans should trust God, whatever happens, it is for our good. Be like a river . . . leave all grudges, expectations aside and go with the flow . . . then life is beautiful and worth appreciating".

Interpreting the Data

This study was carried out with the aim to understand the coping patterns of the elderly as they dealt with the COVID-19 pandemic and identify the factors that influenced their coping and resilience. It was observed that the lockdown imposed to curb the spread of Corona virus brought specific challenges for the elderly as their earlier coping strategies and adaptations failed to address the unprecedented crisis. Senior citizens had to adjust and adapt to their differential vulnerabilities – those living alone compensated with active engagement in social life and taking up roles like being members of management groups in RWAs or *kirtan;* those having chronic ailments took up strict exercise regime and diet control. The lockdown dismantled the state of homeostasis requiring the aged to readjust and readapt.

This challenge may be seen in the framework of "Continuity theory" that postulates that older people prefer to maintain the same life-style and activities as they did in earlier years of life (Atchley, 1999) to have a sense of stability and security. The Corona crisis forced the senior citizens to shed away their preferred way of living, destabilising their "equilibrium" state. However, in this backdrop, the power of resilience is observed among the elderly respondents, about which they themselves were hardly aware.

Resilience may be taken as an individual's ability to withstand stress, overcome difficulty, and find the resources needed to survive in a positive way. Metze et al. (2015) state that resilience is the capacity for successful adaptation despite challenging or threatening circumstances. The factors influencing coping and resilience among older individuals in the study may be discussed as under.

Resoluteness: Most elderly displayed the willingness and firmness to overcome the hardships that cropped up due to the COVID pandemic, as they adapted to the "new normal". Barring a few exceptions, the elderly have shown a proactive approach in maintaining and sustaining healthy life-style by finding ways and means to stick to their exercise and restricted nutrition. As daily routine, they did yoga, walked within the household or corridors, consumed *kadha* (decoctions for treating/preventing cold, Corona infection), drank lukewarm water, and sought online medical advice for health management.

Generativity: It was noted that the elderly who were "helpful" and participated actively in helping and supporting others by trying to contribute meaningfully were more resilient. There were a few older persons in the study area who took initiative to reach out to the deprived and unfortunate social groups like poor stranded migrants while others shared cooked food with security guards and other workers in the society. Moreover, most people reached out to support each other, their friends, and fellow beings by calling them on a regular basis and checking on their health, offering their support in buying household items and medicines. Eric Erickson has mentioned about the notion of generativity in his eighth stage of psycho-social development (see Erickson and Erickson, 1997). Thus, the elderly who were directly contributing in numerous ways within the family, neighbourhood, and community found themselves in a better position to cope with the crisis.

Acceptance and let-go attitude: Apparently, resilience is linked to virtues like patience, perseverance, calm and composed demeanour, let-go attribute, belief in God, acceptance of whatever life offers, attitude of gratitude, forgiveness among the senior citizens. These elderly were able to adjust well with their significant others; they took initiative in helping younger family members in the household work, showed maturity by remaining silent when conflicts emerged, appreciated others for their little gestures of help, and eventually were able to enjoy the love, care, and affection of their family.

Social Support: External support facilitated positive coping and resilience among older adults. Efforts and expressions of care and love by children staying miles away provided fulfilment and contentment to the elderly and they could fight back their vulnerabilities with greater vigour and enthusiasm. Likewise, skills like friendliness, kindness, affability, sociability, among the elderly pay dividends in terms of reciprocating social support.

Maladaptive coping: While most exhibited facilitative or positive coping, a few showed maladaptive behaviour such as perpetuating dependence, passivity, apathy, pessimism, and remaining in victim mode and kept on cribbing about their vulnerabilities. They accepted their defeat against the COVID crisis without fighting and showed lesser resilience.

Conclusion and Suggestions

The COVID-19 pandemic curtailed the active and preferred life-style of the elderly that was characterised by health management measures and meaningful social engagements. It perpetuated health problems, loneliness, death-fear, anxieties and depression, and elder abuse. However, through facilitative coping and resilience, senior citizens successfully adapted to the "new normal". Some of the salient factors influencing resilience were mental strength, courage and firmness, enthusiasm and hope to fight back, generativity, active involvement, social connectedness, participation, taking initiative, maturity, patience, persistence, thankfulness, overt appreciation of others, and remaining calm in conflict-evoking situations. Apathy, passiveness, and pessimism added to dependence, vulnerability, and gloom in old age.

In view of the benefits and power of resilience, efforts should be made to enhance this trait and psychological resource among the senior citizens. All the stakeholders, government and civil society organisations, family and community, and the elderly themselves, in a concerted and coordinated manner need to work towards creating a resilient, peaceful, and enabling environment where the older persons live an active, healthy, happy, and productive life.

Resilience is a critical path to empowerment of the elderly. More research is needed in this area to help design training and capacity building sessions for increasing resilience among older adults. Digital literacy for elderly empowerment is one of the many interventions by HelpAge India that proved highly beneficial during COVID-19 pandemic. These and such other services should be scaled up. At the state level, setting up of geriatric hospitals, wards, and clinics, paper-less and prompt disbursal of pension, medicines, and other benefits should help in creating a conducive environment for positive and resilient living for the senior citizens. Reviving and strengthening informal support system in the form of community care is a must for swift and quality elder care. Alongside, reinforcing familial and intergenerational bonding is another culturally appropriate measure having the potential to activate and enhance resilience among the elderly, facilitating them to effectively deal with most of their problems in normal as well as in crisis situations.

References

Agarwal, P. (2020), "Covid-19: In urban India, the elderly are grappling with hunger and fears of dying alone", *Scroll.in*, 5 May, https://scroll.in/article/961004/covid-19-in-urban-india-the-elderly-are-grappling-with-hunger-and-fears-of-dying-alone, accessed 7 May 2020.

Agewell Foundation (2020), "Elderly are the worst sufferers during COVID-19 lockdown: Survey report", 9 May, www.agewellfoundation.org/?page_id=6103, accessed 3 January 2021.

Armitage, R. and Nellums, L. B. (2020), "COVID-19 and the consequences of isolating the elderly", *Lancet Public Health*, 5(5). https://doi.org/10.1016/S2468-2667(20)30061-X.

Arya, A., Buchman, S., Gagnon, B. and Downar, J. (2020), "Pandemic palliative care: Beyond ventilators and saving lives", *Canadian Medical Association Journal*, *192*, E400–E404. http://dx.doi.org/10.1503/cmaj.200465.

Atchley, R. C. (1999), *Continuity and Adaptation in Aging: Creating Positive Experiences*, Baltimore, MD: Johns Hopkins University Press, pp. 23–51.

Aylaz, R., Pekince, H., Isik, K., Akturk, U. and Yildirim, H. (2020), "The correlation of depression with neglect and abuse in individuals over 65 years of age", *Perspectives in Psychiatric Care*, 56(2), 424–430. https://doi.org/10.1111/ppc.12451.

Banerjee, D. (2020), "Age and ageism in COVID-19: Elderly mental healthcare vulnerabilities and needs", *Asian Journal of Psychiatry*, 51, 102154. Doi: 10.1016/j.ajp.2020.102154.

Brooke, J. and Jackson, D. (2020), "Older people and COVID-19: Isolation, risk and ageism", *Journal of Clinical Nursing*. Advance online publication. http://dx.doi.org/10.1111/jocn.15274.

Daoust, J.-F. (2020), "Elderly people and responses to COVID-19 in 27 Countries", *PLoS One* 15(7), 1–13, e0235590. https://doi.org/10.1371/journal.pone.0235590.

Erikson, E. H. and Erikson, J. M. (1997), *The Life Cycle Completed: Extended Version With New Chapters on the Ninth Stage of Development*, New York: Norton & Comp, pp. 128–134.

Grills, N. and Goli, S. (2020), "Caring for India's elderly during COVID-19", *The Pursuit*. The University of Melbourne, 19 May, https://pursuit.unimelb.edu.au/articles/caring-for-india-s-elderly-during-covid-19, accessed 3 June 2020.

HelpAge India (2020), "COVID-19 emergency response: Situation on ground", www.helpageindia.org/covid-19-emergencyresponse/#:~:text=HelpAge%20India%20is%20reaching%20out,Mobile%20Healthcare%20Units%20%26%20Helpline%20services, accessed 5 March 2021.

Hwang, T. J., Rabheru, K., Peisah, C., Reichman, W. and Ikeda, M. (2020), "Loneliness and social isolation during the COVID-19 pandemic", *International Psychogeriatrics*, 32(10), 1217–1220. https://doi.org/10.1017/S1041610220000988.

Klasa, K., Galaitsi, S., Wister, A. and Linkov, I. (2021), "System models for resilience in gerontology: Application to the COVID-19 pandemic", *BMC Geriatrics*, 21(51), 1–12, https://doi.org/10.1186/s12877-020-01965-2.

Kuiper, J. S., Zuidersma, M., Oude Voshaar, R. C., Zuidema, S. U., van den Heuvel, E. R., Stolk, R. P. and Smidt, N. (2015), "Social relationships and risk of dementia: A systematic review and meta-analysis of longitudinal cohort studies", *Ageing Research Reviews*, 22, 39–57. http://dx.doi.org/10.1016/j.arr.2015.04.006.

Liu, K., Chen, Y., Lin, R. and Han, K. (2020), "Clinical features of COVID-19 in elderly patients: A comparison with young and middle-aged patients", *Journal of Infection*, 80(6), E14–E18. https://doi.org/10.1016/j.jinf.2020.03.005.

Metze, R. N., Kwekkeboom, R. H. and Abma, T. A. (2015), "The potential of family group conferencing for the resilience and relational autonomy of older adults", *Journal of Aging Studies*, 34, 68–81.

Ministry of Health and Family Welfare (2020), "Union health ministry, update: April 5 2020: COVID-19 fatalities in India", 5 April, www.mohfw.gov.in, accessed 5 May 2020.

Monahan, C., Macdonald, J., Lytle, A., Apriceno, M. and Levy, S. R. (2020), "COVID-19 and ageism: How positive and negative responses impact older adults and society", *American Psychologist*, 75(7), 887–896. http://dx.doi.org/10.1037/amp0000699.

Novel, C. P. E. R. E. (2020), "The epidemiological characteristics of an outbreak of 2019 novel coronavirus diseases (COVID-19) in China", *Zhonghua liu xing bing xue za zhi= Zhonghua liuxingbingxue zazhi*, 41(2), 145–151. Doi: 10.3760/cma.j.issn.0254-6450.2020.02.003.

Rosenbaum, L. (2020, May 14), "Facing Covid-19 in Italy – Ethics, logistics, and therapeutics on the epidemic's front line", *The New England Journal of Medicine*, 382, 1873–1875. http://dx.doi.org/10.1056/NEJMp2005492.

Shahid, Z., Kalayanamitra, R., McClafferty, B., Kepko, D., Ramgobin, D., Patel, R. and Aggrawal, C. S. (2020), "COVID-19 and older adults: What we know", *Journal of the American Geriatrics Society*, 68(5), 926–929. https://doi.org/10.1111/jgs.16472.

The Times of India (2020), "Lockdown shrinks donations, charity works", 31 October, https://timesofindia.indiatimes.com/city/nagpur/lockdown-shrinks-donations-charity-works-at-shrines/articleshow/78957788.cms, accessed 4 March 2021.
The Times of India (2020), "What the elderly fear the most in times of COVID-19?" *The Times of India*, 11 May, https://timesofindia.indiatimes.com/india/what-the-elderly-fear-most-in-times-of-covid-19/articleshow/75641568.cms, accessed 3 December 2020.
United Nations (2020), "Policy brief: The impact of COVID-19 on older persons", May, https://unsdg.un.org/sites/default/files/2020-05/Policy-Brief-The-Impact-of-COVID-19-on-Older-Persons.pdf, accessed 15 June 2020.
Van Orden, K. A., Bower, E., Lutz, J., Silva, C., Gallegos, A. M., Podgorski, C. A. and Conwell, Y. (2020), "Strategies to promote social connections among older adults during 'social distancing' restrictions", *The American Journal of Geriatric Psychiatry*. Advance online publication. http://dx.doi.org/10.1016/j.jagp.2020.05.004.
World Health Organization (2020), "Coronavirus disease 2019 (COVID-19): Situation report-72", 1 April, www.who.int/docs/default-source/coronaviruse/situation-reports/20200401-sitrep-72-covid-19.pdf?sfvrsn=3dd8971b_2, accessed 3 May 2020.
Xie, J., Tong, Z., Guan, X., Du, B., Qiu, H. and Slutsky, A. S. (2020), "Critical care crisis and some recommendations during the COVID-19 epidemic in China", *Intensive Care Medicine*, 46, 837–840. http://dx.doi.org/10.1007/s00134-020-05979-7.

Part IV

Regional Narratives

13 Socioeconomic Impact of COVID-19 and Lessons

Bangladesh

Shaheen Anam

Introduction

Bangladesh, with a population of 160 million living in an area of 55,000 square miles, is one of the most densely populated countries in the world (Ritchie, 2019). In the last 50 years since its birth, the country has witnessed innumerable challenges, both natural and manmade. Living with, and overcoming disasters such as cyclones, floods, sea-level rise, river erosion, salinity is a way of life for millions of people. Bangladesh is at the front line of countries facing the worst climate change impacts. It is to the great resilience of the people, pragmatic policies, and civil society efforts that against all odds, Bangladesh is now considered a model of development with improvements in most social indicators such as health, life expectancy, primary school enrolment, and women's empowerment (Human Development Report, 2020). However, there are governance deficits, which need to be addressed urgently.

COVID-19 emerged as a pandemic that nobody was prepared for. It created havoc in the lives and livelihood of people all over the world and Bangladesh is no exception. Riding on a sustained growth rate of 7%, the country was well on its way to becoming a middle-income country. But then came the COVID-19 pandemic, with devastating impact on the economy. With closure of businesses, factories, and restaurants, millions lost their jobs and means of livelihood. The social impact has been as severe. Increase in violence against women and early marriage, rising inequality, and a year of learning lost for children due to closure of educational institutions are some with far-reaching consequences.

As countries are trying to cope with the many challenges faced, studies and research indicate that impact on the poor might be irreversible. "While the rich will recover their losses from the pandemic in one year, it may take a decade for the poor to recover", states an Oxfam (2021) study. As expected, the poorer section of the population – the socially and economically marginalised – are more adversely affected due to their already insecure means of livelihood now made more vulnerable due to the pandemic. The lockdown, which was crucial in decelerating infection rates, came with its unique set of

DOI: 10.4324/9781003282815-18

challenges such as mental trauma, tension in families due to income loss, extra work burden, and violence against women and girls including early marriage. While the virus was raging in other parts of the world, the spread was relatively slow in South Asia. The first case in Bangladesh was identified on 8 March 2020 (TBS News, 2020). As it started to spread with reported daily cases rising steadily, the government ordered a complete lockdown from 26 March 2020, which resulted in huge disruption in the lives and livelihoods of people in every segment of society. As offices, educational institutions, and businesses closed down, people slowly started to adjust to the "new normal", however, with severe social and economic impacts.

Economic Impact

In terms of the number of infections, the United States has topped the list with close to 600,000 deaths so far and 2 million infected, closely followed by the United Kingdom, India, and many countries in Europe (Worldometer, 2021). The overall death globally has crossed 2.2 million while more than 110 million have been infected. To add to the crisis, a second wave in many parts of the world with a new variant of the virus crushed any chance of early recovery. With the world being increasingly interconnected, it is not enough to contain the infection within one's own border and the saying "no one is safe unless everyone is safe" proves to be true. As the pandemic raged in distant Europe, the United States, and the Middle East, its impact is being felt in Bangladesh as it has affected the garment, migrant, and tourism sectors. The closure of construction work and price fall of oil in the Middle East has affected jobs of Bangladeshi migrant workers. Economic slowdown in the United States and Europe has caused cancellation of 50% orders of the readymade garment industry (Reuters, 2021). Tourism has come almost to a halt and flight cancellations have resulted in disaster for the tourism as well as the aviation industry.

The economic impact was most severely felt by the poorer sections of the society, more particularly those who needed to work every day to earn a livelihood and put food on the table. In urban areas, rickshaw pullers, construction workers, and part-time domestic workers became jobless. Due to the absence of social protection schemes for the urban poor, this section of the population found themselves in a precarious situation. In rural areas, agricultural workers became jobless, as did transportation workers. About 85% workers in Bangladesh work in the informal sector (Mujeri, 2020), which is already beset by low pay, job insecurity, and weak and ineffective laws. The pandemic heightened these existing challenges, and a majority of workers found themselves in a hopeless situation risking starvation and consequently long-term malnourishment. Closure of businesses – both large and small – meant job loss for employees. As restaurants, entertainment places, and beauty parlours closed due to lack of customers, employers were forced to offload their employees. The economy of Bangladesh is mostly dependent on four segments, namely the readymade garment industry, remittances from expatriates, small medium enterprise and service sector, and the informal sector. Disruption in any one of these has great impact not only on the overall economy of the country but also on the well-being of workers and their families.

The Readymade Garment Industry

Bangladesh is the second largest readymade garment exporting country in the world and employs 5 million workers, 80% of whom are women (Khatun, 2021). As the world reeled from the economic shock due to the pandemic, European and US buyers started to cancel orders (Reuters, 2021). A huge drop in the shipment of readymade garments due to declining orders in the face of the coronavirus pandemic was the biggest factor behind a 14.57% fall in exports from Bangladesh. New figures from the Export Promotion Bureau reveal that the country's export earnings in 2020 fell to US$33.60 billion from US$39.33 billion in the previous year as the COVID-19 outbreak hit the global economy (Export Promotion Bureau, 2021). The first lockdown caused unprecedented disruption between March and May 2020, when billions of US dollars' worth of exports were cancelled or postponed, threatening the country's garment industry, which is responsible for approximately 84% of the country's exports (Textile Today, 2021).

A number of small and mid-level factories closed down causing job losses for thousands of workers (Mahmood, 2020). The closure of factories from 26 March 2020 was followed by confusion. Manufacturers apprehending missing deadlines announced reopening of factories in April 2020 (Star Correspondent Report, 2020). Garment workers in the thousands started returning only to find that the government had ordered closure of factories till May 2020. This caused considerable suffering to thousands of workers who had to travel long distances using inadequate and unsafe transportation to return to their village homes. It was feared that travel of thousands of workers without maintaining health guidelines would increase infection. Fortunately there has been minimal COVID-19 infection among garment workers (The Daily Star, 2020). However, more workers are at threat of losing jobs if orders do not pick up. There was a sense of optimism when orders started to return slowly but the second wave of the virus, which hit Europe and the United States, has again dampened such expectation (Rahman, 2020). Clothes retailers in Europe and America sit on excess inventory and have cut back on Spring orders. Sourcing agents face late payments. The global apparel industry is seeing its hopes of recovery diminished by a new wave of COVID-19 lockdowns.

Given the importance of the readymade garment sector, the government offered the first stimulus package of BDT 5,000 crore to the industry in soft loans. Although this has given a lifeline to the sector, the threat of more cancellation of orders with job loss of workers is still very much present.

Remittances From Expatriates

An estimated ten million Bangladeshis are currently working abroad, primarily as low-skilled labourers mostly in the Middle East. Only India, Mexico, Russia, and China send out more migrant workers each year according to World Bank (2021). Most Bangladeshi migrants work as gardeners, construction workers, janitors, and house maids. Some also work as mechanics, drivers, or tailors. On average, they earn $400 a month, far more than they would make doing the same jobs at home. The annual $15 billion sent home by migrant workers as remittances is Bangladesh's second-largest source of foreign earnings only next to the readymade garment industry.

Life is not easy for these workers in the countries of their employment. They are often subject to abuse and various kinds of exploitation. However, the necessity to earn and send back money to maintain their families forces them to endure such hardships. The push factor for workers to seek employment abroad is poverty and lack of opportunity at home.

The remittance sent back by these migrant workers helps Bangladesh maintain a healthy foreign exchange reserve. The COVID-19 has hit this sector hard as workers lost their jobs due to the economic downturn in the country of their employment. Many workers who had come home for a holiday could not go back on time as flights were cancelled indefinitely resulting in discontinuation of their employment. Till 18 September 2020, a total of 141,036 migrant workers returned home following the pandemic, while 181,273 migrants managed to go abroad. The government failed to meet the target of sending 700,000 fresh workers abroad this year (Amin, 2020). The fall in the number of migrants going abroad for work will have serious consequences for the economy and for their families. Female migrant workers mostly working as house maids have also been sent back due to COVID-19. Given their immense contribution to the economy, the government has to take immediate steps to rehabilitate these returnee migrants into productive work. However, the present state of unemployment in the country has made it difficult to absorb them into the workforce. The continued economic downturn in the receiving countries might result in more migrant workers returning.

In spite of the global economic fallout, migrant workers continued to send back remittances which showed an increase from last year. In November 2020, Bangladesh received US$19.8 billion as remittance (Tribune Report, 2021). This is attributed to factors. The migrant workers uncertain about their future job security decided to send back home whatever savings they had. They also took loan and sent additional money to their families at home to offset the economic crisis that they were facing during the pandemic. Whatever maybe the outcome of COVID-19, migrant workers will continue to play a crucial role in the economy of Bangladesh and therefore require policy support to sustain them during the present crisis.

Informal Sector (Including Agriculture)

The pandemic and the ensuing lockdown (which was necessary) put workers in the informal sector in the most precarious situation. The informal sector accounts for almost 85% of employment in Bangladesh. They are the rickshaw pullers, agriculture and construction workers, hawkers, rag pickers, and transport and domestic workers (BBS, 2020). Child workers are included numbering around 4.8 million or 12.6% aged from 5 to 14.83% are employed in rural areas for agriculture and 17% work in urban areas. With schools and offices shut, rickshaw pullers had no passengers; construction work came to a halt; therefore, day labourers were sitting idle, and self-employed workers and hawkers, both men and women who earn a living by selling food and other daily use items, had no buyers. As it is, the sector is beset with job insecurity, exploitation, and low pay. COVID-19 has increased their insecurity and vulnerability. Most of their employment depends on the vibrancy of the economy and unless the economy revives, they will only become poorer and fall into the ultra-poor category.

Agriculture is a major economic activity in Bangladesh. It currently employs around 50% of the country's labour force and contributes around 20% of the country's GDP (Raihan, 2012). The agricultural sector faced a number of challenges such as the inability to transport their products, lack of hired labour due to social distancing, and limited capital and inputs to invest further. However, Bangladesh is known and admired the world over for innovations in agriculture and becoming self-sufficient in food. Various innovations were adopted to offset the impacts of COVID-19 and the government was able to keep the supply chair operative (Uddin, 2020).

Small Medium Enterprise and Service Sector

SMEs are the bloodline of Bangladesh's economy creating employment for 7.8 million people directly and providing a livelihood for 31.2 million in total. One of the hardest hits by COVID-19 pandemic is the already vulnerable SMEs due to their dependence on a shorter cash cycle. The sector accounts for 35.49% of the total employment (MTBiz Quarterly Business Review, 2020). In the last 20 years, SMEs have grown exponentially spearheaded by women involved in the small and medium enterprises. The government is trying to revive this sector with stimulus packages but the rate of disbursement is slow, and most small enterprises have not received its benefits (Uddin, 2021).

The service sector, such as hospitals, restaurants, clinics, hotels, beauty parlours, and shopping malls, has also taken a huge beating. Employers had to let off their workers due to low sales and customers. Luckily, this sector is showing signs of recovery after the lockdown started to ease partially since June 2020 (The Business Standard, 2021). After going at half pace in normal times for over three months after the shutdown, the sector has finally made a strong comeback with a 70% recovery, say industry-related people. Private hospitals, non-governmental educational institutions, restaurants, hotels and resorts, and transport have begun to return to normalcy. There is no proper data on how many got their jobs back.

Social Impact

The social impact of COVID-19 is difficult to quantify, is less tangible, and yet much more consequential. Closure of business, and loss of employment and income resulted in severe economic impact but the social impact of COVID-19 is no less critical. Closure of schools, limited access to health facilities, and nonfunctioning public institutions entrusted with protection of vulnerable groups have combined to leave deep and lasting social challenges, which if not addressed now will have long-term consequences even when the pandemic is controlled.

Rising Inequality

COVID-19 has not spared any country or population and is considered a leveller. Yet the impact of COVID-19 is experienced differently by diverse populations divided by class, caste, ethnicity, profession, and level of income. The pandemic has intensified inequality in an already unequal world. In 2018, Oxfam revealed in a report that 82% of the wealth generated in 2017 went to the richest 1% of the global population, while the 3.7 billion people who make up the poorest half of the world saw no increase in their wealth. Again in 2020, Oxfam reported that the world's 2,153 billionaires have more wealth than the 4.6 billion people who make up 60% of the planet's population, going on to say that a CEO of one of the four famous global brands makes in four days what a garment worker in Bangladesh makes in her lifetime. A more recent report states that it will take the poor ten years to go back to their previous state. In Bangladesh, a study conducted by SANEM finds that poverty has gone up to 40% from the previous 20% due to COVID-19 (SANEM, 2020). The 2011 Household Income and Expenditure Survey released by Bangladesh Bureau of Statistics (BBS) found that the income share of the poorest 5% of the population was 0.23% of overall income, a sharp fall from 2010 when it was 0.78%. In contrast, the richest 5% share of income grew to 27.89%, up from 24.61% in 2010. This basically means that the bottom 5% share of national income has decreased, whereas the richest 5% has increased.

Inequality is not only caused by uneven distribution of resources but is also due to social class, ethnic background, caste, and the physical state, such as persons with disabilities. Inequality is in accessing entitlements, services, and rights rendering a set of people voiceless and powerless. The pandemic has increased these inequalities further which if not checked will give rise to new sets of challenges such as social and physical turmoil.

Violence Against Women, Girls, and Children

Women, adolescent girls, and children have faced unique and additional challenges during the lockdown as a result of the pandemic. Globally there has been a rise in domestic violence prompting the Secretary General of UN to request member states to pay attention to the issue and take up preventive measures. Reports suggest a global rise of 20% in domestic violence against women and girls (UN Women, 2020).

In Bangladesh, the rate of domestic violence is already high. A study by BBS in 2010 revealed that 80% women had faced some kind of domestic abuse with 65% experiencing direct physical abuse. In a follow-up study in 2015, the number came down to 65%. As per UNICEF report, 52% girls are married before the legal age of 18 (BBS and UNICEF, 2017).

The current pandemic has exacerbated the already insecure situation for women and girls within families. A six-month survey from April to September 2020 conducted by Manusher Jonno Foundation (MJF) in selected locations revealed that 20% women reported violence not experienced before. The survey was conducted through telephone by 101 Partners of MJF located in 54 Districts and covered 50,000 respondents (Manusher Jonno Foundation, 2020). Women reported various forms of violence ranging from verbal and psychological to economic and physical abuse.

While violence against women and girls cuts across cultures, class, and ethnicity, a BRAC study revealed that women from low-income groups suffered increased violence (BRAC, 2020). Loss of income, male members being forced to stay at home, loss of employment, and inability to provide basic necessities are some of the reasons given for increase in domestic violence. However, as per experience of years of work on women's rights, the primary reason is the unequal power relations within families where men perceive themselves superior to women who have authority to abuse or treat them with disrespect.

Domestic violence and subsequently victims not being able to access assistance due to nonfunctioning public institutions such as police, shelter homes, and local authorities added to the vulnerability of women and adolescent girls. Even citizen groups mandated to monitor homes were unavailable due to the directives on social distancing.

The other challenge women faced was the additional work burden due to the lockdown. Family members remained at home all the time, children were out of school, and male members had no work and therefore stayed at home. Domestic help were also given leave due to the threat of virus spread. The entire responsibility of housework without any help, including cooking several meals every day for the entire family, fell on women. On top of that, husbands took out their frustration of income loss on their spouses through physical, sexual, and other forms of abuse.

Adolescent girls in Asian and African countries faced additional set of challenges and threats. High numbers of early marriages were recorded as

UNICEF has reported that 13 million under-aged girls were married as a result of COVID-19 (UNICEF, 2020). The scenario in Bangladesh is no different. With 52% of girls being married before the legal age of 18, Bangladesh has the highest rate of early marriage in South Asia (UNICEF, 2021). Although a comprehensive study has not been conducted on the present situation of early marriage, reports from the field suggest that it has increased during this time. MJF (2020) survey also confirmed 450 cases of early marriage in May 2020. A rapid assessment of child marriage in selected sample locations revealed that 13,000 early marriages occurred from April to August 2020. The reasons given were poverty in families due to job loss of parents, one less mouth to feed, and deep-rooted cultural, religious, and traditional beliefs and practices. Given the social norm prevailing specially in rural areas, getting a girl married off soon after she reaches puberty is considered the right thing to do. Since insecurity is cited as one of the reasons for high rates of early marriage, parents believe that marriage will provide security.

Children too, especially from low-income families, have suffered disproportionately during the pandemic. With closure of schools, children had limited options to keep themselves occupied in productive ways. They have faced physical and sexual abuse at home and outside (MJF, 2020). Due to financial crisis at home, more and more children have been pushed to labour, often hazardous work.

Marginalised Population

During any crisis, be it cyclone, flood, or health crisis, it is the marginalised and most vulnerable groups who suffer disproportionately. The impact of COVID-19 has been felt acutely by marginalised groups such as persons with disabilities, sex workers, transgender, Dalits. Being already socially discriminated and economically vulnerable, these groups have struggled to survive (Rashid et al., 2020). Hunger, inability to access minimum basic necessities, and the inability to pay house rent due to disruption of their meagre income all compounded to leave them in a state of helplessness. This crisis was felt more acutely among the urban marginalised population who mostly work in the informal sector. Persons with disabilities could not go out of their homes to access food being distributed by government or private groups. Due to social distancing directives, door-to-door services were not available for the sick, infirm, and elderly. Other marginalised groups living in the fringe of society such as sex workers and transgenders had no income and resorted to begging. The cleaners from Dalit and Harijan communities were exposed to the infection as they had no protective gear. The government directive to distribute cash of BDT 2,500 to 5 million of the poorest has only 1.6 million as of July 2020.

Closure of Educational Institutes

In order to contain the spread of infection, most countries around the world imposed strict directives to shut down all educational institutes (WHO, 2020). In Bangladesh, government ordered a complete lockdown and closure of all educational institutes from 26 March 2020. The lockdown was eased by September 2020 and most business, public and private offices started to function. However, schools, colleges, and universities remained shut. Although it was necessary to take such strict measures to contain the spread of the virus, it came with severe disruption to the learning and mental health of children and youth population. The government ordered online teaching from June 2020 but the experiment was not very successful. In a recent survey by Education Watch, it was revealed that 62% children have been left out of online schooling (Alamgir, 2021). Children from the poorest families without access to smart phones, tabs, or Internet connections were left out. A whole year of education lost will have consequences which might be difficult to make up.

Government Stimulus Packages

Since March 2020, the government deployed several stimulus measures to sustain economic activity and protect the most vulnerable. Prime Minister Sheikh Hasina announced a total of 19 stimulus packages amounting to BDT 1.03 trillion, worth 3.7% of the country's gross domestic product, to offset the impact of the coronavirus pandemic on various sectors of the country. As part of this stimulus package, the government expanded the Vulnerable Group Feeding (VGF) and Vulnerable Group Development (VGD) programmes, open market sales of rice at lower prices, and expanding social safety net programmes (Riaz, 2020).

The government also initiated a plan to provide a one-time assistance of BDT 2,500 each to five million families among the most vulnerable sections of society and allocated a total of BDT 1,250 crore for this initiative; BDT 8 crore was allocated to cover the cost of distribution. But as of 7 July 2020, only 1.6 million had received the allocated fund. Some 3.4 million poor are yet to get any support (Wemer and Riaz, 2020). Although well-intentioned, the government's stimulus packages have been beset with multiple problems of mismanagement, corruption, and nepotism.

It is alleged that partisan political considerations were taken in preparing the list of beneficiaries for relief in 82% of the areas included in a survey conducted by Transparency International Bangladesh (TIB). The survey also found incidents of corruption with regard to relief distribution which were reported in the media up to 10 June 2020, where elected representatives (30%), local political leaders (24%), dealers (17%), and business people (14%) were involved (Julkarnayeen et al., 2020).

The government's stimulus package also did not fully reach the most marginalised such as persons with disabilities, LGBTIQ+ groups, ethnic minorities, Dalits, low-income families, and informal and low-wage earners such as daily labourers, transgenders, and sex workers. Data from other rapid assessments shows that 40% of the poor population and 35% of the vulnerable non-poor have already reduced their food consumption to cope with the situation amid the pandemic (Julkarnayeen et al., 2020). The beneficiary lists prepared by the local administrations had many flaws. Those not eligible were listed, such as 3,000 government employees and 7,000 pensioners plus those already receiving support from other social safety programmes.

Civil Society Response

Bangladesh boasts of a vibrant civil society comprising NGOs, academic, human rights, and women activists who have made substantial contribution to the social and economic progress of Bangladesh. Working alongside government, NGOs have been particularly successful in reducing poverty, promoting women's empowerment, and achieving 90% school enrolment. Micro-credit programmes have empowered millions of women economically, and the non-formal education run by BRAC is considered a model globally. The women's movement has brought women's rights issue to centre stage. Although there is a long way to go, today women have made their presence felt in every sector in Bangladesh.

As rates of infections increased, NGOs and civil society organisations, students, and volunteers sprang to action in a bid to save lives. The most important task was to make people aware about the virus and give instructions to take precautionary measures. The lockdown announced by the government was difficult to enforce, particularly the poor, to follow health instructions and maintain social or physical distance. In addition to lack of awareness, the poor had to make a choice between starvation and dying from the virus. Civil society organisations joined government efforts to embark on mass campaigns on hand washing, wearing of masks, and maintaining physical distance. NGOs with support from private sector companies and foreign donors took up food and cash distribution. Research bodies and think tanks gathered evidence on the extent of loss and suffering of people due to the pandemic to assist policy-makers make informed decisions. Women's rights organisations monitored rights violation such as violence against women and girls, early marriage, or other violations. NGOs played an important role in assisting government target the right beneficiaries for the relief operation and distribution of stimulus packages and social safety.

Lessons and Conclusion

No one, neither any country nor society, was prepared for COVID-19. It came with an intensity and speed that could not have been predicted or planned for. However, 13 months after the virus was first detected in Wuhan, China, there is a ray of hope with the arrival of vaccines. No praise can be enough for the scientists who worked day and night to make this miracle possible: miracle, because there is no precedence of a vaccine discovered in such a short time. Collaboration among countries combined with the solidarity and commitment to save the world from the contagion itself has created history.

The global COVID-19 pandemic has left behind a trail of destruction that will take years to overcome – destruction in terms of 2.2 million precious lives lost, millions left jobless, businesses destroyed. Women have faced additional challenges of violence, work burden, and mental trauma; adolescent girls were forced into marriage; and children have lost a year of learning plus the fear that many might never return to school due to financial hardship. As the world gets closer to controlling the virus, we need to reflect on the lessons of the pandemic. One thing is clear; we should not go back to the old lifestyle of unbridled consumerism, destruction of the environment, and skewed allocation of resources. Nobel Laureate Professor Yunus has famously said "going back to that world is equal to committing suicide" (Prof. Yunus on the opportunities presented by COVID (2020). Now is the time to come together in show of solidarity as never before. Countries need to collaborate for the vaccine to be declared a "public good" accessible to the rich and poor countries alike. Rising inequality among nations and within society has to be addressed if we are serious about meeting the overall SDG goal of "Leave No one Behind".

At national level, various health challenges arose, impacting on the physical and mental health of the population. Lack of sexual reproductive services left adolescent girls vulnerable to unwanted pregnancies. Public health services were strained to care for the elderly population with other preexisting conditions. Private hospitals charged extraordinary rates for treatment of COVID-19, causing great suffering, which government failed to monitor. There was also corruption around purchase of PPE, mask, oxygen, and falsification of COVID-19 testing reports.

However, thousands of health workers (both public and private) put themselves on the line to save lives. Local communities, CBOs, and volunteers, not bound to projects, responded quickly to the crisis. They also assisted the government in focused targeting with the private sector joining hands with the government and civil society. There is a need for more research and evidence gathering to comprehensively understand the impact of COVID-19 based on which actions should be taken to be better prepared for next time.

It is likely that Bangladesh might recover from the present crisis given its history of overcoming disasters. However, for that to happen, the economy has to be revived and supported by effective policies with collaboration among all segments of society and strengthening of institutions to a more accountable system catering to the needs of the most vulnerable people.

Recommendations

A number of policy recommendations can be made on the basis of the learnings from the pandemic experience.

1. Proper and authentic data should be collected about the number of adolescent girls and children – both boys and girls who dropped out of schools. Surveys should be undertaken to find out the reason for drop out. Education and Labour Ministries should put forward action plans on how to bring children back to schools.
2. Small and petty enterprises destroyed due to the pandemic should be given cash support.
3. Widening inequality should be addressed with special incentive packages for the extremely poor and marginalised population.
4. The long-term social and economic impact of the pandemic on the lives of the most vulnerable population such as children, minorities, persons with disabilities, and trans-gender should be assessed though scientific surveys, and research and plan of action developed accordingly so that Bangladesh is able to meet the lSDG Goal of "Leave No one Behind".
5. Campaign and awareness-raising on mask wearing, following health guidelines, and taking of vaccination should be continued by government and civil society organisations to prevent a second surge.
6. Finally, the Task Force set up to monitor the pandemic should be strengthened with inclusion of civil society experts from diverse fields reflecting different segments of the population.

References

ACT alliance appeal: Global response to the Covid-19 Pandemic – Act201 – SUB-APPEAL – Act 201-BGD – COVID-19 response to refugees and HOST communities in Bangladesh – BANGLADESH (2020), 19 June, https://reliefweb.int/report/bangladesh/act-alliance-appeal-global-response-covid-19-pandemic-act201-sub-appeal-act-201, accessed 10 February 2021.

Admin, Y. (2020), "Going back to that world is equal to committing suicide. – Professor Muhammad Yunus on the opportunity presented by COVID-19", *Yunus Social Business*, 26 May, www.yunussb.com/blog/ 2020/5/20/professor-muhammad-yunus-opportunity-covid-19. (It is within the text according to author- Page 15).

Alamgir, M. (2021), "Education during pandemic: Digital divide wreaks damage", *The Daily Star*, 19 January, www.thedailystar.net/frontpage/news/education-during-pandemic-digital-divide-wreaks-damage-2030637, accessed 10 February 2021.

Amin, M. A. (2020), "Remittance record AMID Covid-19 Pandemic unveils magnitude of illegal transactions", *Dhaka Tribune*, 3 October, www.dhakatribune.com/bangladesh/2020/10/03/remittance-record-during-pandemic-unveils-magnitude-of-illegal-transactions, accessed 15 February 2021.

Bangladesh Bureau of Statistics, Statistics Division, Ministry of Planning (2011), "Report of the household income and expenditure survey 2010", December, http://203.112.218.65:8008/WebTestApplication/userfiles/Image/LatestReports/HIES-10.pdf, accessed 9 February 2021.

Bangladesh Bureau of Statistics, Statistics and Informatics Division, Ministry of Planning, Government of the People's Republic of Bangladesh (2016), *Report on Violence Against Women Survey 2015*, Dhaka, Bangladesh.

Berkhout, E., Galasso, N., Lawson, M., Morales, P., Taneja, A. and Pimentel, D. (2021), "The inequality virus", *OXFAM*, 25 January, www.oxfam.org/en/research/inequality-virus, accessed 14 February 2021.

BRAC (2020), "Rapid perception survey on COVID19 awareness and economic impact", May, www.brac.net/program/wp-content/uploads/2020/09/080920-Covid19-economy-impact-vol.2.pdf, accessed 9 February 2021.

Business recovery confidence grows stronger: SANEM survey (2021), *The Business Standard*, 16 February, https://tbsnews.net/economy/business-recovery-confidence-grows-stronger-sanem-survey-202591.

Correspondent, S. (2020), "Survey on RMG workers DURING Pandemic: 99.8pc say they're not covid-infected", *The Daily Star*, 4 October, www.thedailystar.net/frontpage/news/survey-rmg-workers-during-pandemic-998pc-say-theyre-not-covid-infected-1972481, accessed 13 February 2021.

Export promotion BUREAU (2021), http://epb.gov.bd/site/view/epb_export_data/-, accessed 16 February 2021.

"Going back to that world is equal to committing suicide" (Prof. Yunus on the opportunities presented by COVID). Talk/Speaking at a special panel hosted by Yunus Social Business Brazilian Arm, 20 May 2020. https://www.oxfam.org/en/press-releases/mega-rich-recoup-covid-losses-record-time-yet-millions-will-live-poverty-leastes.

Impacts of COVID-19 on the Bangladesh Economy (2020), *MTBiz Quarterly Business Review*, 11(2), April–June, www.mutualtrustbank.com/wp-content/uploads/mtbiz/2020/MTBiz_April-June%202020.pdf, accessed 13 February 2021.

Julkarnayeen, M., Akter, M., Akter, T. and Khoda, M. E. (2020), "Governance challenges in tackling corona virus", *COVID Response Track, Transparency International Bangladesh*, September, www.ti-bangladesh.org/beta3/images/2020/report/covid-19/Covid-Resp-Track-ES-Eng-15062020.pdf, accessed 9 February 2021.

Khatun, F. (2021), "Women's work during pandemic in the Bimstec region", *ORF Online*, 15 January, www.orfonline.org/expert-speak/womens-work-pandemic-bimstec-region/, accessed February 2021.

Labour Force Survey 2016–2017 (2020), "Bangladesh bureau of statistics", 15 October, http://data.bbs.gov.bd/index.php/catalog/200#metadata-identification, accessed 10 February 2021.

Mahmood, M. (2020), "Covid-19: Economic challenges facing Bangladesh", *The Financial Express*, 13 June, https://thefinancialexpress.com.bd/views/covid-19-economic-challenges-facing-bangladesh-1592064588, accessed 14 February 2021.

Manusher Jonno Foundation (MJF) (2020), "Violence against women and children: COVID 19 A telephone survey: Initiative of Manusher Jonno foundation survey period", June, www.manusherjonno.org/wp-content/uploads/2020/03/Final-Report-of-Telephone-Survey-on-VAW-June-2020.pdf, accessed 10 February 2021.

March and Report, T. (2020), "First coronavirus cases detected in Bangladesh", *TBS News*, 8 March, https://tbsnews.net/bangladesh/health/3-tested-positive-coronavirus-bangladesh-iedcr-53476, accessed 14 February 2021.

Migration and remittances data (2021), *World Bank*, www.worldbank.org/en/topic/migrationremittancesdiasporaissues/brief/migration-remittances-data, accessed 15 February 2021.

Mujeri, M. (2020), "Informal economy and economic inclusion", *The Daily Star*, 17 February, www.thedailystar.net/supplements/29th-anniversary-supplements/digitisation-and-inclusivity-taking-everyone-along/news/informal-economy-and-economic-inclusion-1869601, accessed February 2021.

Oxfam (2018), "Richest 1 percent bagged 82 percent of wealth created last year – poorest half of humanity got nothing" [Press release], 25 April, www.oxfam.org/en/press-releases/richest-1-percent-bagged-82-percent-wealth-created-last-year-poorest-half-humanity, accessed 12 February 2021.

Oxfam (2020), "World's billionaires have more wealth than 4.6 billion people" [Press release], 20 January, www.oxfam.org/en/press-releases/worlds-billionaires-have-more-wealth-46-billion-people, accessed 12 February 2021.

Rahman, M. (2020), "Second wave could inflict bigger damage to economy", *The Daily Star*, 9 November, www.thedailystar.net/business/news/second-wave-could-inflict-bigger-damage-economy-1991765, accessed 13 February 2021.

Raihan, S. (2012), *Economic Reforms and Agriculture in Bangladesh: Assessment of Impacts Using Economy-wide Simulation Models*, ILO, 31 December, www.ilo.org/wcmsp5/groups/public/ – asia/ – ro-bangkok/ – ilo-dhaka/documents/publication/wcms_204089.pdf, accessed 12 February 2021.

Rashid, Sabina, Theobald, Sally and Ozano, Kim (2020), "Towards a socially just model: Balancing hunger and response to the COVID-19 pandemic in Bangladesh", *BMJ Global Health*, 5, e002715. Doi: 10.1136/bmjgh-2020-002715.

Remittance: Why was it the highest amid a pandemic? (2021), *Dhaka Tribune*, 17 January, www.dhakatribune.com/business/2021/01/17/remittance-why-was-it-the-highest-amid-a-pandemic, accessed 15 February 2021.

Report, S. O. (2020), "Factories to reopen gradually: BGMEA", *The Daily Star*, 25 April, www.thedailystar.net/business/news/factories-reopen-gradually-bgmea-1896640, accessed 14 February 2021.

Reuters (2021), "What recovery? Clothes retailers cut orders while factories fight to survive", *The Daily Star*, 8 February, www.thedailystar.net/business/news/what-recovery-clothes-retailers-cut-orders-while-factories-fight-survive-2041609, accessed 14 February 2021.

Riaz, A. (2020), "A tale of misplaced priorities", *The Daily Star*, 15 July, www.thedailystar.net/opinion/black-white-grey/news/tale-misplaced-priorities-1928729, accessed 9 February 2021.

Ritchie, H. (2019), "Which countries are most densely populated?" *Our World in Data*, 6 September, https://ourworldindata.org/most-densely-populated-countries, accessed 2 February 2021.

RMG export earnings contribution to national export declined in 2020. (2021), *Textile Today*, 7 January, www.textiletoday.com.bd/rmg-export-earnings-contribution-national-export-declined-2020/#:%7E:text=Bangladesh's%20economic%20backbone%2C%20its%20readymade,Export%20Promotion%20Bureau%20(EPB).&text=While%20woven%20exports%20declined%2010.22%25%20to%20%247.01%20billion, accessed 15 February 2021.

A Scoping Analysis of Budget Allocations for Ending Child Marriage in Bangladesh (2017), Bangladesh Bureau of Statistics and UNICEF Bangladesh 2017, Dhaka, Bangladesh. ISBN: 978-984-8969-29-8.

South Asian Network on Economic Modeling (SANEM). (2020), "SANEM researchers assess poverty impacts of covid-19", *SANEM*, 1 May, https://sanemnet.org/sanem-researchers-assess-poverty-impacts-of-covid-19/, accessed 11 February 2021.

Uddin, A. (2021), "Small enterprises, farmers still languish in neglect", *The Daily Star*, 6 February, www.thedailystar.net/business/news/small-enterprises-farmers-still-languish-neglect-2040517, accessed 11 February 2021.

Uddin, J., Shoaib, M. and Arafat, M. F. (2020), "Impacts of COVID-19 on agriculture in Bangladesh", *World Overview of Conservation Approaches and Technologies (WOCAT)*, 1–4, www.wocat.net/documents/1042/Impact_of_Covid_in_Bangladesh.pdf, accessed 12 February 2021.

UN Women (2020), "Press release: UN women raises awareness of the Shadow pandemic of violence against women during covid-19", *United Nations*, 27 May, www.unwomen.org/en/news/stories/2020/5/press-release-the-shadow-pandemic-of-violence-against-women-during-covid-19, accessed 9 February 2021.

UNDP (2020), *The Next Frontier: Human Development and the Anthropocene*, Human Development Report, http://hdr.undp.org/sites/default/files/Country-Profiles/BGD.pdf, accessed 16 February 2021.

UNICEF (2020), "Pandemic-induced poverty pushing up child marriage", *UNICEF*, 13 September, www.unicef.org/bangladesh/en/stories/pandemic-induced-poverty-pushing-child-marriage, accessed 10 February 2021.

UNICEF (2021), "Child marriage", www.unicef.org/rosa/what-we-do/child-protection/child-marriage#:~:text=India%20has%20the%20largest%20number,for%20both%20boys%20and%20girls, accessed 11 February 2021.

United States Coronavirus: 29,370,705 Cases and 529,214 Deaths – Worldometer (2021), *Worldometer*, 3 March, www.worldometers.info/coronavirus/country/us/, accessed 3 March 2021.

Wemer, D. and Riaz, A. (2020), "Bangladesh's COVID-19 stimulus: Leaving the most vulnerable behind", *Atlantic Council*, 22 December, www.atlanticcouncil.org/blogs/new-atlanticist/bangladeshs-covid-19-stimulus-leaving-the-most-vulnerable-behind/, accessed 14 February 2021.

WHO (2020), "Coronavirus disease (covid-19) situation reports", www.who.int/emergencies/diseases/novel-coronavirus-2019/situation-reports, accessed 9 February 2021.

14 A Neighbour's Anguish

Myanmar's Response to the Pandemic

Reshmi Banerjee

Introduction

The land of the Shwedagon like its regional neighbours has struggled to protect its citizens from the deadly COVID-19 virus. Although the number of infected persons has been much less than India, the country's apparently inadequate medical facilities have been a perennial cause of immense worry. The pandemic has exposed (like in other countries) the pre-existing fault lines within Myanmar with its adverse impact experienced by its vulnerable marginalised communities. Corona-related restrictions/closures in Myanmar have impacted many: from the garment manufacturing sector to tourism; from health workers to refugees. Distress faced by the common masses is similar to the challenges faced across the border in India but each country has its own story to tell and lessons to share.

The chapter attempts to capture the unfolding of the Corona crisis in Myanmar[*] and its socio-economic impact. The chapter is a reflection on the impact of the COVID-19 virus on the country from March 2020 to January 2021 under the erstwhile NLD (National League for Democracy) government. It attempts to understand the challenges faced due to Coronavirus and the resilience of the people in tackling it.

The Calamity and Its Impact

In late August 2020, Sittwe (Rakhine's state capital)[**] went into semi-lockdown with night-time curfew imposed as cases of infections surged. The battle against the virus was on even after five months (Myanmar reported its first case in March 2020) [***] (Lynn, 2020a). Disasters are not new for Myanmar as it has been hit before by severe cyclones (Nargis in 2008), floods, and landslides (2015). But the impact of the restrictions imposed by the arrival of the pandemic has been massive. According to the World Bank, Myanmar's GDP decreased by 2%–3% because of COVID-19 with net profits of private banks going negative in a decade for the first time. The Union Myanmar Federation Chambers of Commerce and Industry pointed out the high vulnerability of three sectors of tourism, cut-make-package (CMP),

DOI: 10.4324/9781003282815-19

and small medium enterprises (SMEs). Asia Foundations' telephonic survey further revealed that businesses had laid off 16% of their employees (on an average) with 64% of the businesses expected to face financial (cash flow) problems. The Confederation of Trade Unions of Myanmar also stated that 16 factories were shut down (Flanders Investment and Trade, 2020).

Incomes among the rural households displayed a notable short-term decline with non-farm jobs nationally falling by 5.3 million. While industry witnessed output decline by 52% (manufacturing fell by 40%), output declined by 56% in the services sector and agriculture overall fell by 14%. Falling consumer demand and exports, problems faced by agri-businesses, loss of remittance incomes all compounded the problems faced. Within the agricultural food sector, the food service component fell by 71% on account of closures of food catering services and restaurants. The COVID-19 Economic Relief Plan (CERP), which was published by the government on 27 April 2020, included goals of easing the impact on households, labourers and works, and private sector along with increasing access to COVID-19 response financing. The plan implementation is expected to cost a minimum of 2.8 trillion Kyat or US$2 billion (IFPRI, 2020).

A publication titled "Six Charts on Myanmar's Economy in the Time of COVID-19" by the IMF stated that the key engines of growth were badly hit and noted the sharp decline in exports, remittances, and tourist arrivals (Chinese tourists account for 25% of the tourist flow). The Myanmar Trade Promotion Organization's (MTPO's) report also reiterated the fact that tourism had been hit the hardest followed by the garment industry. Small-scale rubber industries (the country produces around 200,000 tonnes of rubber each year with 90% exported to other countries like China, Malaysia, Indonesia, and Singapore) and sea food industry have taken an unfortunate hit. One million people were estimated to lose their jobs in the fisheries industry in Myanmar (Nortajuddin, 2020).

A survey conducted by the Luxembourg Aid and Development and the Luxembourg Agency for Development Cooperation (supported by the Ministry of Hotels and Tourism-MOHT) observed that almost 90% of MSMEs (micro, small, and medium enterprises) related to tourism saw a decline in revenues. The MOHT in April 2020 declared that hotels, tours, and travel businesses would be exempt from license fees for one year (Lwin, 2020). But the eerie silence in the Inle Lake region reveals not only the idle workless boatmen but the uncertainty lying for the future. Susan Bailey recalls how the residents of the area were happy with the lack of pollution and noise yet yearning for tourists to return (Bailey, 2020). Thus, people experienced paradoxical feelings in unprecedented pandemic times!

The garment industry where over 500,000 people are estimated to be employed has faced serious challenges. Clothing factories were forced to shut down (90% of supplies came from China) with demands drying from Europe and Japan. Many foreign factories (majority of them are owned by the Chinese) closed down with the employers leaving without at times paying salaries to the employees like five garment factory managers in the Shwepyithar industrial zone left without paying salaries. Myanmar has witnessed a 50% demand reduction for its clothing, handbags, and footwear on account of international closure (San Myo, 2020).

The pandemic and its resultant challenges have been provided as reasons to also dismiss unionised workers in Myanmar like Rui-Ning factory in May 2020 lay off 324 workers of which 298 were union members. Myan Mode factory also dismissed workers, many of whom were union members. However, the factory union workers have relentlessly fought to get back their rights. An agreement was reached on 30 May 2020, whereby Myan Mode reinstated 75 fired unionised workers and recalled hundreds of other union members once operations were to return to normal. Similarly on 17 July, the Rui-Ning factory union was successful in reinstating 298 fired union members including the union president (Business and Human Rights Resource Centre, 2020). Araddhya Mehtta, Country Director of Action Aid Myanmar, observed that the worst affected were the informal migrant workers, which included the garment factory workers (Action Aid, 2020).

The economy has been adversely impacted but the impact on society has been no less. The level of country-wide infections was quite low between March and August 2020 but the second wave erupted in August 2020 with Rakhine being the epicentre and infections quickly spreading to Yangon and Mandalay region's Myingyan Township. The Rakhine province became the epicentre of challenges with a local media outlet *The Voice* running a cartoon showing a Rohingya man crossing the border carrying COVID-19 with the label "illegal interloper". Although all ethnic communities have personal and business links across borders and find themselves crossing it, some communities seem to have apparently faced discrimination from the public (shops not wanting to sell anything to them) and unnecessary stigmatisation (Nachemson, 2020).

Daw Aung San Suu Kyi's public statements did not ease the tensions. She not only reprimanded careless nightclub owners and rule flouting Yangon citizens but also warned disobliging citizens with legal action. She also stated that anybody entering the country illegally as well as those who protect such undocumented people will be severely dealt with. Tactics of shaming and strict government control was exercised (ibid.).

Each city within the country seems to have seen its own unique local circumstances generating its specific responses: some Yangon residents made barricades around their own neighbourhoods without taking permission from the local authorities to protect themselves, thus triggering social media users to call these "mini republics" (Oo Zaw Naing, 2020). On the other hand, many street vendors of the same city continued with their trade as they needed to earn to survive, thus exposing themselves to the virus as they had no alternative choices (Al Jazeera, 2020). Mandalay City Development Committee declared that opening of businesses will be based on their priority to the public like clothing, beauty salons, and construction materials (Mann and Aung, 2020).

Border towns of Myanmar were at the receiving end of stricter controls imposed by regional neighbours to check the spread of the virus. The vice mayor of Ruili (a town in western Yunnan province bordering Muse town in Myanmar) stated in a press conference that people with no fixed residence and no fixed place of work will be repatriated (Medical Xpress, 2020). This was evidently targeted at Burmese migrants who had tested positive in China's border town. The border town of Wanding in Dai-Jingpo Autonomous Prefecture Yunnan hardly saw any tourists including daily crossings (Pang Sai in Myanmar is connected to Wanding with many people having relatives/family living on either side). Only trucks carrying seasonal harvests of Myanmar farmers to China (watermelons and sugarcanes) were allowed to ply. Also China provided face masks and protective gear in northern Myanmar with some doctors in the northern parts communicating with their counterparts in China too (Jie, 2020).

Similarly Thai military started sending Myanmar nationals back with tightening of border restrictions. Medical supplies have been limited in the border areas with halting Internet facilities, which in turn have limited the flow of useful information regarding COVID-19. The quarantine centres were overcrowded with many forced to leave, thus raising the possibilities of community transmission (Howell, 2020). The ethnic armed groups like the United WA State Army ordered night clubs and casinos to close (Onishi and Nitta, 2020). The reluctance of civil society organisations and residents to house migrants (more than a hundred) returning from Manipur in North East India in Tamu's sports hall (as a quarantine centre) is telling (Htwe, 2020). The fear of the virus was paramount exerting its influence on cross-border socio-economic interaction especially impacting border economies and border trade.

Other marginalised categories like women, refugees, IDPs, and senior citizens seem to have suffered too. All over the world, women faced increasing domestic and sexual abuse with nowhere to escape as lockdown measures kept them stranded with the abuser at home. Many lost their jobs (a huge number works in the garment industry in Myanmar) with lack of financial independence adding to their poverty and vulnerability.

The Karen Women's Empowerment Group (KWEG) was informed by community members that increase in alcohol and substance abuse was fuelling violence inside homes and within the community with the KWEG documenting both rising intimate partner violence (on account of income insecurity) and fighting between family members, neighbours, and young people from neighbouring villages. The KWEG also noticed increasing debt, rising theft, threats to women's safety with women facing the triple work burden: domestic, community, and income-generating work. Also regions with overlapping authorities (of the government and the Ethnic Armed Organizations/EAOs) had dual guidelines, which made life difficult for the common people as they had to negotiate constantly through two different sets of sometimes contradictory COVID-19 restrictions. This increased the levels of anxiousness among people including their difficulty in accessing their farms, markets, and jobs especially during the harvesting period. Also decision-making seems to have been entirely in the hands of men, thus women's issues were not sufficiently factored in (Saferworld, 2020).

The UN has described domestic violence against women as a "shadow pandemic". COVID-19 has deeply impacted the IDPs of which majority are women (77% of the IDPs are women and children). Sexual slavery, human trafficking, harassment, and discrimination are some of the gender-related risks that these women face (Neranjan and Shetty, 2020). The lockdown has also restricted the accessibility of women and girls to contraception. The loss of jobs, added pressure of looking after the family including children, and school closures all have reduced the earning capability of women to pay for and access health services including contraceptives (Oo and Davies, 2020). Many women (nearly 800,000) in Myanmar are working overseas as migrant workers with women constituting 90% of garment workers and 60% of workers in the food and accommodation services within the country. Even within the critical health sector, women constitute more than 75% of Myanmar's health workers and first responders (Balakrishnan and Burniat, 2020).

The condition of refugee women in camps like that in Cox's Bazaar in Bangladesh is very challenging with social distancing not possible although volunteers have been trying to spread the message of hygiene and disease prevention (Rayburn, 2020). The older refugees (almost two-thirds of them) felt anxious most of the times as essential services were being provided with limited delivery of age-specific support systems (Qureshi, 2020).

Large sections of the country's population are very poor and the lockdown restrictions have hit them the hardest. According to the Living Condition Survey by the UNDP and the World Bank, nearly 30% of the population in the country was surviving on less than 1,600 Kyat per day (just US$1.2) in 2017. The survey pointed out that the poorest 40% earned less than 22% of the total income in Myanmar and among the poorest 40%, landless labourers were in the worst condition. People in the border areas of Shan, Mon, and Karen states feared that their lives were going to be changed forever on account of rising job insecurity. Big cities like Yangon have also seen the plight of street hawkers who have been badly affected (Khine, 2020).

Schools have been shut with disruption to the daily education routine for thousands of children. This can have devastating consequences for the younger generation as many might never see the face of schools again especially those from the poorer communities. The UN Secretary General Antonio Guterres' statement that school closures "could waste untold human potential, undermine decades of progress, and exacerbate entrenched inequalities" holds special relevance in this context (Newey, 2020). These extremely dire circumstances will have a dreadful impact on the mental health of individuals in the future. Older people have suffered from intense isolation and loneliness (social and religious gatherings have been prohibited). Pillars of connectivity like community networks and interaction have been thrown into disarray. Many of the community organisations dependent on overseas support have suffered from decline in international donations (Khan and Wai, 2020).

Initiatives From Civil Society

Dissemination of useful health safety information/protocols on time is critical in a pandemic. Although ethnic news providers faced challenges in 2020, the local community media in the Chin State realised the usefulness of disseminating information in the local language and thus promoted it. This can make a huge difference especially in the ethnic minority areas where accessing information is poor. In Falam Township, audio material on COVID-19 was posted on the community media Facebook page with people responding. Although the 2016 Broadcast Law in Myanmar opened up the country for community media, the bye-laws required for licensing rules are still not in place (Jacobsson, 2020).

The people of Myanmar have always trusted their social networks including friends, social figures, and religious leaders in times of any crisis. Buddhism was also a factor, which influenced people's responses. Richard C. Paddock observed the promotion of some non-medical remedies by some Buddhist figures. Some doctors even felt that the pandemic would pass over Myanmar without causing much damage on account of its Buddhist religious practices (Paddock, 2020). Myanmar is not an exception in taking recourse to religion to tackle unprecedented dire conditions. Many countries have experienced this form of intense faith from citizens in the face of adversity and unending uncertainty.

The Buddhist monks, churches, and Muslim leaders offered their premises for quarantine centres as civil society organisations were overburdened (Seinn, 2020). Buddhist monasteries distributed food and used their premises in the slums of Yangon to home returning migrant workers from Thailand and Malaysia. Dhama Duta College in Yangon (the meditation centre of monk Ashin Sakeinda) changed itself into a temporary quarantine centre for up to 400 people. Monk Sitagu Sayadaw Ashin Nyanissara in Mandalay donated US$10,000 to the COVID-19 Emergency Fund that Pope Francis launched. The Buddhist Sangha not only closed the Shwedagon Pagoda in Yangon with most other monasteries also closing as safety measures but the Thingyan Buddhist Festival marking the New Year was also cancelled (Bara, 2020).

Gerard McCarthy has analysed the role of Myanmar's "informal mechanisms of reciprocity" (based on Buddhist social morality) like the charitable events and neighbourhood funeral associations in cementing social ties within the overall language of merit making (McCarthy, 2016: 319–320).

These associations will continue to play a crucial role in building the country in the post-pandemic phase.

The KNU (Karen National Union) was the first EAO (ethnic armed organisation) to call for cooperation between the erstwhile NLD government and the EAOs. Several EAOs set up the Community Health and Development Network (CHDN), which included six Karenni EAOs like the Karenni National Progressive Party and the Kayan New Land Party. However, the situation of the displaced population in Myanmar in the face of the pandemic remains vulnerable (Progressive Voice, 2020). Loss of land and resources by communities (in zones of conflict) has made the lockdown restrictions even more strenuous to bear.

Initiatives have been taken by NGOs for connecting people and keeping them safe and secure. In Yangon, the NGO Clean Yangon (since March 2020) has been trying to raise awareness about the disease and has been helping the squatters, daily wage earners, and elderly vendors to lessen the impact of the virus. Their volunteers have helped the healthcare workers and supplied food including multivitamin pills to hospitals and quarantine centres. They also assisted the Yangon Public Health Department in data collection on the overseas returnees. They distributed basic food packages (containing rice, cooking oil, canned fish, salt, beans, and vitamin pills) not only to 1,500 poor families in East and South Dagon, Hlaing Tharyar, and Kawhmu Townships but also to those living on the streets including the municipal staff (Aung, 2020).

The Freedom Fund's emergency response fund has been providing immediate small-scale funding to its hundred or so frontline partners so that vulnerable communities can be provided assistance (India, Nepal, Brazil, Thailand, and Ethiopia are also being helped through this fund) (Bond, 2020). The Kachin Baptist Convention (KBC) has been working with IDPs in the camps to provide clean water and better hygiene. The installation of a network of hand washing stations with soap across 15 camps is a case in point (OCHA, 2020).

A psychosocial counselling programme is being funded by the Livelihoods and Food Security Fund (LIFT). This is part of the "Aye Chan Thaw Ein" project implemented by PIN (People in Need), its Alliance 2015 partner Helvetas, and other local NGOs. The service provider Call Me Today is helping to implement the COVID-19 Phone Line Counselling helpline whereby people (500 workers and their families) in the industrial district of Shwe Pyi Thar Township can access free counselling sessions (each session lasts one hour to handle anxiety and depression). Call Me Today has also started a private Facebook group to spread information regarding social psychology and mental health support. About 8,000 migrants and host community households in the region are also being provided with soaps and hand sanitisers by PIN, which is supported by the Community Development Association (CDA). Ward administrative committees in the area have also been provided by PIN with sound systems and megaphones to spread the message of health (People in Need 2020). The launching of the "Radio-Rights for Information" by the community-based group Rakhine Ethnic Congress (REC) showcases the critical need to pass on valuable information (they provided radios to each of the camps in the state, which has more than 100 camps) (Arab News, 2020).

In 2016, the erstwhile NLD government's National Health Plan formally recognised the role of ethnic health providers for the first time, whose services could be useful in the future. A committee in April 2020 led by chief peace negotiator Tin Myo Win to coordinate with armed groups on information sharing on issues such as return of migrant workers, suspected cases, and treatment protocols, and contact tracing was seen as a welcome step. Tackling the COVID-19 virus requires a combined approach, and building a joint partnership in these trying times can eventually help in building longstanding personal relationships (International Crisis Group, 2020).

Meanwhile initiatives have continued like the Ministry of Planning, Finance, and Industry along with the Japan International Cooperation Agency (JICA) aiming to provide 64 billion Kyat in funds to micro, small, and medium enterprises. The Myanmar Investment Commission also approved 11 new projects in April 2020 in the manufacturing, construction, and other sectors with the commission trying to create 3,200 job opportunities in the labour-intensive projects (Lynn, 2020b). Action Aid Myanmar has been supporting 150,000 garment workers in five industrial areas of Yangon, Bago, and Ayeyarwaddy (giving public health information in the local languages) (Action Aid, 2020).

The Gender Equality Network in Myanmar has released several briefs related to gender advocacy and domestic violence along with resources for women in the context of COVID-19. The Karen Women's Organisation (KWO) has helped in sewing of thousands of masks and creating emergency food packets, whereas UN Women has helped certain communities to digitally market their products by providing them with Internet accessibility (Neranjan and Shetty, 2020).

The Thandaunggyi Women Group in partnership with the Department of Social Welfare organised a ten-day mask training course in the Myine Gyi Ngu IDP camp in order to support the State's Cloth Mask Campaign (Balakrishnan and Burniat, 2020). The Voluntary Service Overseas in partnership with the Mon National Education Committee distributed back-to-school kits (containing milk, soap) for 10,000 children and provided nutrition support (including rice, oil, and beans) for 744 teachers (Hodges, 2020). Artists have also contributed in their own ways to create awareness as evident by the exhibition titled "COVID-19" by MPP Yei Myint, which ran from 8 to 14 August 2020 at the Yangon Book Plaza (Myint, 2020).

Conclusion

Myanmar, like other countries of the world, has struggled with the deadly COVID-19 virus, which has adversely impacted its economy and society. The resilient and enterprising people of the land of the Irrawaddy have risen to the occasion to contribute to their country in whatever form they can to alleviate the hardships triggered by the pandemic lockdown. Civil society organisations including religious ones have provided support along with everyday hope that people have consciously cultivated to face the storm generated by the pandemic.

What will happen in the future (in terms of policies to tackle the impact of COVID-19) will depend on how much importance is given to economic rejuvenation and social transformation – critical for all countries as they emerge out of this long, dramatic, and forced hibernation from normalcy created by the devastating pandemic. One can only hope for better times to unfold for a nation which has always faced turbulent times with an endearing spirit of courage and conviction.

Notes

* Myanmar is a country in Southeast Asia, which is bordered by countries like India and Bangladesh in its north west, China in its north east and Thailand to its south east. It has Arabian Sea in its south and the Bay of Bengal in its south-west. With its capital in Naypyidaw, it is a country which is well known for its rich cultural history, amazing natural beauty, unique biodiversity, and ethnically diverse population. It is home to various tribes like the Chins, Kachins, Mons, Shans, and Karens.

** Rakhine is a state in Myanmar situated on the west coast of the country.

*** The first two cases in Myanmar were declared in March 2020 when two men (Myanmar citizens) returned from the United States and the United Kingdom, respectively. For details, please see Myanmar announces first Coronavirus cases (2020), *Myanmar Now*, 24 March, www.myanmar-now.org/en/news/myanmar-announces-first-coronavirus-cases, accessed 21 August 2021.

References

12 ways NGOs are helping the world's poorest during COVID-19 (2020), *Bond*, 9 June, https://bond.org.uk/news/2020/06/12-ways-ngos-are-helping-the-worlds-poorest-during-covid-19, accessed 8 October 2020.

Aung, San Yamin (2020), "Myanmar volunteers help Yangon's hungry during COVID-19 outbreak", *The Irrawaddy*, 23 April, https://irrawaddy.com/news/burma/myanmar-volunteers-help-yangons-hungry-covid-19-outbreak.html, accessed 8 October 2020.

Bailey, Susan (2020), "Inle Lakes Boats go quiet during COVID", *Myanmore*, 14 August, https://myanmore.com/2020/08/inle-lakes-boats-go-quiet-during-covid/, accessed 29 September 2020.

Balakrishnan, Ramanathan and Burniat, Nicolas (2020), "Women can help Myanmar emerge stronger from COVID-19 if they are given a chance", *United Nations Myanmar*, 3 July, https://myanmar.un.org/en/51819-women-can-help-myanmar-emerge-stronger-covid-19-if-they-are-given-chance, accessed 30 September 2020.

Bara, Thibaut (2020), "Religious leaders unite to face pandemic in Myanmar", *UCA News*, 20 May, https://ucanews.com/news/religious-leaders-unite-to-face-pandemic-in-myanmar/88042#, accessed 7 September 2020.

Cheesman, Nick and Farrelly, Nicholas (eds) (2016), *Conflict in Myanmar – War, Politics, Religion*, Singapore: ISEAS.

China locks down city on Myanmar border over coronavirus (2020), *Medical Xpress*, 15 September, https://medicalxpress.com/news/2020-09-china-city-myanmar-border-coronavirus.html, accessed 28 September 2020.

Conflict, Health Cooperation and COVID-19 in Myanmar (2020), *International Crisis Group*, 19 May, https://crisisgroup.org/asia/south-east-asia/myanmar/b161-conflict-health-cooperation-and-covid-19-myanmar, accessed 8 October 2020.

Coronavirus – The Situation in Myanmar (2020), *Flanders Investment and Trade*, 23 September, https://flandersinvestmentandtrade.com/export/nieuws/coronavirus-situation-myanmar, accessed 28 September 2020.

COVID-19 crisis: Myanmar's garment workers at greater risk of domestic violence (2020), *Action Aid*, 1 May, https://actionaid.org/news/2020/covid-19-crisis-myanmars-garment-workers-greater-risk-domestic-violence, accessed 29 September 2020.

Diao, Xinshen, Aung, Nilar, Lwin, Wuit Yi, Zone, Phoo Pye, Nyunt, Khin Maung and Thurlow, James (2020), "Assessing the impacts of COVID-19 on Myanmar's economy: A Social Accounting Matrix (SAM) multiplier approach", Strategy Support Program Policy Note 05, *International Food Policy Research Institute (IFPRI)*, May, https://ifpri.org/publication/assesing-impacts-covid-19-myanmars-economy-social-accounting-matrix-sam-multiplier-O, accessed 29 September 2020.

Gender and COVID-19: Economic impacts in northern Karen State, Myanmar (2020), *Saferworld*, 27 September, https://safterworld.org.uk/resources/news-and-analysis/post/907-gender-and-covid-19-economic-impacts-in-northern-karen-state-myanmar-, accessed 29 September 2020.

Helping Workers affected by COVID-19 in Myanmar (2020), *People in Need*, 27 May, https://clovekvtisni.cz/en/helping-workers-affected-by-covid-19-in-myanmar-6759gp, accessed 8 October 2020.

Hodges, Charlotte (2020), "How marginalised Myanmar children are getting back to school during the pandemic", *Independent*, 4 September, https//www.independent.co.uk/news/education/back-to-school-children-myanmar-coronavirus-a969, accessed 24 August 2022.

Howell, Owen (2020), "Myanmar sees major coronavirus outbreak after a month of zero cases", *World Socialist Web Site*, 18 September, https://wsws.org/en/articles/2020/09/18/myan-s18.html, accessed 28 September 2020.

Htwe, Zaw Zaw (2020), "India-Myanmar border town opposes quarantine center amid COVID-19 fears", *The Irrawaddy*, 16 June, https://irrawaddy.com/news/burma/india-myanmar-border-town-opposes-quarantine-center-amid-covid-19-fears.html, accessed 28 September 2020.

Jacobsson, Agneta Soderberg (2020), "Myanmar: Community media stops COVID-19 panic", *IMS (International Media Support)*, 2 April, https://mediasupport.org/community-media-stops-covid-19-panic-in-myanmar/, accessed 6 October 2020.

Jie, Shan (2020), "China-Myanmar border sounds highest alarms to avoid imported COVID-19 cases", *Global Times*, 15 April, https://globaltimes.cn/content/1185702.shtml, accessed 28 September 2020.

Khan, Samia C. Akhter and Wai, Khin Myo (2020), "Can COVID-19 move Myanmar in the right direction? Perspectives on older people, mental health, and local organizations", *Elsevier Public Health Emergency Collection*, 12 June, https://ncbi.nlm.nih.gov/pmc/articles/PMC7291977/, accessed 30 September 2020.

Khine, Nwet Kay (2020), "Hitting where it hurts: Impacts of COVID-19 measures on Myanmar poor", *TNI*, 6 July, https://tni.org/en/article/hitting-where-it-hurts-impacts-of-covid-19-measures-on-myanmar-poor, accessed 30 September 2020.

Lwin, Nan (2020), "Myanmar tourism sector needs more government support during COVID-19: New survey", *The Irrawaddy*, 27 May, https://irrawaddy.com/specials/myanmar-covid-19/myanmar-tourism-sector-needs-govt-support-covid-19-new-survey.html, accessed 29 September 2020.

Lynn, Kyaw Ye (2020a), "COVID-19: Myanmar records highest single day cases", *AA*, 26 August, https://aa.com/tr/en/asia-pacific/covid-19-myanmar-records-highest-single-day-cases/1953539, accessed 28 September 2020.

Lynn, Kyaw Ye (2020b), "Myanmar's Rakhine state fears worsening virus outbreak", *Arab News*, 29 August, https://arabnews.com/node/1726231/world, accessed 8 October 2020.

Mann, Zarni and Aung, San Yamin (2020), "Myanmar's major cities to ease some COVID-19 business restrictions", *The Irrawaddy*, 14 May, https://irrawaddy.com/specials/myanmar-covid-19/myanmars-major-cities-ease-covid-19-business-restrictions.html, accessed 28 September 2020.

McCarthy, Gerard (2016), "Buddhist welfare and the limits of big 'P' politics in provincial Myanmar", in Nick Cheesman and Nicholas Farrelly (eds), *Conflict in Myanmar – War, Politics, Religion*, Singapore: ISEAS.

Myanmar: Garment workers allege factories are using COVID-19 to dismiss union members; Incl. Company responses (2020), "Business & human rights resource Centre", 12 May, https://business-humanrights.org/en/latest-news/myanmar-garment-workers-allege-factories-are-using-covid-19-to-dismiss-union-members-incl-company-responses, accessed 29 September 2020.

Myint, Lae Phyu Pya Myo (2020), "Fear of COVID-19, in art", *Myanmar Times*, 17 August, https://mmtimes.com/news/fear-covid-19-art.html, accessed 12 October 2020.

Nachemson, Andrew (2020), "Racism is fueling Myanmar's deadly second wave of COVID-19", *The Diplomat*, 11 September, https://thediplomat.com/2020/09/racism-is-fueling-myanmars-deadly-second-wave-of-covid-19/, accessed 28 September 2020.

A Nation Left Behind – Myanmar's Weaponization of COVID-19 (2020), *Progressive Voice*, June, https://progressivevoicemyanmar.org/wp-content/uploads/2020/06/Final_PV-COVID-19_Report-2020.pdf, accessed 13 October 2020.

Neranjan, Kassandra and Shetty, Sakshi (2020), "Women and COVID-19 in Myanmar", *Tea Circle*, 15 June, https://teacircleoxford.com/2020/06/15/women-and-covid-19-in-myanmar/, accessed 30 September 2020.

Newey, Sarah (2020), "A 'generational catastrophe': 24 million children will never return to school post-COVID, UN warns", *The Telegraph*, 4 August, https://telegraph.co.uk/global-health/climate-and-people/generational-catastrophe-24-million-children-will-never-return/, accessed 30 September 2020.

NGOs at the forefront of COVID-19 efforts with OCHA's pooled funds (2020), *OCHA* (United Nations Office for the Coordination of Humanitarian Affairs), 8 May, https://unocha.org/story/ngos-forefront-covid-19-efforts-ocha's-pooled-funds, accessed 8 October 2020.

Nortajuddin, Athira (2020), "Virus – Hit sectors in Myanmar", *The Asean Post*, 24 July, https://theaseanpost.com/article/virus-hit-sectors-myanmar, accessed 29 September 2020.

Onishi, Tomoya and Nitta, Yuichi (2020), "Coronavirus fears haunt Vietnam and Myanmar border towns", *Nikkei Asian Review*, 29 January, https://asia.nikkei.com/Spotlight/Coronavirus/Coronavirus-fears-haunt-Vietnam-and-Myanmar-border-towns, accessed 28 September 2020.

Oo, Phyu Phyu and Davies, Sara E. (2020), "The impact of COVID-19 on women's sexual and reproductive health and rights in Myanmar", *Griffith Asia Insights*, 24 July, https://blogs.griffith.edu.au/asiansights/the-impact-of-covid-19-on-womens-sexual-and-reproductive-health-and-rights-in-myanmar/, accessed 30 September 2020.

Oo, Zaw Naing (2020), "Myanmar residents barricade city streets as coronavirus cases rise", *Reuters*, 12 September, https://reuters.com/article/us-health-coronavirus-myanmar-idUSKBN2630QL, accessed 28 September 2020.

Paddock, Richard C. (2020), "Having brushed off Coronavirus threat, Southeast Asia begins to confront it", *The New York Times*, 17 March, https://nytimes.com/2020/03/17/world/asia/coronavirus-southeast-asia.html, accessed 7 September 2020.

Qureshi, Yasmin (2020), "Three years since the Rohingya crisis, the coronavirus is robbing refugees of hope for a brighter future", *Independent*, 25 August, https://independent.co.uk/voices/rohyngya-crisis-anniversary-coronavirus-refugees-myanmar-bangladesh-a9685906.html, accessed 30 September 2020.

Rayburn, Athena (2020), "Opinion: COVID-19 and the Rohingya refugee crisis", *Thomson Reuters Foundation*, 24 March, https://news.trust.org/item/20200324151746-iv3m4/, accessed 30 September 2020.

San, Myo Pa Pa (2020), "Myanmar's Garment sector facing implosion as orders slump with COVID-19", *The Irrawaddy*, 15 July, https://irrawaddy.com/news/burma/myanmars-garment-sector-facing-implosion-orders-slump-covid-19.html, accessed 29 September 2020.

Seinn, Kyi Kyi (2020), "The Coronavirus challenges Myanmar's transition", *United States Institute of Peace*, 26 May, https://usip.org/publications/2020/05/coronavirus-challenges-myanmars-transition, accessed 7 September 2020.

Yangon under strain as Myanmar coronavirus cases surge (2020), *Aljazeera*, 27 September, https://aljazeera.com/news/2020/9/27/yangon-under-strain-as-myanmar-coronavirus-cases-surge, accessed 28 September 2020.

15 Social Dimension of COVID-19 Outbreak in Nepal

Madhusudan Subedi and Prativa Subedi

Introduction

COVID-19 pandemic is an unprecedented health emergency of the globe. During the COVID-19 pandemic, policies and preparedness have been aimed at reducing morbidity and mortality related to infections through early diagnosis and appropriate treatment, and preventing disease transmission and spread. It has also been focused on preservation of healthcare resources and preparation for patient surge including management of essential equipment such as personal protection equipment (PPE) and ventilators, and mobilisation of human resources with due consideration on safety protocols. To tackle the COVID-19 pandemic, countries across the world have implemented a range of stringent policies, including stay-at-home "lockdowns"; school and workplace closures; cancellation of mass events and public gatherings; and restrictions on public transport (Subedi and Subedi, 2020; Rayamajhee et al., 2021). These measures were implemented in Nepal as well to slow the spread of the virus by enforcing physical distancing between people.

In Nepal, the first case of COVID-19 was officially confirmed on 23 January 2020. This is quite early as the global case of COVID-19 was also reported only a month prior to it (around the end of December, 2019). The Government of Nepal, like other countries, was in a state of confusion, Nepal being a neighbour to China (the epicentre of the disease) and India (one of the hard-hit countries by the virus), the infection curve rose steeply in Nepal too. The effect of this pandemic is undoubtedly immense but on the flip side of the coin, this pandemic has also been an eye-opener to the weaknesses in the current healthcare system; and the challenges coming forth if taken as a lesson, can open a window to a huge set of opportunities (Subedi and Subedi, 2020; Marahatta and Paudel, 2020).

Analytical Framework

The COVID-19 pandemic and its response have created various challenges in Nepal. The pandemic has highly impacted the sectors of health,

DOI: 10.4324/9781003282815-20

education, economy, tourism, transport, and remittance. The framework of analysis of this chapter focuses on two main domains – governance and service delivery. Under the governance domain, leadership, coordination at different levels of government, policy and legal framework, coordination and collaboration, financing, transparency, and accountability issues are focused. The service delivery theme covers quarantine management, case identification and management, testing and isolation, contact tracing, diagnosis and case management, transportation management, lockdown and travel restriction, delivery of essential services, human resources, communication and coordination supplies and logistics management, infrastructure, community engagement, dead body management, and vaccination.

The first author had frequent meetings and discussions with authorities of the Ministry of Health and Population, Nepal Health Research Council, Mayors of various municipalities and the doctors of various hospitals who were mainly focused on the treatment of COVID-19 patients. Furthermore, the teaching hospital of the Patan Academy of Health Sciences where the first author is the Chair of the Department of Community Health Sciences and Coordinator of the School of Public Health had to play an important role for the prevention and control of COVID-19. As a medical officer, the second author has played an important role for the implementation of the government policies and guidelines to control the infections and provide hospital services for the infected persons. The experiences of both the authors have been very useful to write this chapter.

Activities Carried by the Government of Nepal

The Government of Nepal declared a nationwide lockdown on 24 March 2020 and implemented the general guidelines on how to prevent the spread of the virus including closing of schools and colleges, restaurants and bars, and closing of public services and provisioning lockdown. The pandemic disrupted its health, economy, education, society, and culture.

On a macro scale, mitigation strategies such as "physical distancing" and "lockdown" entailed high cost for the national and household economy. Daily wage workers, travel and tourism sector, movie industry, and hotels were among the most hard-hit sectors during the pandemic (UNDP, 2020). On the other hand, there has been a significant surge in online business and service delivery mechanisms that has in a way boosted entrepreneurship and innovation. There has also been a shift of paradigm from traditional lecture method to virtual classes and e-learning (Paudel, 2021).

On a micro scale, panic and fear increased. There has been a substantial rise in mental health illness like anxiety and depression, and suicide rates have increased after the COVID-19 pandemic (Pokhrel et al., 2020). This could be attributed to factors like loss of job, disruption and delay in academic sessions, rise in intimate partner violence, and physical distancing leading to decreased social support from peers and loved ones.

The Government of Nepal developed numerous policies, guidelines and directives for the control of the disease since the identification of the first case of COVID-19 in Nepal. Due to the scarcity of masks, sanitisers, and PPEs and blockade of supply from outside, a lot of organisations and hospitals started producing them locally. Despite the guidelines from the government about physical distancing and hygiene measures, the implementation part was equally challenging. Owing to the low literacy level, many people, especially in the rural areas, were not aware of the importance of such measures. At the same time, many did not know the right technique to follow such measures (proper way of using masks and sanitisers). Thus, for the better and easy dissemination of this information, government collaborated with the leading mobile network companies of Nepal.

Governance

Governance is important for effective regulation, attention to the system design, and accountability. Leadership provides the basis for overall policy regulation (WHO, 2010). Nepal adopted a federal democratic structure in 2017 and currently has seven provinces. At the beginning, the Government of Nepal designated three public hospitals located in Kathmandu, the capital city of Nepal, for the treatment of COVID-19 cases. Later with the rise in case load, all the central hospitals, provincial hospitals, medical colleges, academic institutions, and hub-hospitals were designated for its treatment. A high-level coordination committee for COVID-19 prevention and control in Nepal was formed under the coordination of honourable deputy prime minister and defence minister on 1 March 2020. The committee included Ministry of Health and Population, Ministry of Home Affairs, Ministry of Foreign Affairs, Ministry of Finance, Tourism and Civil Aviation, Ministry of Culture, Ministry of Urban Development, Nepal Army, Nepal Police, and Armed Police Force (MoHP, 2021). This committee has been chaired by the deputy prime minister and restructured as the Corona Crisis Management Center (CCMC). Furthermore, to make this more effective, district level crisis management centres (DCMC) were also established.

Leadership and governance in building health system for COVID-19 response were facilitated by the formation of District CCMC in each district. The district CCMC was responsible for making major decisions related to COVID-19 response and crisis in the district. The members of CCMC were political leaders, bureaucrats, and some medical experts. The committee did not realise the importance of the disciplines like public health and social sciences (Nepal Health Research Council, 2020). Due to intra-party conflict among the members of the ruling party, leadership, and governance were criticised by the academia and civil society members (Rai, 2020).

For case investigation and contract tracing, most of the cases were from the local levels, so all the responsibility was under the local government. Therefore, the major work was to be done by the local government, and the health ministry was supposed to support the local government and strengthen them by providing them the required training, technical support, equipment, and funds.

The Ministry of Social Development and Province Health Directorate were leading the COVID-19 management under the direct involvement of the Chief Minister and other line Ministers in coordination with local governments. While clear direction, policy choices, and central management of the crisis are paramount, delivery mainly occurred at the provincial and local levels. Local government established quarantine facilities and isolation centres and the necessary resources for the target population (Gautam, 2020). However, there was inadequate intersectoral coordination and the lack of clarity in the roles of the three tiers of government (MoHP, 2021).

Due to the open border system between India and Nepal, many migrant workers returned to Nepal due to COVID-19 and lockdown imposed by the Government of India. The local government of bordering districts faced challenges to manage quarantine and isolation centres in the initial phase (Democracy Resource Center, 2020). Furthermore, the quality of the quarantines and isolation centres was compromised due to inadequate financial, technical, and human resources available at the local level (Nepal Health Research Council, 2020).

The Ministry of Health and Population developed plans and policies. There was lack of legal framework to implement the plan and policies issued at the local level. Additionally, all the plans, policies, and the guidelines were difficult to follow in the local context as it was not always possible to meet all the standards (MoHP, 2021). In such cases, some of the local governments also formulated their own policies and programmes for effective management of the COVID-19 pandemic such as quarantine and isolation centre management, treatment, and distribution of relief material (Nepal Health Research Council, 2020).

Coronavirus is a novel virus, and little was known about it. New information unfolded with continuous research. Thus, the guidelines of WHO also changed frequently, thereby subsequently changing the national policies too. For example, the initial discharge criteria for infected patients required two negative RT-PCR test results (WHO, 2020). Later, repeat PCR was considered unnecessary and patients could be discharged from isolation after ten days (for asymptomatic cases) and ten days after symptom onset, plus at least three additional days without symptoms (for symptomatic cases). Likewise, initial recommendation was health facility-based isolation strictly for all positive cases. The policy later shifted to home isolation for asymptomatic and mild cases (MoHP, 2021). Frequent change in policies and guidelines increased the confusion of people and the health workers working at the periphery levels and also decreased public trust towards the government (Nepal Health Research Council, 2020).

The policy of the Government of Nepal has clearly mentioned that collaboration with public, non-governmental organisations, private sectors, development partners, academia, and professional societies will be promoted for capacity building, logistic supplies, expansion, and upgradation of hospital infrastructure, supply chain management, community engagement and risk communication, human resource mobilisation and capacity building, community-based risk mapping, referral services including ambulance services, and management of quarantine where necessary. However, in practice, coordination among the various stakeholders was very low (see Rayamajhee et al., 2021).

The Ministry of Health and Population had signed a memorandum of understanding for collaboration with hotels and restaurants, transportation, and private hospitals to provide services based on approved cost reimbursement modality. However, the poor and the marginalised who had lost their jobs in the current place of work and wanted to return from the gulf countries were struggling to manage airfare and quarantine costs (Nepali Times, 2020).

Along with coordination and collaboration with the private sector, there was need to involve academicians for research purposes, as the research produced by academicians can serve as an authentic source of information and can be helpful in generating evidence for policy-making purpose. However, the government hardly took advice from the academia, and could not utilise the knowledge and skills of bio-medical, public health, and social scientists who could have given better advice during the pandemic (Nepal Health Research Council, 2020).

The Nepal government partnered with international humanitarian assistance and formulated a high-level coordination mechanism to combat COVID-19 disease in Nepal. The financing of COVID-19 response was done through budgetary support from provincial level and reallocating development budget at local level. The development budget was diverted to the Corona crisis funds for effective COVID-19 response. The federal government has been financing the provincial and local governments for quarantine management, logistic management, and upgrading of health facility. The local government played an important role in preparation of quarantine and isolation centres and management (Adhikari and Budhathoki, 2020). The representatives of the local government were found to be more responsive (Adhikari et al., 2021). Some municipalities had an up-to-date record of total infected cases, recovered cases, the number of deaths, people currently in quarantine and admitted in hospital, total expenses for the COVID-19 control, and management. The local leaderships were found to be accountable towards their citizens and records were transparent.

Several challenges were faced by the local governments in their work and efforts to control and prevent the spread of COVID-19. These challenges were related to the lack of priority given to the health sector by the three levels of government, poor coordination in the decisions taken by the federal and provincial governments to prevent and control the spread of

COVID-19, cure the coronavirus infected persons and issues related to the adjustment of health workforce (Democracy Resource Center, 2020).

In March 2020, the Government of Nepal had given the responsibility of managing the bodies of those who died of COVID-19 to the Nepal Army. The army kept the detail records of each body managed. Some journalists found that the daily update of the death cases by the Ministry of Health and Population due to COVID-19 and the actual dead body managed by the Nepal Army did not match (Poudel, 2020). Initially, the government ignored this issue and indicated that there was no such discrepancy. Later, after several evidences presented in daily newspapers, the ministry formed a committee to investigate the variation in data on the deaths. The committee found that the number of people who died from the virus were more than the reported cases by the ministry (MoHP, 2021). More than one-fourth of the total deaths were found to be under-reported. The vast discrepancies in the data of the death cases between the Health Ministry and the Nepal Army showed the poor level of coordination among different government agencies during the pandemic.

Public health depends on people's participation, and this is even truer during the pandemic. Trust in the government and health authorities is a necessary condition for people to abide by restrictive rules. Low trust in authorities led to widespread conspiracy theory. Political contradictions within the ruling party and frequent change of guidelines have been questioned by the opposition party leaders and civil society members. Likewise, the hefty budget expenditure that was attributed to COVID-19 management by the government was also questioned by the opposition party and civil society members (Ganguly, 2020). For transparency and accountability, all the information such as details of expenses and details of patient's type were expected to be transparent and easily accessible to public. Such practice would help trusting the state mechanism.

Service Delivery

Strengthening service delivery is a crucial function of a health system. Important guidelines are prepared for maintaining essential health services during the public health pandemic. The Government of Nepal recommended use of facemasks by the public when in confined public spaces, public transport, in hospitals and maintain physical distancing. The government used media to promote the policy and exhibit its seriousness on the issue. The media briefing was focused on the number of infected cases and deaths. However, the government did not have any policy of providing facemasks for those who could not pay for it. Likewise, the government introduced a policy of public transport safety measures to be taken including limiting the number of passengers in a vehicle and allowing odd and even number plate vehicles to run alternately but it was not implemented seriously (Shrestha, 2020).

All the quarantine centres were primarily managed by the local government with partial involvement of private organisations. Various committees were formed for handling various issues including logistics arrangement monitoring and supervision of day-to-day activities related to quarantine.

Initially, there were only few quarantine centres; therefore, the standards were maintained. But eventually, as the number of cases rose rapidly and many of the health workers also got infected, the exhaustion of resources (including human resource) and lack of adequate budget led to poor logistic management, inadequate space for the people in quarantine, inadequate water, poor hygiene and sanitation facilities, and inadequate healthcare support for the infected ones (Nepal Health Research Council, 2020).

The District Public Health Officer was the main stakeholder for the establishment and management of quarantine in all districts. Likewise, federal and provincial governments provided financial support for the establishment and management of quarantine (MoHP, 2021). The Nepal police provided security support for public quarantine, and health workers were involved in managing the facilities. In many quarantine centres, there were problems of electricity, water, toilet facility, and waste management (Democracy Resource Center, 2020). Gradually the quarantine conditions were improved and managed with the support of the provincial and local government.

Although quarantine centres at the community level were managed by local governments, most of the local level and provincial stakeholders were found in less compliance with the quarantine management guidelines and basic criteria that were issued by the federal government (Nepal Health Research Council, 2020). They focused on basic needs like food, beds, water, light, toilets, bathrooms, and Internet. Due to the inadequate knowledge on quarantine management and constraints of resource and time, most of the quarantine centres were less friendly in preventing and controlling the COVID-19 transmission.

Maintaining quarantine facilities was a little bit difficult in places due to late reporting of PCR results. It was difficult to segregate the isolation rooms for the positive ones and suspected cases awaited results owing to financial and resource constraints. While accommodating the suspects with the general patients (COVID negative) imposed a risk to the general patients if they turned out to be positive, accommodating the suspects with infected ones (COVID positive) would be potentially risky to them if they turned out negative. This problem was especially paramount in the areas where there was a surge of patients with acute respiratory infections and asthma. It was difficult to distinguish clinically if the exacerbation was due to COVID infection. Since PCR testing and reporting took time, it was difficult to adjust and manage the patients in the period in between (MoHP, 2021).

The major challenges faced regarding the management of quarantine facilities were unavailability of adequate quarantine centres, sharing common rooms and toilets, convincing people to follow quarantine guidelines and safety precautions, decrease immunity of the people in quarantine due to lack of nutrition and daily increment of COVID-19 positive cases. Location of the quarantine was also a challenging factor. Due to the establishment of quarantine centres in human settlement areas, people in some municipalities were making complaints, which was difficult to manage (Nepal Health Research Council, 2020). Initially, as the academic classes were halted to abide by the physical distancing norms, schools and colleges were designated as quarantine and isolation centres. Later when the academic sessions resumed, it was difficult to manage the quarantine and isolation centres. Additionally, excessive fear among people and health workers created more havoc during the initial days (Singh and Subedi, 2020). The quality of quarantine was improved but they still did not fully comply with the guidelines issued by the federal government.

Lack of polymerase chain reaction (PCR) testing capacity during the early days was a big challenge, which led to difficulty in testing. After the testing capacity was improved, case identification became relatively easier. There was good provision of virus collection and transport kits, swab collection and testing materials in Kathmandu Valley and other urban areas. However, many districts still have to wait for 4–5 days to get PRC test results.

In the initial days, where PCR facility had not been well expanded, government decided to increase Rapid Diagnostic Testing (RDT) tests as much as possible as a screening tool for COVID-19. A large number of RDT kits were thus bought in different districts. However, within a short span of time, a new guideline was put forth, which considered RDT as an unnecessary and unreliable screening test. This created a state of confusion and incredibility among the general public towards the government policy.

Active participation of the local governments and health facilities was found in case identification and management. In some areas, infected people faced some security issues because some of the community/people intentionally tortured the infected people and their families as well (Singh and Subedi, 2020).

Local- and district-level health facilities collected swabs of suspected people, which were sent to the nearest laboratories. Transportation issue was a major challenge, especially in the hilly and mountain areas where it took hours or even a day to transport the collected swab to the nearest laboratory. This increased the expenditure on transport on one hand and increased the chances of false negative results on the other. Even though the PCR test was done as per the protocol set by the government, still there was delay in the reporting of the test results.

As the cases were increasing day by day, there were more problems in providing services to the people, such as problems in availability of beds, intensive care units, oxygen, and ventilators in the COVID-19-dedicated hospitals. In such cases, the patients and their family members faced problems in receiving free treatment. Those who were able to afford the care went and admitted themselves and their families in private hospitals. The poor and the marginalised COVID-19 positive patients stayed at home (Singh et al., 2021).

Additionally, people were unable to get treatment in time due to inadequate human resources and inadequately trained health workers. The reason being, most of the health workers got infection and they had to isolate themselves or stay in quarantine (MoHP, 2021). All the resources supplied were not provided as per demand either from the province or from the federal government (Nepal Health Research Council, 2020).

While COVID-19 had impacted the lives of all, health workers had to face its double brunt. Firstly, they had to risk their lives and also the lives of their family while working in the diagnosis and management of infected patients (Singh et al., 2021). But on top of that, instead of appreciating and acknowledging their contribution, the public treated them with stigma and discrimination. Health workers were rejected residence in many of the houses and hotels. In contrary to other countries, where health workers were provided special incentives and facilities while combating the pandemic, the health workers in Nepal did not even receive the risk allowance that they were promised by the government at many places (Tiwari, 2021). This kind of situation decreased their morale and motivation to serve at the time of crisis (Baral, 2021).

The gender implications of COVID-19 cannot be denied, with women being disproportionately affected. Loss of job, increased burden of household work, and increased gender-based violence have significantly affected the psychological and reproductive health of women during the pandemic (Nepal Research Institute and CARE Nepal, 2020).

For proper testing of the cases, swabs were collected from both the suspect and the confirmed cases so that it would help in the identification of the cases. Along with the laboratory workers, medical officers were also involved in swab collection. However, there was problem in swab collection due to unavailability of equipment, testing kits, and PPEs.

The cost of test was high in the initial stage of the pandemic, which came down in subsequent days. Few people who were aware of COVID symptoms and could afford the cost were voluntarily getting themselves tested. But those not meeting the testing criteria of the government and not being able to afford to get tested in private remained untested, which clearly shows that the number of reported cases is just the tip of the iceberg.

Initially, the Government of Nepal brought the provision of insurance system for COVID-19 patients that would provide a reimbursement of up to NPR 100,000 in the management of COVID patients. When the Coronavirus insurance scheme was introduced in April 2020, Nepal had very few cases. Various private insurance companies launched their schemes as a good business. There was an arrangement for the insured to get the full amount immediately after being diagnosed positive. As the number of positive cases rose steeply and the hospital started getting full, the companies were reluctant to pay stating lack of required documents and other reasons.

Later they stopped promoting their insurance package (Banskota, 2020). The government could not sustain the insurance programme and changed the criteria of COVID-19 insurance. The infected person would get only NPR 25,000, and the remaining amount would be provided on the basis of the hospital treatment bill (Banskota, 2020).

Every municipality had made the provisions of isolation centres. Isolation centres were prepared with the active involvement of local leaders, local, provincial, and federal government, Nepal Red Cross Society, Nepal Army, Nepal Police, and local organisations. Treatment facilities were provided in isolation centres. Along with this, home isolation centres were also promoted. Although home isolation centres were promoted, it was quite difficult to manage the minimum standards and rules for those who live in slum areas or in rented rooms. Some municipalities had taken such issue seriously and managed them in community isolation centre. Others could not manage. Those who were staying in rented rooms faced challenges to manage themselves in home isolation. They had to share room with family members and toilet with other members staying in the same house. Furthermore, they also faced stigma, exclusion, and discrimination in the community (Democracy resource Center, 2020).

Contact tracing is one of the indicators to identify the cases. There is the prescribed guideline of WHO for case investigation and contact tracing (CICT), and the same guidelines are adopted in the context of Nepal too. Epidemiology and Disease Control Division (EDCD) is the main organisation currently working in contact tracing. The contact tracing guideline has mentioned the need to form CICT teams in each local level in coordination with the CICT coordinator of the district. Likewise, the province has formed the required number of CICT team members in each local level. Initially, when there were few reported positive cases, the teams were active through telephone calls.

Contact tracing was not a problem in the beginning because most of the cases were detected in quarantine facilities. The health workers however had to face problem in contact tracing because some people who were infected did not give their contact numbers correctly. This might be due to the fear of stigma and discrimination at the community level. Later as cases started to be seen in the community, contact tracing although required had not been prioritised well mainly because of two reasons: lack of adequate human resources/testing kits and lack of commitment of the government. The entire contact tracing was done by the government in the initial stage through mobilisation of their health workers as it was easy because of less number of cases (MoHP, 2021). The Government of Nepal did not have adequate plan for contact tracing; hence, it was stopped without any specific reasons.

The Ministry of Health and Population on 12 May 2020 directed the local governments to form Case Investigation and Contact Tracing Team (CICTT) consisting of public health officers with at least Bachelor's Degree in Public Health and nurses and lab technicians to conduct contract tracing and investigation at every local level. Most of the local levels did not have public health officers with public health degree. The ones who were in government jobs prior to implementation of federal set-up are now designated at federal and provincial levels. Even in this, there was debate over these decisions as Community Medicine Assistants (CMAs) who were working at the local level thought that someone is going to replace them. Due to high population density in urban areas, it was difficult for CICT teams to function properly without a clear activity plan.

The transportation of COVID-19 patients was done by ambulance drivers who were given proper PPE. Private vehicles and other public transport vehicles were not allowed to carry COVID patients. Most of the places had ambulances available for 24 hours. Along with the government institutions, the municipalities, other institutions, and organisations were active locally to make the ambulance service available. However, not all the standard criteria were met. Though the government had a clear travel guideline, the guidelines for transportation management had not been followed. Also, the ambulance drivers were not aware of guidelines.

Lockdown and travel restrictions declared by the Nepal government became one of the effective interventions to control the transmission of COVID-19. However, its impacts were multifold and especially the impact on the economy was highly significant (Baniya et al., 2020). In a country like Nepal, where people have meagre savings and need to work daily to make their ends meet, people could hardly afford to stay at home for months. Due to lockdown, the poor and marginalised section of the population at risk could not get daily wages work and faced difficulty to feed their family members (Gautam, 2020). A survey conducted by the International Labour Organization has shown that between 1.6 million and 2 million people in Nepal either lost their job or reduced working hours resulting in decreased wages (ILO, 2020). Government employees received their salary even during the lockdown but the employees in most of the private sectors were forced to live on an unpaid leave. Social isolation and financial pressure created mental stress especially for economically poor families. Further, the suicide cases in Nepal also increased (Himalayan Climate Initiative, 2021).

The Ministry of Federal Affair and General Administration issued a circular to all local governments to provide necessary relief material to families and persons that were in need of special support. In order to select needy persons, many local governments conducted rapid need assessment but the implementation to reach relief material to unreached was found to be unjust and unfair (Gautam, 2020).

The phrase "social distancing" used by the western scholars was understood differently in the Nepali context. "Social distancing" could not emphasise adequately the distance to be maintained from one individual to another. Rather, some people understood the possibility of infection through the use of technology like the mobile phone or from all kinds of health workers. Health workers were publicly humiliated and threatened by landlords and neighbours who suspect them of being carriers of the virus. They were forced to isolate within hospital boundary (Himalayan Climate Initiative, 2021).

The lockdown lasted for a certain period but when it was ending, proper and adequate precautions were not taken. Due to the haphazard end of the lockdown, most of the public vehicles were operated without taking proper measures to prevent COVID-19. The unplanned ending of the lockdown and travel restrictions washed away all the measures taken during the lockdown which in turn resulted in the tremendous increase in positive cases. Lockdown was done for preventing the mobility of transmission and for controlling the spread of the disease but it also affected the socio-economic life of the people at the same time. That's why it could not be imposed for a long period of time.

The lockdown was effective due to the efforts of the elected representatives and the administration in the initial days. People would comply with the lockdown regulations either because they were aware and scared that the disease would spread in the community or were scared of the security maintained by the police.

Nepali people who were working in India lost their jobs in India due to COVID-19, and came to Nepal through prohibited routes rather than through the border check posts and thus could not be screened for quarantine. This was a great challenge due to which cases have increased. Those who came through the provisioned border were kept in quarantine, but the quarantine facility was mismanaged. Powerful people misusing the vehicle travel pass were common. The important point about the lockdown was that it was unable to halt the movement of people. There was considerable movement of people on foot even during the lockdown especially those returning home and at night. Strict provision of lockdown was not made. Lack of support and coordination was the cause for the unsuccessful lockdown. The travel restrictions were followed as per protocol in the beginning but with the increasing number of cases, local people got infected as well which decreased the fear of COVID-19 in people. Henceforth, they didn't follow the rules of lockdown properly, thereby making it even more challenging.

Nepal Army is responsible for managing dead bodies in collaboration with the local government. Initially family members were not allowed to see the dead body (deceased) person. Family members were unable to pay their respects and follow their own cultural practices. Later, the policy was changed with the nearest family members given the permission to see the dead body and pay respect by maintaining the distance using preventive measures (Kamat, 2020).

Conclusion

Nepal's public health system is underfunded. The current public health policy and healthcare systems are inadequate to deal with the challenges. The role of local government, healthcare workers, and security persons for the control of transmission of COVID-19 was very important. The key players for policy-making were a handful of medical experts and politicians. Social scientists, public health professionals, and civil society members have a responsibility to draw the attention of political leaders to prevent and control pandemic. The Government of Nepal has focused its policy on hospital care but COVID-19 pandemic has economic, social, and cultural consequences. These consequences are not adequately recognised as part of policy discussion. It requires multi-disciplinary collaboration. The interplay between health, technology, and socio-political economy in a more holistic way should be discovered and managed when dealing with new emerging infections. The possibility for more dangerous pandemics in the future is high. The Government of Nepal should be ready to save lives and livelihoods of people.

References

Adhikari, B. and Budhathoki, S. S. (2020), "Silver-lining in the time of Mayhem: The role of local governments of Nepal during the COVID-19 pandemic", *JNMA: Journal of the Nepal Medical Association*, 58(231), 960.

Adhikary, P., Balen, J., Gautam, S., Ghimire, S., Karki, J. K., Lee, A., . . . Van Teijlingen, E. (2021), "COVID-19 pandemic in Nepal: Emerging evidence on the effectiveness of action by, and cooperation between, different levels of government in a federal system", *Journal of Karnali Academy of Health Sciences*, 3(3), 1–11.

Baniya, J., Bhattarai, S., Pradhan, V. and Thapa, B. J. (2020), "Visibility of invisible: Covid-19 and Nepal-India Migration", *Tribhuvan University Journal*, 101–114.

Banskota, R. (2020), "Nepal tries to ensure COVID-19 insurance", *Nepali Times*. 12 October, www.nepalitimes.com/latest/nepal-tries-to-ensure-covid-19-insurance/.

Baral, P. (2021), "Health workers deprived of risk allowance in Baglung", *The Kathmandu Post*. 5 April, https://kathmandupost.com/gandaki-province/2021/04/05/health-workers-deprived-of-risk-allowance-in-baglung.

Democracy Resource Center (2020), *Role of Local Governments in COVID-19 Prevention and Quarantine Management*, Kathmandu, Nepal: Democracy Resource Center.

Ganguly, Meenakshi (2020), "Don't let Nepal's COVID-19 relief be squandered", *Human Right Watch*, 16 April, www.cipe.org/resources/stalling-the-pandemic-of-corruption/.

Gautam, D. (2020), *The COVID-19 Crisis in Nepal: Coping Crackdown Challenges*, Kathmandu: National Disaster Risk Reduction Centre.

Himalayan Climate Initiative (2021), "COVID-19 & the new normal for women in the economy in Nepal", https://asiafoundation.org/wp-content/uploads/2021/03/Covid-19-The-New-Normal-for-Women-in-the-Economy-in-Nepal.pdf.

ILO (2020), "COVID-19 labour market impact in Nepal", www.ilo.org/wcmsp5/groups/public/ – asia/ – ro-bangkok/ – ilo-kathmandu/documents/briefingnote/wcms_745439.pdf.

Kamat, R. K. (2020), "Protocol for disposal of COVID dead changed", *The Himalayan*, 19 October, https://thehimalayantimes.com/nepal/protocol-for-disposal-of-covid-dead-changed.

Marahatta, S. B. and Paudel, S. (2020), "Tackling COVID-19 in Nepal: Opportunities and challenges", *Journal of Karnali Academy of Health Sciences*, 3.

MoHP (2021), *Responding to COVID-19: Health Sector Preparedness, Response and Lessons Learnt*, Kathmandu: Ministry of Health and Population.

Nepal Health Research Council (2020), *Rapid Assessment of COVID-19 Related Policy Audit in Nepal*, Kathmandu: Nepal Health Research Council.

Nepal Research Institute and CARE Nepal (2020), *Rapid Gender Analysis Report on COVID-19 Nepal, 2020*, Lalitpur: CARE Nepal.

Nepali Times (2020), "Nepali workers stuck in no-man's land", *Nepali Times*, 19 September, www.nepalitimes.com/here-now/nepali-workers-stuck-in-no-mans-land/.

Paudel, P. (2021), "Online education: Benefits, challenges and strategies during and after COVID-19 in higher education", *International Journal on Studies in Education*, 3(2), 70–85.

Pokhrel, S., Sedhai, Y. R. and Atreya, A. (2020), "An increase in suicides amidst the coronavirus disease 2019 pandemic in Nepal", *Medicine, Science and the Law*, 0025802420966501.

Poudel, A. (2020), "Number of COVID-19 deaths far higher than what the government claims, officials say", *The Kathmandu Post*, 18 November, https://kathmandupost.com/health/2020/11/18/number-of-covid-19-deaths-far-higher-than-what-the-government-claims-officials-say.

Rai, S. (2020), "Nepal ruling party feud affecting COVID-19 response", *Nepali Times*, 10 July, www.nepalitimes.com/here-now/nepal-ruling-party-feud-affecting-covid-19-response/.

Rayamajhee, B., Pokhrel, A., Syangtan, G., Khadka, S., Lama, B., Rawal, L. B., . . . Yadav, U. N. (2021), "How well the government of Nepal is responding to COVID-19? An experience from a resource-limited country to confront unprecedented pandemic", *Frontiers in Public Health*, 9, 85.

Shrestha, S. (2020), "Public transport health safety a must", *The Rising Nepal*, 23 October, https://risingnepaldaily.com/detour/public-transport-health-safety-a-must.

Singh, D. R. and Subedi, M. (2020), "COVID-19 and stigma: Social discrimination towards frontline healthcare providers and COVID-19 recovered patients in Nepal", *Asian Journal of Psychiatry*, 53, 102222.

Singh, D. R., Sunuwar, D. R., Shah, S. K., Karki, K., Sah, L. K., Adhikari, B. and Sah, R. K. (2021), "Impact of COVID-19 on health services utilization in Province-2 of Nepal: A qualitative study among community members and stakeholders", *BMC Health Services Research*, 21(1), 1–14.

Subedi, M. and Subedi, P. (2020), "Lesson from COVID-19: Restructuring the current health system and policies in Nepal", *Applied Science and Technology Annals*, 1(1), 183–186.

Tiwari, A. (2021), "Health workers deprived of risk allowance warn of halting service", *The Kathmandu Post*, 24 January, https://kathmandupost.com/province-no-3/2021/01/24/frontline-workers-deprived-of-covid-19-risk-allowance-warn-to-halt-service.

UNDP (2020), *Rapid Assessment of Socio-economic Impact of COVID-19 in Nepal*, Lalitpur, Nepal: United Nations Development Programme.

World Health Organization (2010), *Monitoring the Building Blocks of Health Systems: A Handbook of Indicators and Their Measurement Strategies*, Geneva: World Health Organization.

World Health Organization (2020), "Criteria for releasing COVID-19 patients from isolation: Scientific brief", www.who.int/news-room/commentaries/detail/criteria-for-releasing-covid-19-patients-from-isolation.

16 The Crown and the Corona

A Close-up on Bhutan's Successful COVID Response Led by the King

Sonam Kinga

Introduction

When Mrs. Kanni Wignaraja, the UN Assistant Secretary General, met Dr. Lotay Tshering, Bhutan's Prime Minister, in Thimphu on 12 March 2021, she stated, "If only there were 193 avatars of His Majesty The King of Bhutan, the world would be a much better place" (Chencho, 2021). Her reference was to leaders of 193 UN members and in the context of Bhutan's successful response to the pandemic. Bert Hewitt, a 76-year-old American tourist had become Bhutan's first positive case on 5 March 2020 (Office of the Prime Minister and Cabinet, 2020). Exactly a year later, there were 867 confirmed cases but only one death with 866 recoveries.

Bhutan's remarkable success in the fight against the pandemic has earned her international accolade. As early as 18 May 2020, Baroness Buscombe, the UK Under-Secretary of State for Works and Pensions stated in the House of Lords during a session on "COVID-19: International Response" thus: "My Lords, I pay tribute to the King of Bhutan and his people for their amazing fortitude and smart response to the virus" (Ugyen Penjore, 2020). Krishna (2020) wrote, "Landlocked Bhutan has managed to keep its Coronavirus cases contained so far". News reports and articles have pointed out the central role played by the King of Bhutan. Turner (2020) wrote, "The leadership triumvirate of the Prime Minister, Health Minister and King played a major role in this success story".

Likewise, Drexler wrote

> Bhutan had trusted, smart, and hands-on direction from its king, whose moral authority carries great weight. He explicitly told government leaders that even one death from COVID-19 would be too much for a small nation that regards itself as a family, pressed officials for detailed plans covering every possible pandemic scenario, and made multiple trips to the front lines, encouraging health workers, volunteers, and others.
>
> (Drexler, 2021)

DOI: 10.4324/9781003282815-21

Kugelman (2021) reiterated similar arguments in a news story he wrote for Arab News. CNN's Zakaria (2021) attributed strong leadership besides rapid early actions and stringent public health response: "The King also played an active role, visiting the frontlines and fostering a sense of cohesion".

Bhutan's success is indeed an outcome of the unified response of multiple actors including the government, monastic bodies, civil society, volunteers, and people from all walks of life. But this was possible due to the leadership of the King.

In this paper, I will discuss the key directions and strategic interventions which he provided by framing them within Bhutan's geo-political context and cultural perspective of Buddhist kingship, which are either missing or inadequate in these journalistic accounts. My approach is ethnographic drawing from my engagement as a member of a special Task Force and also from my experiences of having served as a front-liner.

The Geo-Political Context

In order to appreciate the content, scale, and diversity of responses, it is necessary to contextualise them within Bhutan's overall geo-politics and political economy. Bhutan is small and land-locked, surrounded by India and China. The geographic, demographic, economic, and military sizes of the two neighbours and the nature of their relationship further exacerbate the Bhutanese perception, experience, and consciousness of smallness as well as vulnerability.

In the Bhutanese national psyche and historical consciousness, the threat perception of Coronavirus cannot be isolated from the larger discourse of national security. The King shared to members of the Special Task Force after the first lockdown in August 2020 about what the fourth King said concerning the pandemic; "I never thought that your generation will have to fight a war. But the pandemic is your war. You are fighting an invisible enemy". He stated during a televised address on 10 April 2020 that "ensuring national security is of paramount importance, especially in these uncertain times" (Bhutan Broadcasting Corporation [BBS], 2020 a). During another address on 12 April 2020, he said, "the possible focus of the world will be on security" during the pandemic. On 23 June 2020, he shared to a large audience that the pandemic can disrupt our stability and survival as a nation. In another address on 12 September 2020, he said that "[t]he enemy that we are confronting is invisible" (BBS, 2020 b).

During the National Day Address on 17 December 2020, he stated that "we will make sure we are victorious in the present battle" (His Majesty King Jigme Khesar Namgyel, 2020, 22.03). These statements underscore the fact that the pandemic continues to be perceived from Bhutan's national security perspective within the geo-political context. Observers of Bhutan also share similar perspective. By 9 April 2021, Bhutan ranked No.1 in terms of the share of population (61.4%) who received at least one dose of COVID vaccine.[1] The free doses of 550,000 AstraZeneca provided by the Government of India is seen as part of vaccine diplomacy to counter Chinese influence in the region. An analyst commented that

> New Delhi has made Bhutan a major target of its vaccine diplomacy . . . This effort may be grounded in humanitarian concerns, but it's also a way to consolidate Indian influence at a moment when China's footprint is deepening around the region.
>
> (Wallen, 2021)

Patient Zero

When Bert Hewitt became Bhutan's first confirmed case, the King, the prime minister, the health minister, and a host of officials remained awake monitoring his situation throughout the night (Slater, 2020). As news broke the following morning, the whole country was in prayers. People sent him letters and flowers.

At the King's command, he was moved to the VIP room of the hospital. The King chose a doctor to attend to him and also sent him a set of silk pyjamas. A new TV set was also installed in his room. The King's personal care and attention gave him immense psychological boost (Yonten Tshedup, 2021). A few weeks later, he was evacuated. The US Secretary of State Mike Pompeo praised the evacuation exercise as he expected the patient to die. Despite having many co-morbidity conditions, the patient recovered (Slater, 2020).

Hewitt shared a message on the King's birthday on 21 February 2021. "I'd like to wish His Majesty a very happy birthday, and would like to thank him personally for his involvement and kindness" and

> To the people of Bhutan, I'd like to say thank you for the cards and flowers you sent me in the hospital. You could so easily have thought of me as harbinger of disease, but instead, you all expressed concern for the welfare of a complete stranger.
>
> (Younten Tshedup, 2021)

The Bodhisattva Vow

At 9:15 p.m. on 9 March 2020, the King was addressing the COVID Task Force of the southern district of Samtse. Owing to the urgency of the situation and worsening threat perception, he had left behind his queen, Her Majesty Jetsun Pema Wangchuck, who was soon expecting the birth of a prince.

He said that Bhutan simply cannot waste time and must prepare for worst-case scenarios. He was deeply worried about the pandemic situation unfolding particularly in the neighbourhood. His thoughts were with the

Bhutanese working and studying abroad who may be exposed to the virus. The danger of cross-border transmission, which would trigger a local transmission, was high. "Our country cannot take this lightly. Don't wait for orders from Thimphu". He encouraged all protocols to be put in place and test them. I can never forget what he said next. "Don't spread panic to the people. Let us worry and panic so that our people can sleep better!" (personal notes, 9 March 2020). In another audience in Thimphu soon after, he said that he would not allow a single Bhutanese to succumb to COVID-19.

On hearing these words, what came to my mind were the stories of the legendary vows of Bodhisattvas. They commit to keep working until samsara is emptied of sentient beings and achieve liberation. The essential quality of Boddhisattvas and their vows is unqualified compassion and courage. In order to understand the centrality of the King in the fight against COVID, it must also be seen within the framework of Buddhist kingship of a Bodhisattva ideal driven by the quality of compassion and courage. As the Indian ambassador to Bhutan Ruchira Kamboj put it, "His Majesty has not only prevented the depths of the pandemic from entering Bhutan but has also stood as an emblem of hope within the world. An example of courage and compassion" (Tshering Palden, 2021).

Ten days after that audience, Gyalsey Ugyen Wangchuck was born. The news gave great comfort to the Bhutanese who were yet to reconcile to the first COVID case detected two weeks earlier. On 23 March 2020, the King delivered a short but powerful televised address to the nation announcing the closure of Bhutan's international borders. He said:

> Starting tomorrow, our land borders will be sealed. We are compelled to take this drastic measure in light of the COVID-19 pandemic. As you have been made aware through various government bulletins, the virus is spreading, causing immense disruption worldwide, and drawing closer to us each day. At such a time, the health and safety of the people of Bhutan is of the greatest priority, and as such, we are putting in place every measure necessary to safeguard the people of Bhutan.
>
> (Ministry of Foreign Affairs [MoFA], 2020)

His speech reflected genuine concern for his people. He spoke about children whose education must continue despite the closure of schools. He said we must take care of the elderly people who are at the greatest risk. To Bhutanese abroad who wished to return home, he assured help. His speech set the tone of Bhutan's response to the pandemic.

> A day after this address, His Majesty left behind His four-day old prince and Her Majesty The Gyaltsuen at the palace and embarked on a nationwide tour to meet local authorities, frontline workers, and to see first-hand the mitigation measures against the pandemic.
>
> (Tshering Palden, 2021)

In 2020, his constant travels throughout the country to address COVID challenges took a total of five months and 21 days.

The Hit

The decision to close the international border was bound to hit Bhutan's small economy with a GDP of Nu.178 billion (US$2.5 million). In his address, the King said "COVID-19 will cause great disruptions to the global economy, and Bhutan will not be an exception. The economic repercussions will not just impact a select few sectors, but each and every one of us" (MoFA, 2020). As predicted, economic growth has plummeted since then. From an earlier forecast of negative 2.1% growth for 2020, it was being revised to decelerate to negative 6.1%. The economy was in a state of stagflation with unemployment rate increasing from 2.7% in 2019 to 14.3% in 2020. Inflation has risen from 2.2% in October 2019 to 8% in September 2020 forecast (Lotay Tshering, 2020).

Bhutan's economy is strongly tied to India. For example, trade with India in 2019 constituted about 84% of exports and 82% of imports. India and China rank first and second in terms of being sources of Bhutan's imports (National Statistics Bureau [NSB], 2020a, pp. 266–269). The border closure had severely impacted exports and imports. Within nine months, total trade volume reduced by 30%.

Tourism is one of the most important sectors of the economy. Although it contributes only about 2.61% to the GDP, it is the top earner of foreign currency. There are two categories of tourists: regional and international. The international tourists pay in dollars as well as the mandatory daily sustainable development fee of $65 compared to the concessional $16 for regional tourists. In 2019, Indians topped the list at 230,381 (73%) from a total of 315,599 tourists (Tourism Council of Bhutan [TCB], 2019: 30). Among the dollar-paying tourists, the Chinese were second at 7,353 following the Americans at 10,602 (TCB, 2020: 21). The border closure saw tourists dwindle from 28,937 in 2020 to zero soon. Direct revenue went down from $27.3 million in 2019 to $2.63 million in 2020. More than 50,737 employees were impacted (Lotay Tshering, 2020: 84).

A very important sector is the Construction Industry, which contributed about 11.48% to the economy in 2019 (NSB, 2020b: 349). Government construction accounted for 23.60%, while that of private and public corporations accounted for 76.40% in 2019 (NSB, 2020b, p. 18). This sector depends tremendously on expatriate labour from India. From a total of 40,174 foreign workers by 28 February 2020, it was down to 8,292 by 17 March 2021 (Secretary Sonam Wangchuk, personal communication, 17 March 2021).

All schools and educational institutes were closed from 18 March 2020. They re-opened in July 2020 only for those studying between grades IX and XII while remaining closed for others till the commencement of 2021 academic sessions. Although various online and alternative learning modes were instituted, children lost valuable time for education.

Movie theatres, karaoke bars, and entertainment centres remained closed for a very long time. Then there were two national lockdowns triggered first by a suspected case and the second by a confirmed case of local transmission between August 11 to September 2020 and 19 December 2020 to 30 January 2021, respectively.

The Relief

On 10 April, the King delivered another televised address announcing the launch of Nu.30 billion National Resilience Fund (NRF) to support individuals and businesses (His Majesty The King, 2020). To the Task Force, His Majesty shared that the pandemic was an emergency and a crisis. During this period, he said that it is not about raw economics but about giving people the confidence as well as dignified means to livelihood. As he said, "The state must leave no stone unturned to support the people. Even if the state must bleed, we must take on the challenge whatever the cost. If the state bleeds, people will sleep well" (Personal notes, April, 2020). He also commanded that the relief support must be "swift, efficient and impactful" as well as "substantive, timely and inclusive".

A robust and yet simple procedural system was instituted to enable people apply for relief support.[2] Known as the Druk Gyalpo's Relief Kidu (DGRK), it has provided Nu.2.10 billion between April 2020 and February 2021 as direct income support to 45,762 people who were displaced by the pandemic. For families with children, additional relief grant was provided. As of February 2021, a total of Nu.65.59 million was provided to over 6,000 children every month.

The NRF also supported interest payment of Nu.7.5 billion for 139,096 loan account holders from 14 Financial Service Providers between April and December 2020 (Lotay Tshering, 2020: 30). Interests on loans were fully waived for the first six months (April–September 2020) followed by 50% waiver for the next six months. The interests were paid by DGRK with financial institutions paying 50% for the first three months. The 19,126 non-performing loan accounts of which hotel and construction sector accounted for about 30% also benefited from the waiver (Tshering Palden, 2021: 2). Support was also granted to more than 5,000 unemployed Desuups who have been deployed as frontline workers.

In his annual State of the Nation Address to the Parliament in 2020, the prime minister stated:

> The Royal *Kidu*, a uniquely Bhutanese institution, provided immediate financial support to distressed individuals affected by the pandemic.

> Besides defraying cost of living expenses and sustaining demand for goods and services, the Royal *Kidu* has also boosted morale and provided assurance and hope in these difficult times.
>
> (Lotay Tshering, 2020: 31)

During the two national lockdowns, the royal secretariat provided separate support to the most vulnerable sections of the society. I served as a frontline worker during the first lockdown. I was one of the 96 volunteers entrusted in delivering meals to different groups of volunteers enforcing the lockdown protocols in the capital city. Additionally, I had to deliver supplies to volunteer groups located further away. On a few occasions, I had the opportunity to help deliver support from the royal secretariat to needy families. The following is a message I sent concerning a delivery.

Dasho,

> Another kidu applicant. Name: Karma Wangmo. CID:11513002276 Contact:17103576[3] Camp: RBP Camp. From: Punakha. Came for child delivery to JDWNRH [Jigme Dorji Wangchuck National Referral Hospital]. After being discharged, put with a host at RBP camp with an acquaintance from village. Next day, lockdown initiated. She is with three children including the newborn. Her rations exhausted and dependence on humble host has been difficult. Request for kidu.

His response: "If not today, tomorrow laa but already included in the list as per our SOP, they should reach latest by next day" (Dy. Chamberlain, Tashi, personal communication, 28 August 2020). The ration support was delivered the next day. To a single mother of two children aged 6 and 11 and her two nephews stranded with her during the lockdown, I delivered royal support on 22 August.

During the National Day Address, the King reassured the people and private businesses that support will be extended as much as possible to help them overcome their difficulties. He said that the costs will indeed be substantial but they can be recovered. This will be critical to safeguard Bhutan's economic foundations which have been built over many decades.

The People's Response

The King's call for unity and resilience had deeply touched the people. Even more moving was the sight of the King on TV who looked frail after weeks and months of travels in different parts of the country. Many people wanted to come forward and do their part.

On 16 April 2020, I accompanied my cousin, who wanted to contribute to His Majesty's Fund. He wrote a letter to the Royal Chamberlain. It read:

> Kindly accept it as a very humble expression of my family's profound gratitude for His Majesty's unconditional love and care for us, His

> people, especially during a most difficult time in our country and elsewhere . . . It is only proper that humble, proud and loyal subjects like us thank His Majesty during times like this.

He received a letter on 20 April from the Royal Chamberlain thanking him for the contribution. It stated:

> The Welfare Fund was created due to the response received in the form of contributions from across the country and abroad. The donations are being efficiently utilised to meet expenses that address critical issues identified in our country's on-going response measures against the spread of the disease.
>
> (Samten, personal communication, April 16 and 20, 2020)

By March 2020, 7,077 individuals and 738 organisations had contributed to the fund.

Just below the office where the Deputy Chamberlain accepted the donation was a sizeable tent pitched. We saw many rural farmers who had come from far-flung areas bringing rice, vegetables, and other in-kind contributions. Records show that farmers have contributed 83,308 *dreys* (1 drey = 1.5 kg) of rice and 21,222 kgs of assorted vegetables (Dy. Chamberlain Kunzang Dorji, personal communication, 18 March 2020). These would later be granted as part of food supplies to front-liners.

When the first lockdown was announced in the early hours of 11 August 2020, I reported, as a Desuup, to my pre-assigned base. Most of us did not know we cannot return home till the lockdown was relaxed. So, there was a lot of uncertainty about accommodation for Desuups. Even as we were contemplating classrooms of nearby schools, many hoteliers came forward offering their hotels free of charge. A fellow Desuup, Ugyen Tenzin, opened the doors of his yet-to-be inaugurated Thimphu Residency and accommodated more than 40 of us for over a month at no cost. Likewise, others were accommodated in nearby hotels.

In a show of solidarity, people shared what they could for others who did not have access to essentials due to the sudden lockdown. Kuenzang Choki, a homemaker and owner of a shop in Olakha in Thimphu, went beyond her ways. On many occasions, I collected her contributions of snacks and beverages for Desuups as well as vegetables and even an LPG cylinder for other people who needed them. On 14 August 2020, a couple, Tshewang Tashi and Tshering Denkar, contacted me to celebrate their son's third birthday by cooking delicacies for nearly 100 Desuups deployed at Thimphu hospital.

On 17 August 2020, I went to a village to collect loads of fresh vegetables, particularly green chillies. My Facebook post that day read:

> Lop. Dorji Kinley and his family from Wang Simu contributed fresh vegetables for the Desung kitchen, which prepares and delivers meals to

> Desuups on duty at various locations in Thimphu. He works for Bhutan Power Corporation. We thank him and his family!
>
> (Sonam Kinga, 2020)

On 19 August, I received an sms message. It read:

> Kuzuzangpola Dasho. Hope all is keeping well amidst COVID19. Just to apprise dasho that I have 1 unit Isuzu Hilux and I am ready to join the nation and frontliners. I couldn't find other ways of expressing my interest and concerns. If there is any possibilities I can be of help, I am ready to come forward with my Hilux. Kindly provide me with the opportunity to help as a son of this motherland la (Ugyen Dorji, personal communications, 19 August 2020).

The national mood was singular, focused, and united. What these anecdotes show are articulation of genuine concern and support of people from all walks of life to be part of the larger national fight inspired by the King.

The Entertainment

I wrote this paper while spending a seven-day quarantine since such measures were made mandatory for people travelling from high-risk areas of southern Bhutan bordering India to low-risk areas. The quarantine measure has been one of the most successful strategies. It was in quarantine facilities that most imported COVID cases were detected.

Another system of 21-day mandatory quarantine had been put in place as early as 2020 in government-sponsored facilities for people returning from abroad despite WHO's recommendation of two weeks.

As of 19 March 2021, there were 3,199 people in 131 quarantine facilities, five in home quarantine, and one in isolation ward. A total of 44,842 people had completed the quarantine by then. Throughout the country, a total of 50,274 people had been discharged from quarantine facilities. The cumulative number of people who were in and had been through quarantine was 53,479 (Director Chencho, Prime Minister's Office, personal communications, 19 March 2020).

Upon the King's command, the royal guest house in Mongar was transformed into COVID-19 hospital in April 2020 with 24 beds for isolation cases (BBS, 2020c). Records show that a total of 110 people have been quarantined in the guest house as of 25 January 2021 (Governor Ugyen Sonam, personal communications, 4 April 2021).

Everybody wondered how a person can survive sequestered for three weeks. The King went deep-diving to this level of concern about people's mental and psychological well-being. Minutes of the meeting held on 10 April 2020 between Bhutan's only TV broadcaster and representatives of the entertainment industry reveal that the King's command was received the previous month to launch an entertainment programme called "Chikthuen" or "Unity" on Bhutan Broadcasting Service (BBS) by including all entertainers. Its objectives were two-fold: entertain the public, especially those in quarantine and provide some income to non-salaried performers.

The Royal Secretariat had financed a series of programmes which BBS aired since March 2020. A two-hour daily show ran till mid-August airing over 70 episodes. With many popular artists performing, it became a much-awaited entertainment. A popular dance group called Gokab produced eight 30-minute episodes of fitness routines, and 25 episodes of various yoga exercises were aired.

For children, a ten-part series of 30-minute episode called "Chey Chey's Tree House" was broadcast. To teach them art, the Voluntary Artist Studio produced the Co-Beat Art Show. There were eight episodes with each being 15 minutes long. A programme called E-learning was launched for students in various grades. With the collaboration between Voluntary Teachers Organization of Bhutan and BBS, 420 teaching programmes were broadcast.

With funds from the Royal Secretariat, BBS invited proposals and approved production of 45 short movies. Besides entertaining those in quarantine or lockdown, it created works for those in the film industry during the pandemic.

Moreover, 21 local films were purchased for broadcast at a cost of Nu.2.035 million. The total financial support from the Royal Secretariat was Nu.16 million. The secretariat further purchased 83 Bhutanese movies and handed them to BBS. During the two lockdowns, BBS aired two films a day, one each in the morning and afternoon.[4]

The Orange Force

On 8 September 2020, I left Thimphu for the south-eastern district of Samdrup Jongkhar. At Tashigang, I was joined by 99 Desuups. We had volunteered to serve for a month and half for the Southern Border Deployment. Our details were three-fold: guard border outposts and point of entries, enforce lockdown protocols of the Samdrup Jongkhar town where a recent positive case was detected, and provide escort services for vehicles coming through the international checkpoint bringing in essential supplies and ferrying out export items. We were to work under the supervision of local police force and in partnership with local Desuups.

These Desuups were mostly from the 38th to 41st batches trained after April 2020. After the King's televised address in April, thousands of youths volunteered for Desuung training, which was initially launched on 14 February 2011. It is a value-based personal development programme intended to encourage active citizenry in the process of nation-building. Founded on the spirit of volunteerism and community service, they serve during disaster operations and participate in social services. I had trained in September 2014. Till the 37th batch, there were only 4,557 Desuups trained over nine years. Responding to their enthusiasm to serve during the pandemic, the training was accelerated in 2020. When the 44th batch completed training on 6 March 2021, there were 20,090 Desuups making it Bhutan's largest voluntary organisation.[5]

> His Majesty visited desuup centres around the country more than 50 times in the past year alone, and every one of the 20,000 desuups has heard the heartfelt appreciation, encouragement, and guidance from His Majesty in person. Desuups around the country could have been addressed through video calls. . . . But every time a new batch was trained, at six to nine different locations around Bhutan, His Majesty visited them in person.
>
> (A Royal Example, 2021)

I was privileged to be in audience when he addressed the 44th batch. He thanked them for answering the call of duty. He said the country was going through tremendous pressures: psychological, social, and economic, and it is deeply impacting the security of the nation. He said: "You could have stayed at home but you chose to come forward . . . Your love, dedication and effort to make a difference by being there in person is more important than anything else" (Personal notes, 5 March 2021).

Such encouragement from the King has profound impact on the way Desuups see their identity, personhood, and sense of duty. He visited Samdrup Jongkhar in September–October 2020, met with COVID Task Force, and reviewed the situation providing advice and guidance. He spent time talking to Desuups at the Indo-Bhutan gate, and many border outposts. During each stop, he repeated his message, "I am very proud of you all. The nation is very thankful for your service" (personal notes, 30 September 2020).

To lead by example, he observed every protocol prescribed by health officials during his numerous travels and meetings. Every time, he returned to Thimphu, he quarantined himself for a week, for example, on 9 March 2021 and ended it to be in time for the first birthday of Gyalsey Ugyen Wangchuck on 19 March 2021.

On 2 September 2020, a driver sent me a voice message sharing his deep sense of guilt at not being able to serve. He asked for my guidance on how 300 truck drivers can immediately avail Desuung training and go to the frontlines. I shared the message with an official of the royal secretariat.

The Desuups' orange uniform became the defining colour of the fight against the pandemic. As of March 2021, there were 5,064 Desuups on active duty throughout the country. Among them, 1,021 were guarding Bhutan's international borders (Director General Tashi Tobgye, personal communication, 20 March 2021).

The Bhutanese Beyond

While the first COVID patient in Bhutan was an American, it was in America that Bhutanese nationals first began to test positive. Thousands of Bhutanese live and work in New York. Since 27 March 2020, ten Bhutanese had tested positive. During the second peak period in New York, 32 tested positive. To provide better care and support, the King commanded Bhutan's Permanent Mission in New York to rent two apartments for use as quarantine facility and extend financial support. A seven-member Task Force created among the Bhutanese community and a practicing Bhutanese nurse supported and monitored the quarantine facility.

> During the Second Wave, His Majesty The King had made a personal contribution to the community task force to support the establishment of additional quarantine facilities, and to extend logistic and material support to all Bhutanese nationals seeking such assistance.
>
> (Ambassador Doma Tshering, personal communication, 25 March 2020)

In early 2021, the King also commanded that the cost of vaccination even for Bhutanese overseas would be borne by the state. All Bhutanese in New York have recovered.

Closer home was the high risk to more than 5,000 Bhutanese who lived in the Indian town of Jaigaon right across Bhutan's commercial town of Phuntsholing. Just before the border closure, the King commanded and facilitated an unprecedented operation to bring them in. On 28 March 2020, the construction of 1,000 units of temporary shelters began. On the King's command, the Royal Bhutan Army deployed about 1,300 soldiers and officers for the construction (The World News, 2020). These were completed within 28 days. On 15 May, the first 40 families totalling 164 people moved in (His Majesty returns, 16 May 2020). By March 2021, 1,074 families consisting of 3,042 people were living in these rent-free homes (Dy. Governor Karma Rinchen, personal communication, 20 March 2021).

There are many Bhutanese working in the Gulf countries, who returned home through special repatriation flights organised by the government. But a significant number chose to stay back. The DGRK extended relief support to over 600 Bhutanese in Gulf countries. The grant of $130 every month from July–September 2020 translated to a total of $0.23 million.

The Other Interventions

In his first televised address, the King pointed out the COVID risk to elderly people. To more than 51,000 elderly people throughout the country, who were above 70 years, he sent free packages of multi-vitamins. Between 23

March 2020 and 25 January 2021, five rounds of essential food supplies and vitamins were distributed. On average, essential food supplies were provided every month to 2,400 people. Vitamins were provided every month to 31,480 people at a cost of Nu.15 million (Dy. Chamberlain Chiteem Tenzin, personal communication, 20 March 2021).

"As the streets are empty due to the lockdown, the dogs, which usually depend on scraps from hotels or food left by passers-by, may go hungry and become feral (De-suup Choki Tshomo, personal communication, March 19, 2021)". The King commanded that some 45,000 stray dogs in the country be fed during the lockdown. The uniformed personnel supported by Desuups undertook the task. In Thimphu, the cooking of rice and lentils took place at the army mess. Leftover foods were also collected from the common Desuup kitchen. At one point, there were around 7,000 chickens unfit for human consumption in Thimphu. It was delivered to the army kitchen to be cooked and mixed with rice and lentil soup. Between 24 December 2020 and 30 January 2021, 4,598 kgs of rice and 3,049 kgs of lentils were cooked and fed to 42,154 dogs.

Conclusion

To the small, land-locked and resource-strapped nation, the pandemic came as the most daunting threat to its society, economy, and security. Despite the gravity of the threat, the Bhutanese people were able to lead a normal and dignified life. Due to the guidance, pre-emptive and strategic interventions of the King, the situation has been what the prime minister said: "it is as if we don't have COVID-19" (Rai, 2020).

What made this possible? National unity was at the heart of the King's rallying point. He said that if the King, government, and people worked like members of one family, we can emerge unscathed from any adversity. During the meeting at Samtse, he had no illusions of what was coming ahead. "The pandemic will put us to the test. It will test the people's resolve to serve and take responsibility" (personal notes, 9 March 2020). The government and the people rose up to this challenge. The King acknowledged them time and again saying that when it comes to national interests, no Bhutanese needs any lesson. They demonstrated their love for the country in exceptional ways. There is this natural instinct and native intelligence to unite in the face of adversity. These are rooted in the Bhutanese historical consciousness for national survival.

But for the consciousness to remain alive or be activated, visionary and charismatic leadership matters. What goes into the making of such leadership? Undoubtedly, it is indomitable courage. And that courage, as I have shown, is founded on the King's genuine love and compassion for his people. Only an unqualified and unconditional compassion can sustain the willpower and courage to deal with a menace that has brought the richest and most powerful nations to their knees.

The other defining characteristic of visionary leadership is the ability to anticipate and pre-empt unexpected situations. Courage founded on genuine compassion and aided by the intellect to anticipate the future translated into a series of diverse, timely, effective, and strategic interventions. The COVID-19 situation became a defining socio-political framework for a Buddhist King to express his innate Bodhisattva quality.

The pandemic also became a defining geo-strategic framework for Bhutan's security and survival. His Majesty was clear early on that this indeed was the fight of our generation. He frequently spoke about the need for Bhutan to come out stronger, more unified, and resilient at the end of the pandemic. The pandemic is far from over. Nationwide vaccination has begun on 27 March 2021. Yet, looking at Bhutan's success in the last one year, the fight against COVID-19 will remain as a defining and lasting legacy of His Majesty the King.

Notes

1 See https://ourworldindata.org/covid-vaccinations.
2 See https://royalkidu.bt/ for information and application procedure concerning the DGRK as well as information on the amount of relief support and number of beneficiaries.
3 In order to protect the identity of the beneficiary, I have changed the name, identity, and contact numbers.
4 I would like to thank General Manager Tashi from BBS for providing detailed information about entertainment during lockdown and quarantine periods.
5 See https://desuung.org.bt/de-suung-training-conducted/ for details of number of De-suups and training dates.

References

Bhutan Broadcasting Corporation (2020a), "His Majesty the king addresses the nation", 11 April, www.bbs.bt/news/?p=130945, accessed 18 March 2021.

Bhutan Broadcasting Corporation (2020b), "His Majesty the king's address to the people of Bhutan – 12 September 2020", 14 September, www.bbs.bt/news/?p=136367, accessed 18 March 2021.

Bhutan Broadcasting Corporation (2020c), "COVID019 hospital in Monggar ready to handle outbreak in the eastern region", April 8, www.bbs.bt/news/?p=130813, accessed 18 March 2021.

Chencho (2021), *Felt Really Proud!* [Facebook status update], 12 March, www.facebook.com/pg/UNDPBhutan/posts/, accessed 17 March 2021.

Drexler, M. (2021), "The unlikeliest pandemic success story", *The Atlantic*, 28 February. www.theatlantic.com/international/archive/2021/02/coronavirus-pandemic-bhutan/617976/?utm_source=pocket-newtab, accessed 18 March 2021.

His Majesty The King addresses the nation (2020), *Kuensel*, 11 April, 1.

His Majesty King Jigme Khesar Namgyel (2020), *His Majesty's National Day Address to the Nation* [Video], 17 December, Facebook, www.facebook.com/King Jigme Khesar/videos/173229924517176/, accessed 19 March 2021.

His Majesty returns from the tour of the south (2020), *Kuensel,* 16 May, https://kuenselonline.com/his-majesty-returns-from-the-tour-of-south/, accessed 17 March 2021.
Krishna, S. V. (2020), "Bhutan: A coronavirus success story", 21 May. https://carnegieindia.org/2020/05/21/bhutan-coronavirus-success-story-pub-81856, accessed 19 March 2021.
Kugelman, M. (2021), "The Covid-19 success story you never knew about", *Arab News*, 28 February. www.arabnews.com/node/1817311, accessed 19 March 2021.
Lotay Tshering (2020), *State of the Nation* [Speech], 12 December, Fourth Session The Third Parliament of Bhutan, Thimphu, Bhutan.
Ministry of Foreign Affairs (2020), "English translation of his Majesty's address to the people of Bhutan on 22 March 2020", 24 March, www.mfa.gov.bt/?p=7747, accessed March 2021.
National Statistics Bureau (2020a), *Statistical Yearbook of Bhutan 2020*, Thimphu: Author.
National Statistics Bureau (2020b), *National Accounts Statistics 2020*, Thimphu: Author.
Office of the Prime Minister and Cabinet (2020), "First confirmed COVID-19 case in Bhutan", 6 March, www.cabinet.gov.bt/first-confirmed-covid-19-case-in-bhutan/, accessed 15 March 2021.
Rai, R. (2020), "Recipients of temporary shelters express gratitude to His Majesty the king", *Kuensel*, 16 May, https://kuenselonline.com/recipients-of-temporary-shelters-express-gratitude-to-his-majesty-the-king/, accessed 19 March 2021.
A Royal Example (2021), *Kuensel*, 10 March, https://kuenselonline.com/a-royal-example/, accessed 15 March 2021.
Slater, J. (2020), "A king, a ventilator, an 8,000-mile journey: One American's coronavirus rescue from Bhutan", *The Washington Post*, 14 May, www.washingtonpost.com/world/asia_pacific/bhutan-coronavirus-american-tourist-evacuation/2020/05/13/2f43f1e6-8f16-11ea-9322-a29e75effc93_story.html, accessed 11 November 2020.
Sonam Kinga (2020), "Lop. Dorji Kinley and his family from Wang Simu contributed fresh vegetables for the Desung kitchen [Facebook update]", 17 August.
Tourism Council of Bhutan (2019), *Bhutan Tourism Monitor 2019*, Thimphu: Author.
Tourism Council of Bhutan (2020), *Bhutan Tourism Monitors 2020*, Thimphu: Author.
Tshering Palden (2021), "The North Star in the Covid-19 storm", *Kuensel*, 21 February.
Turner, M. (2020), "Bhutan's decisive response to Covid-19", *East Asia Forum*, 6 November, www.eastasiaforum.org/2020/11/06/bhutans-decisive-response-to-covid-19/, accessed 17 March 2021.
Ugyen Penjore (2020, May 22), "UK Baroness lauds Bhutan's effort in fighting Covid-19", *Kuensel*, 1.
Wallen, J. (2021), "How Bhutan managed to vaccinate more than half its citizens in a single week", *The Telegraph*, 7 April, www.telegraph.co.uk/global-health/science-and-disease/bhutan-managed-vaccinate-half-citizens-single-week/?fbclid=IwAR2NTxTi8WEz-AfVWg6bojF6v3rXHBqmseu4DMvaMnDnoQZmq-gyNt4FSjI, accessed 11 April 2021.
The World News (2020), "His Majesty in south to inspect preparedness plan", https://theworldnews.net/bt-news/his-majesty-in-south-to-inspect-preparedness-plan, accessed 26 March 2021.
Yonten Tshedup (2021), "A king to a tourist's rescue", *Kuensel*, 21 February, 5.

17 Risks, Livelihoods, and Family Life

Negotiating the COVID-19 Pandemic in Urban Pakistan

Faiza Mushtaq

The COVID-19 pandemic has played itself out across Pakistan in fits and starts, threatening to develop into a full-blown public health crisis at times but so far steering clear of a large-scale loss of life unlike some of its regional neighbours. The first confirmed case of COVID-19 was reported in the country on 26 February 2020, and most early transmission was linked to travellers coming in from Iran, the United Kingdom, and other places. It was in July 2021 that the number of officially recorded cases hit the 1 million mark, with just over 23,000 deaths recorded nationwide by the end of that month.

Given a population of 225 million people, a resource-poor state, and a weak healthcare system, Pakistan's Coronavirus outbreak has remained relatively mild. Yet the impact has been profound across many areas of social, political, and economic life. It still poses risks to the well-being of individuals, families, and communities amid the ongoing fourth wave of the pandemic. Lockdowns and other government-imposed public health restrictions have led to lost jobs and incomes, food insecurity, and increased economic precarity especially among marginalised sections of the population. The education sector has faced severe disruptions over the last one and a half years, with children and youth left struggling with the demands of online schooling, unequal access to opportunities, and adverse mental health outcomes. Changes in the workplace and the increased burden of care work within the home have disproportionately affected women and are exacerbating already existing patterns of gender inequality.

This chapter looks at the policy responses of the Pakistani government as it has managed the twin public health and economic challenges posed by the COVID-19 pandemic, and examines how the crisis has shaped state-society relations. In addition, it presents early findings from a qualitative research study that has gathered longitudinal data from a cross section of families in Karachi, the largest urban centre of Pakistan. A team of researchers (including the chapter author) for the project "Families and Communities in a Time of COVID-19", or FACT Pakistan,[1] has used digital ethnographic methods including interviews and diary entries to track 27 households, with 57 individual study participants, between August 2020 and July 2021. These

DOI: 10.4324/9781003282815-22

responses provide an in-depth insight into the experiences and perceptions of urban dwellers from diverse ethnic, occupational, age, gender, and social class backgrounds as they lived through the ups and downs of the pandemic.

From the First to the Fourth Wave

Coronavirus cases first started being reported in Pakistan in February and on 23 March 2020, the federal and provincial governments implemented a strict lockdown that closed schools, businesses, and public facilities, imposed domestic and international travel restrictions and border closures, and instituted social distancing guidelines. Many of these measures, especially those affecting economic activity, began to be lifted gradually in April but the number of new daily cases kept climbing steadily until they hit a peak of 6,533 on 19 June 2020.[2] The first wave of the pandemic began to subside over the summer months and by September, a cautious re-opening of schools and colleges followed a resumption of most other normal activities.

The number of cases began to rise again in November 2020 and by early December, the country was seeing a second wave of infections with more than 3,000 new cases being recorded daily. This time around the mitigation measures were less restrictive and, instead of implementing widespread shutdowns, the federal government adopted the strategy of targeted "smart lockdowns" in the hardest hit urban localities coupled with a closure of educational institutions and public events. Following a brief respite in the early months of 2021, the third wave hit hard and by April, the number of new daily cases had once again reached nearly 6,000.[3] The COVID-19 vaccine reached Pakistan in February 2021 and a limited rollout began with the vaccination of frontline healthcare workers. In March 2021, the public vaccination campaign got off to a slow start with an initial focus on the elderly and at-risk population and gradually expanded to other segments. Most restrictions on travel, recreation, and business were being lifted in May 2021 as the number of infections once again began to climb down, and it was believed that the vaccination campaign would now effectively prevent virus transmission rates from going too high again.

However, by early July there were alarm bells ringing about a potential fourth wave being ushered in with the more easily transmissible, deadlier, and vaccine-resistant Delta variant of the virus having entered the country. By the end of July 2021, the number of new daily cases being reported had reached 5,000 and the total number of confirmed Coronavirus cases in Pakistan stood at 1,034,837. The total number of deaths caused by the virus, as officially recorded, had reached 23,422 at that time.[4] Rates of transmission as well as fatalities have not been distributed evenly across Pakistan, with the provinces of Sindh and Punjab having the highest tallies and a majority of cases being concentrated in some of the country's large urban centres such as Karachi, Lahore, Islamabad, and Peshawar.

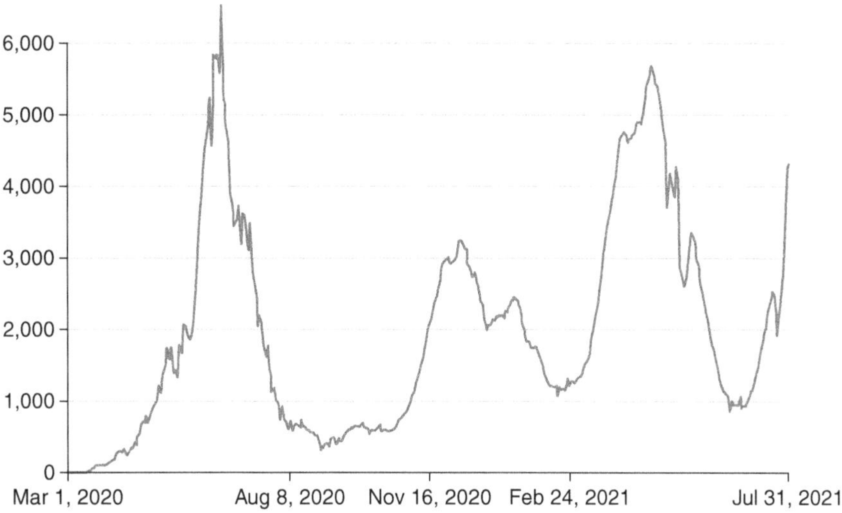

Figure 17.1 Daily New Coronavirus Cases Reported in Pakistan

Source: Our World in Data, *Pakistan: Coronavirus Pandemic Country Profile* based on data from Johns Hopkins University CSSE

The number of daily average fatalities has increased with each new surge in infections in Pakistan, corresponding to the global trend whereby new COVID-19 deaths are doubling at a higher rate than earlier in the pandemic.[5] There has been persistent scepticism about official reporting of the number of deaths, and anecdotal evidence abounds about families not disclosing COVID as the cause of death when it occurs at home or not even getting tested due to the stigma attached to a positive diagnosis, as well as hospitals recording cause of deaths inaccurately. One estimate from the Institute of Health Metrics and Evaluation places the actual number of COVID-related deaths in Pakistan as being 4.1 times higher than the reported figure.[6]

A big issue in gauging the reliability of case and fatality figures in Pakistan, and one of the weaknesses in the government's response and management of the pandemic, has been the low rate of testing for COVID-19. According to Our World in Data, there were daily 0.23 tests per 1,000 people being carried out in Pakistan in July 2021, far below the world average and lower than most comparable middle-income countries. This number peaked at 0.29 tests per 1,000 people on 20 April 2021.[7] The government has made attempts to increase testing capacity and protocols in private as well as public health facilities, and also to encourage greater voluntary testing, but with limited success. As a result, the government remains hampered in its ability to monitor the spread of the outbreak and devise adequate containment strategies.

Rates of vaccination have remained similarly low. In early 2021, Pakistan faced shortages of vaccine supply and delays in procurement, but the situation improved with Chinese donations, support from the COVAX facility, and government allocation of funds to purchase vaccines from China. The Government of Pakistan opened up the free-of-cost vaccination campaign for everyone aged 18 and above in May 2021 and plans to vaccinate 70 million people by the end of 2021.[8] By 31 July 2021, the total number of people who had received both doses stood at 6.3 million, meaning that a mere 2.91% of the total Pakistani population has so far been fully vaccinated.[9]

Mixed Messages and the Trust Deficit

The COVID containment measures imposed by the government have only been intermittently successful and have not received widespread compliance among the public in Pakistan. The complete lockdown that was initially implemented in March 2020 had a devastating impact on the economy and led to serious resistance among traders and the business community. Subsequent closures of markets have been brief and ill-enforced, while industry has remained mostly exempt from shutdowns. It is common to see bustling marketplaces, little to no social distancing, and very sporadic mask wearing behaviour among large chunks of the urban public, especially in periods leading up to major festivals like Eid, even when COVID cases have been recording a steep increase. Clamping down on congregational prayers in mosques, religious gatherings, and large wedding parties has been especially difficult for authorities across the country. Schools and universities often end up being the easiest sector to regulate and enforce mandatory shutdowns for, and developing a plan to keep educational institutions safe and open has not been the government's priority.

This resistance to social distancing measures and deep-rooted scepticism about the threat posed by the Coronavirus as well as vaccine hesitancy has to be understood against the backdrop of pre-existing patterns of state-society relations in Pakistan. The current public health crisis is playing out in a context where government spending on the healthcare infrastructure and social services is abysmally low, citizens' perceptions about the performance and credibility of state institutions are largely negative, and the population is fragmented along bitterly fought ethnic, religious, sectarian, and class divisions. Making individual-level behavioural adjustments and sacrifices for the sake of an imagined collective benefit requires not only a certain level of social cohesion but also the belief that "the state is acting for the common good and that the lives of all citizens are valued equally".[10] Equally damaging has been the decades-long neglect of the educational system and the systematic undermining of scientific research and enquiry, leaving very little public understanding or trust in scientific explanations of disease prevalence and prevention.

This government's handling of the pandemic has not helped. Public messaging around the health emergency and social distancing guidelines has been inconsistent, and has not adequately conveyed the risks of the Coronavirus. Early in February, the National Health Ministry in Islamabad issued a detailed "National Action Plan" for COVID-19 preparedness, outlining coordination mechanisms at the national and provincial levels, screening and surveillance, case management and testing protocols, fund allocations, and communication plans.[11] However, the actual roll-out of the government response was not as swift and organised, soon falling victim to all too familiar political bickering, turnover of key personnel in leadership positions, and institutional weaknesses.

The confusion began from the highest levels of political leadership at the centre, with Prime Minister Imran Khan underplaying the seriousness of the virus and any fears around it, comparing it to the ordinary flu and suggesting that most patients recover without any medical treatment.[12] Khan's government resisted calls for a nationwide lockdown even as the number of cases continued to spiral upward in March 2020, claiming he could not risk the livelihoods of millions of working class citizens and instead advocating voluntary compliance with SOPs (standard operating procedures). It was eventually the country's powerful military that ended up forcing the civilian government's hand. In a televised press conference on 23 March 2020, the military spokesperson declared the pandemic an unprecedented threat and announced the military's support in enforcing a government lockdown.[13] The prime minister was rarely seen wearing a mask during his public appearances through much of the pandemic's early months, until he himself tested positive for the virus in March 2021.

Tussles between the centre and the federating units over containment and mitigation strategies have also marred Pakistan's COVID response. Political rivalries between Imran Khan's government at the centre and the opposition Pakistan People's Party (PPP) government in the province of Sindh have led to the most visible battles. The Government of Sindh received local and international praise for mobilising quickly and imposing strict precautionary measures, which led to dismissive statements from Khan and his allies about "elites" locking down the country and not caring for the suffering of daily wage earners who end up going hungry.[14] More recently, the Sindh government once again instituted a province-wide lockdown at the end of July 2021 as the rising fourth wave cases fill up hospital beds in Karachi and stretch the provincial healthcare system to its limit. The prime minister and his spokespersons continue to criticise the leadership in Sindh for not following the federal government's lead and going against the COVID policy advocated by the National Command and Control Centre (NCOC).

The Pakistani government routinely claims that its management of the Coronavirus pandemic, focused on the strategy of targeted smart lockdowns, has resulted in low fatality and positivity rates. Others, especially doctors and health experts, in the country are not convinced of the effectiveness of state interventions or the quality of data gathering, and continue to worry about a false sense of security that the government's narrative has instilled without a full understanding of the scale of the virus's spread. In contrast to business groups, trade unions, and religious leadership – all of which have successfully persuaded Khan's government to keep the economy as well as places of worship open – the medical establishment has been issuing desperate pleas for the government and the public to take the disease more seriously, follow social distancing guidelines, and not ease restrictions prematurely.[15]

A strategy that relies upon micro-lockdowns of select neighbourhoods and infection hotspots also requires rigorous testing and tracing in order to successfully contain the spread of the virus. Yet, voluntary testing rates remain woefully inadequate in Pakistan, with large numbers of asymptomatic carriers and those who recover from mild symptoms at home without requiring medical treatment never getting detected. If a suspected case tests positive, the benefits mostly "accrue to others" rather than to her or himself, while the "costs" of getting tested can often be prohibitive: self-isolation, loss of earnings, the social stigma of being a carrier, fears of involuntary quarantining, loss of privacy, and of contact tracing that will invite opprobrium from one's social networks.[16] The Pakistani government failed to come up with a clear and compelling communication plan that would inform the public about the benefits of testing, masking or getting vaccinated, quell rumours and misinformation, and instil faith in public health services as well as governmental guidelines. Senior government spokespersons, and the prime minister himself, issue confusing and contradictory signals while passing the blame on to the public for not voluntarily following precautionary measures.

During the first wave of the pandemic, the Ministry of Health collaborated with the UNDP to develop an awareness and prevention strategy relying on a low-cost mass communication channel used by 90% of the Pakistani population, that is mobile phones. A pre-recorded ringtone message plays each time someone places a call, some emphasising the need to wash hands properly or avoid public gatherings, getting replaced with updated health-related content over the months. The messages reached more than 113 million listeners,[17] but it is harder to calculate what impact they had on changing perceptions and behaviours. At the same time, misinformation, conspiracy theories, and irresponsible statements by government ministers and other public figures keep getting amplified through coverage on mainstream media and circulation through social media channels.

The list of these dangerous beliefs and fallacies is long.[18] In April 2020, the influential religious scholar and leader of the Tablighi Jamaat, Maulana Tariq Jameel, sat beside Prime Minister Imran Khan in a telethon and commented that COVID-19 is God's punishment for a society where women's immodest clothing choices and immorality are rampant. Other religious clerics have insisted that congregational prayers in mosques are not to be interrupted by social distancing guidelines, that their faith protects them against the virus, and that the virus and/or the vaccine are part of a Western conspiracy to weaken Muslims. A Gallup survey in October 2020 found that 55% of the Pakistani population believes the COVID-19 threat is exaggerated.[19] Some believe that the government is interested in showing inflated numbers of infections in order to receive foreign aid, while others believe hospitals get paid for every COVID patient they treat and every COVID death they report. In November 2020, a video of former senator Faisal Raza Abidi surfaced where he declared the COVID pandemic a hoax perpetrated against Pakistan and Iran to get them to recognise Israel.[20] In June 2021, health minister of Punjab province, Yasmin Rashid, was quoted as saying people should get vaccinated against COVID-19 "at their own risk" and linking some side effects of vaccines to deaths.[21] Rumours that vaccines cause infertility, or were being promoted due to sinister motives of China, Russia, Western donor countries or individuals like Bill Gates, freely circulated among the urban literate elite as well as among the rest of the public.

The COVID-19 vaccination campaign is linked to the digital database of national identity cards, making it easy to track and verify vaccination status. It also builds upon Pakistan's experiences with the extensive polio vaccination campaign and the organisational as well as information infrastructure built up for it. For instance, the 1166 telephone helpline was originally set up for polio and other immunisation campaigns with the help of UNICEF and other international partners, but has since been converted into the COVID-19 helpline centre where it offers a vital information and support service. The uptake of the vaccine, however, remained frustratingly slow in the absence of any concerted media awareness campaign. The demand for vaccinations only began to register a sharp increase in late July 2021 after provincial and federal governments announced a series of incentives and penalties linked to the vaccination status of individuals: allowing domestic travel and tourism only for those who are fully vaccinated, stopping salary payments of government employees who are unvaccinated, blocking mobile phone connections of unvaccinated people, and making vaccination mandatory for educational and corporate sector employees.

The Economic Impact of the Pandemic

COVID-19 hit Pakistan at a time when the country was making a shaky recovery from an economic crisis with the assistance of an IMF bailout package. Over the course of the 2020 financial year, most economic indicators worsened and the overall economic growth rate plunged to negative 0.5%.[22] On 24 March 2020, the prime minister announced a relief and stimulus package worth PKR 1.2 trillion that included cash grants for daily wage workers and low-income families, as well as subsidies, tax incentives, and non-cash initiatives for emergency economic support. The government has not released a full audit report of how these funds were utilised, but by the end of 2020 only 34% of disbursements from this package had actually taken place.[23] The federal government also sought debt relief and suspended the IMF programme, while provincial governments introduced measures to expand the social safety net and increase spending on health services in their respective budgets.

The Pakistan Bureau of Statistics (PBS) conducted a survey in October 2020 to assess the impact of COVID-related shocks on economic well-being.[24] These are the only comprehensive nationwide figures that are available to date and show that 20.7 million people lost their jobs during the first wave of the pandemic until July 2020. Job losses, inability to find work, and a decrease in income affected 49% of the working population across the country due to COVID-related closures in that time period. Those working in the informal urban economy were most badly affected, including construction workers, casual labour, small vendors and shopkeepers, and those in the transport/storage and retail/restaurant sectors. Fifty-three percent of households across urban and rural Pakistan faced reduced income due to the April–July 2020 lockdowns and 59% of households reported some degree of concern about not having adequate access to food supplies. The increase in severe food insecurity from 3% to 10% of households during this period is one of the most worrying indicators. The most common coping strategy across households in response to these uncertain circumstances was reported as a reduction in non-food expenditures.

The PBS survey notes that the re-opening of manufacturing and construction sectors after July 2020 contributed to the recovery process and nearly 18 million people were re-absorbed back into the labour force. In other words, 35% of the working age population was employed pre-COVID, and this number dipped to 22% during the crisis period, with a 33% employment rate recovered by October 2020. These findings are echoed in the Economic Vulnerability Assessment conducted through a survey of households in the Punjab province by the Centre for Economic Research in Pakistan (CERP).[25] Between July and October 2020, the fraction of unemployed individuals fell from 34% to 21%.

However, Round 3 of the CERP survey, which was carried out in December 2020–January 2021, finds that labour market recovery has stagnated and the unemployment rate continues at 21%, while the partial income recovery earlier being reported has stalled in urban areas and experienced a reversal in rural areas. Spending levels have returned to pre-COVID standards, but 30% of rural households and 23% of urban households continue to experience some form of financial distress (measured as the inability to pay bills). This assessment also notes that individuals with higher levels of education suffered disproportionate income losses as a result of COVID-related shocks, but their recovery has been faster and more robust than the continuing struggles of lesser-educated individuals.

The start of the 2021 financial year saw an overall improvement in Pakistan's macroeconomic indicators, and the government was loudly proclaiming a successful recovery with an economic growth rate of 3.9%. Sales and corporate profitability recorded steep increases, yet the picture was less rosy when it came to the economic realities faced by the bulk of the population. Salaried employees of large companies fared better than those employed by small and medium enterprises, while daily wage earners were hardest hit and experienced negative wage growth – "real wages for skilled and unskilled workers have fallen sharply through the year 2020 and are refusing to pick up, even as inflation eats away their meagre purchasing power, month after month".[26] The benefits of the government's aggressive stimulus and economic inducement efforts, coupled with enhanced public expenditures, have accrued to the country's elites while the most marginalised segments of the population continue to face high risks of impoverishment.

Disparities Within and Across Families

Public discourse around the pandemic has been filled with political debates about saving lives versus livelihoods, the ups and downs of the national economy or performance of various levels of government, and numbers tracking new Coronavirus cases, positivity ratios, and death rates. How these developments translate into the lived practices and perceptions of urban households and the evolving uncertainties of living through this unprecedented crisis can be glimpsed through the findings of the FACT Pakistan digital ethnography. It also helps us understand how individuals' positions within the household (as determined by age and gender, for instance) and families' positions relative to other households (e.g. by social class, ethnicity, and locality) provide different resources through which they can mitigate risks and negotiate their well-being.

Both male and female participants spoke about their anxieties relating to work and fluctuating incomes, with multi-generational families containing more than one earning member being better positioned to weather these changes. A female community health worker was without a job for months, while another young family experienced a temporary increase in their household income thanks to the boom in online shopping which helped the husband's small leather garment business gain expanded access to international buyers. For a large number of female respondents, however, the actual or threatened loss of paid work outside the home was stressful because it also implied a loss of their financial and inter-personal autonomy. Those who were fortunate enough to continue working from home or return to well-paying jobs spoke about their work as a source of meaning and value in addition to being a source of income.

Participants from across all ages, genders, and occupational backgrounds were keen to resume their work activities outside the home as soon as restrictions were lifted. For urban professionals across Pakistan, there has not been the kind of large-scale structural shift towards work from home or remote employment opportunities as we find in other countries and employers have not been keen to put such arrangements in place. Few companies or urban neighbourhoods have a digital technology infrastructure well-developed enough to support such a shift, but part of the reason also has to do with family dynamics and what working at home means in this context.

Male participants in the study spoke about enjoying family time together in the early periods of confinement, making some robust contribution to childcare, cooking and domestic chores in this duration, but also made it clear that they had used any available opportunity to spend time outside the house. In some cases this meant using free time to volunteer for community service and welfare activities, especially in neighbourhoods where ethnic and other networks of solidarity were already strong, while in other cases it meant seeing friends, running errands, or fulfilling job responsibilities even when that meant taking on health risks. Many more female participants, in contrast, reported stricter compliance with social distancing guidelines for themselves and their children and feeling anxiety for male family members who were more exposed to the virus. The mandate of enforcing hand washing, masking, checking up on loved ones near and far, dealing with illness when COVID struck a family member at home, keeping children entertained, and other additional burdens of care work fell disproportionately on female members of these households. Some of these women reported that being confined at home allowed them to give more attention to self-care through practices such as yoga, meditation, prayer, or physical exercise, but almost all reported spending a larger amount of time on cooking, cleaning, and other time-consuming household activities, sometimes enlisting the help of older children. A few, especially younger women, spoke candidly about the toxic environment at home and the unwelcome presence of certain male family members during periods of lockdown that contributed to stress and conflict.

Many of these patterns of isolation, stress, and anxiety were exacerbated for adolescents (12–18 years old) and young adults (19–24 years) within these households. The loss of socialisation opportunities and access to peer networks were the most common factors cited when they described their experience of the pandemic. These young people are adept users of digital technologies and found many online venues for entertainment and for virtually connecting with friends and family members, but also felt exhausted and consciously cut back on their usage of social media at times. Many school and university students spoke about the pressures of online schooling and the difficulty of being productive in the home setting, and at least one family in the study experienced a mental health breakdown of a teenager who then had to get professional help and withdraw from school temporarily. Experts have been pointing out that Pakistan is not prepared for the mental health-related aftermath of the COVID-19 pandemic and the shortage of facilities as well as trained professionals is especially dire when it comes to meeting the requirements of the youth.[27]

Schools, colleges, and universities in most parts of the country have been closed for one and a half years, with some limited campus openings for in-person classes or exams before being forced to shut down again due to rising COVID cases. The majority do not have access to computers or the Internet and have not been afforded the luxury of online schooling at all. Many parents with young children in the FACT study had the education of their children as one of their highest priorities and the massive disruptions to schooling were a constant source of worry and frustration. For university students and recent graduates, uncertainties about career prospects and the resumption of any form of normal life routine loomed large.

Some participants praised the swift response of the Sindh provincial government where Karachi is based; others expressed ambivalence towards lockdown and quarantine requirements in light of continuously changing guidelines from the national government. Many reported lax attitudes towards distancing measures within their communities, especially after the first wave of infections had subsided and the death toll had remained low. Cynicism about the government and distrust of official figures also shaped participants' mixed response towards the vaccination campaign, with those who had prior positive experiences with the healthcare system or any form of state services being the most ready to believe information about the virus and vaccines. By the time the fourth wave of the pandemic rolled around, some noted feeling a sense of fatigue and a disjuncture between alarmist official pronouncements on the media and the scenes from daily life they see in marketplaces and streets around them. A few referred to the devastation wrought by COVID in neighbouring India in May 2021 as a sobering reminder that we have been lucky on this side of the border and start taking the risks of the pandemic more seriously.

Future Directions

The disruptions to family life, and the turmoil within many social institutions that families are embedded in, will not simply vanish if and when the COVID-19 pandemic winds down, in Pakistan as in the rest of the world. The government might well weather any criticisms over its handling of the pandemic but families and communities will have to continue dealing with the long-term impacts of death and illness, emotional and mental health vulnerabilities, disarray in educational activities and outcomes, and reordered networks of solidarity. Career paths, incomes, and aspirations, especially for groups that already struggled against accumulated disadvantages, are likely to be altered significantly. The pandemic threatens to undo some hard-fought gains in female participation in the labour force and higher education, as well as the increased primary school enrolments of recent years for children across gender in Pakistan.

There are some obvious lessons for how the Pakistani government can better deal with such a pandemic in the future. The government's response to a public health crisis has to be led by public health professionals, using scientific data and medical advice, and not be driven by political expediency or pandering to interest groups. We saw this happen repeatedly when lockdowns got lifted prematurely, certain sectors of public activity received preferential treatment at the cost of others, or the provision of vaccines did not get the kind of dedicated planning and resources that were required. When there is a lack of transparent information-sharing about number of cases and fatalities and when mask mandates and other guidelines don't get enforced, cynicism about the government deepens and public compliance becomes harder to secure in each round. A consistent and coordinated public messaging campaign can go a long way towards combatting rumours and conspiracy theories, removing stigmas around the illness, and making people understand the risks of the virus as well as its modes of transmission.

Future planning by the government also needs to take into account a deeper understanding of who the most vulnerable social groups are and what kinds of interventions need to be targeted specifically towards them. This includes the elderly who require special types of assistance and access to healthcare, women and young people who are at risk of domestic abuse, and the urban poor who lack a social safety net. Instead of ill-planned experiments, such as the prime minister's rallying of volunteers to form a Corona Relief Tiger Force,[28] strengthening existing public institutions and making long-term investments in the education and healthcare sectors (including mental health) has to be a priority.

Notes

1 Faiza Mushtaq, Ayesha Khan, and Shama Dossa are the lead researchers. The study received ethics clearance from the National Bioethics Committee (NBC) Pakistan. Ref: No.4–87/NBC-COVID19–23/20/ dated 5 July 2020.
2 The following sources were consulted for figures about the officially reported Coronavirus cases and deaths: Government of Pakistan https://covid.gov.pk/; Johns Hopkins University https://coronavirus.jhu.edu/region/pakistan; Our World in Data https://ourworldindata.org/coronavirus/country/pakistan
3 https://covid.gov.pk/
4 https://coronavirus.jhu.edu/region/pakistan
5 Dagia, 2021.
6 www.healthdata.org/sites/default/files/covid_briefs/165_briefing_Pakistan.pdf
7 https://ourworldindata.org/coronavirus/country/pakistan; Junaidi, 2021.
8 The government allowed 50,000 doses of the Sputnik-V vaccine to be imported and sold through the private sector, but has not permitted any further private distribution of vaccines after this initial chaotic experiment, marred by allegations of corruption and disputed pricing mechanisms (Shahid, 2021).
9 https://coronavirus.jhu.edu/region/pakistan
10 Mushtaq, 2020.
11 http://shcc.org.pk/public-docs/National_Action_Plan_COVID19.pdf
12 Saleem, 2020.
13 The News, 2020
14 Khattak, 2020
15 Dawn, 2020a.

16 Gazdar, 2020.
17 Masood and Taj, 2020
18 Khattak, 2020; Saleem, 2020; Ur-Rehman and Schmall, 2020.
19 Saleem, 2020.
20 Ur-Rehman and Schmall, 2020.
21 Geo News, 2021.
22 IMF, 2021.
23 Rana, 2021.
24 www.pbs.gov.pk/sites/default/files//other/covid/Final_Report_for_Covid_Survey_0.pdf
25 www.cerp.org.pk/updata/news/files/96_20210308040608.pdf
26 Husain, 2021.
27 Mian et al., 2020.
28 Dawn, 2020b.

References

Centre for Economic Research in Pakistan (2021), *Economic Vulnerability Assessment: Round 3 Findings*, www.cerp.org.pk/updata/news/files/96_20210308040608.pdf.

Dagia, Niha (2021), "Why Isn't Pakistan's COVID-19 death rate falling as quickly as infections?" *The Diplomat*, 21 June.

Dawn (2020a), "Doctors demand strict lockdown, urge religious scholars to review decision to open mosques", 22 April, www.dawn.com/news/1551370.

Dawn (2020b), "Tigers unleashed", 14 October, www.dawn.com/news/1584954.

Gazdar, Haris (2020), "Testing times: The only way to fight corona is through rigorous testing", *Dawn*, 27 May.

Geo News (2021), "Vaccinate against coronavirus 'at your own risk', says Punjab health minister citing 'side effects' ", 1 February, www.geo.tv/latest/332823-vaccinate-against-coronavirus-covid-19-at-your-own-risk-says-punjab-health-minister-citing-side-effects.

Husain, Khurram (2021), "The economy is growing, but for whom?" *Dawn, Eos,* 6 June.

Institute for Health Metrics and Evaluation (2021), "Covid-19 results briefing: Pakistan", 30 July, www.healthdata.org/sites/default/files/covid_briefs/165_briefing_Pakistan.pdf.

International Monetary Fund (2021), "Policy responses to Covid-19: Pakistan", www.imf.org/en/Topics/imf-and-covid19/Policy-Responses-to-COVID-19.

Junaidi, Ikram (2021), "Record tests for Covid-19 conducted in day", *Dawn*, 16 April.

Khattak, Daud (2020), "Pakistan's confused COVID-19 response", *The Diplomat*, 9 June.

Masood, Javeria and Taj, Umar (2020), *Innovative Ringtone Messages Positively Impact Knowledge, Perceptions and Behaviours Related to COVID-19 in Pakistan*, UNDP Pakistan, www.pk.undp.org/content/pakistan/en/home/blog/2020/innovative-ringtonemessages-positively-impacts-knowledge – perce.html.

Mian, Ayesha, Lodhi, Momin Iqbal, Khan, Mahrukh Nadeem, Chachar, Ayesha Sanober and Siddiqui, Sana Asif (2020), "Mental health in Pakistan: Policymakers need to act now", *Learners' Republic*, 2 June, https://learnersrepublic.com/mental-health-in-pakistanpolicymakers-need-to-act-now/.

Ministry of National Health Services, Regulation and Coordination, Pakistan (2020), "National action plan for preparedness & response to corona virus disease (Covid-19) Pakistan", http://shcc.org.pk/public-docs/National_Action_Plan_COVID19.pdf.
Mushtaq, Faiza (2020), "A sociological perspective on the Covid-19 crisis in Pakistan", *IBA Business Review: Short Notes on the Economy during the Covid-19 Crisis*, 6 April, 3.
The News (2020), "Coronavirus an unprecedented danger, best defence is 'cooperation', says DG ISPR", 23 March, www.thenews.com.pk/latest/633425-dg-ispr-confident-of countering-coronavirus-with-support-from-nation.
Pakistan Bureau of Statistics (2020), *Special Survey for Evaluating Socio-Economic Impact of Covid-19 on Wellbeing of People,* Islamabad: Government of Pakistan, Ministry of Planning Development and Special Initiatives, www.pbs.gov.pk/sites/default/files//other/covid/Final_Report_for_Covid_Survey 0.pdf.
Rana, Shahbaz (2021), "66% of Covid-19 relief package remains unutilized", *The Express Tribune*, 17 January.
Saleem, Aasim (2020), "How denial and conspiracy theories fuel coronavirus crisis in Pakistan", *DW*, 23 June.
Shahid, Ariba (2021), "The urban upper middle classes are desperate for the vaccines of their choice. Why don't we let them pay for it?' *Profit*, 13 June.
Ur-Rehman, Zia and Schmall, Emily (2020), "A Covid-19 surge and conspiracy theories roil Pakistan", *The New York Times*, 19 December.

Websites

Government of Pakistan, "Official covid portal", https://covid.gov.pk/.
Johns Hopkins University and Medicine, "Coronavirus resource Center: Pakistan", https://coronavirus.jhu.edu/region/pakistan.
Our World in Data, "Pakistan: Coronavirus pandemic country profile", https://ourworldindata.org/coronavirus/country/pakistan

18 “New Normal” in Sri Lanka

The Impact of Local Reaction to a Global Pandemic in Shaping Everyday Lives of the Citizens

Anton Piyarathne

Introduction

During the first lockdown in March 2020, I got a WhatsApp message alert from Dasith[1] who lives at the top of the 11th Lane in Malabe, a suburban town in Colombo, informing that a “vegetable lorry is coming”. During the total lockdown in the country, in our neighbourhood, we always got updates about the various food supply lorries, trucks, vans, and three wheelers approaching the lane so that residents in the inner areas could be ready to purchase their daily essentials. When we got the message, we came up to the road and stayed in front of our respective houses, maintaining physical distancing but closely connecting socially to each other. This daily reality contradicts, and pinpoints inappropriateness of the term “social distance” introduced to denote physical distance to prevent the spread of COVID-19 virus from one person to another. On such occasions, we who always lived indoors with shut gates and gardens covered with hedges or parapet walls came up to the roads and got updates on deaths and rumours about the spread of the virus; worked online from home; and got daily essentials through online shopping.

During this time, we had a vegetable lorry operated by a family where the father served as the driver, the mother was the cashier while the daughter measured and distributed the vegetables to the people in waiting. To me, this was a fascinating story of survival of a family while helping others. Moreover, they also shared with us various information they gathered from other areas when they went around to sell essential food stuffs. Basically, these mobile sellers were the nexus between us and the society at large since we could not go out for about three months under the curfew condition in the western province.

I kept daily records for 80 days from the first day that the country was locked down on 12 March 2020, covering three themes: the impact of the virus on family, country, and the world. I developed further my arguments by critically analysing the reports in newspapers and other media, having discussions with my extended family members and the others in my workplace, and by referring to the relevant literature on the pandemic.

DOI: 10.4324/9781003282815-23

Though it is scientifically and officially identified as COVID-19, people in their everyday conversation referred to it as "Corona" in Sinhala (hereafter S:) කොරෝනා (korōnā) and in Tamil (hereafter T:) as கொரோனா (Korōṉā) a language used by (inter-intra) ethnic Tamils, Muslims, (some) Malays, and (some) Burghers. I decided to use the term "Coronavirus" considering its everyday shape of usage. The country is currently experiencing the third week of the nationwide lockdown at the beginning of the fourth wave of the Coronavirus and severe economic strain fearing shortage of essential items.

Conceptual Background

People's daily life struggle against the threats posed by Coronavirus within an ethno-politically divided and socially stratified country where state welfare mechanism is shaped by party loyalty (see Höglund and Piyarathne, 2009) can be explained by using the phrase "constructing commongrounds" (Piyarathne, 2018). Concepts introduced by Pierre Bourdieu and Michael Jackson were used within the broader framework of anthropology of everyday life. Bourdieu refers to embodied dispositions that inform everyday practices while Michael Jackson talks about the existential and intersubjective lives of human beings. In his discussion of interaction between individuals in a society, Jackson values the "interplay of subject and object, ego and alter" as subject for ethnographic analysis (Jackson, 1998: 6). For Bourdieu, peoples' habitus is comprised of systems of perception and common values and assumptions, "which generate and organize practices and representations that can be objectively adapted to their outcomes without presupposing a conscious aiming at ends or an express mastery of the operations necessary to attain them" (Bourdieu, 1990: 53).

Using both these ideas, I understand commongrounds as inhabitants' continuous and creative efforts to live in and relate to each other in fields of common endeavour informed by embodied (conscious or unconscious) understandings of the social and material world.

The Gradual Spread of Coronavirus in Sri Lanka

In the month of January 2020, Sri Lankan health authorities took actions to screen passengers for symptoms at the Bandaranaike International Airport (BIA) considering the origin of the disease as "foreign" or "outside" the country. Sri Lanka also has a huge Chinese population who are involved in various capacities from labourer to highly technical staff in the Chinese-funded projects. Since Coronavirus originated in China initially, there has been panic among the Sri Lankans about the Chinese workers in Sri Lanka with the government and the Chinese authorities agreeing to confine Chinese workers to their own workplaces and lodgings to avoid possible discriminations against the Chinese in Sri Lanka. Proving the accuracy of the steps, the first confirmed case of Corona impacted person was a 44-year-old Chinese female tourist who came from Hubei province in China as reported by the National Institute of Infection Diseases. This was a novel experience for local doctors and politicians. By then there were a total of 194 Corona patients in the hospital out of which 148 were Sri Lankans and 56 were foreign nationals (Epidemiology Unit, 2020). The gradual increase of Corona cases in the country grew the demand for face masks which initiated the authorities to introduce a price control for masks by the country's drug regulatory agency via Pricing of Medical Devices Regulations, No. 1 of 2020 (The Gazette of the Democratic Socialist Republic of Sri Lanka, 2020).

In the meantime, Sri Lankan Airlines, the national carrier, was able to successfully evacuate 33 Sri Lankan students and families from Wuhan on 1 February 2020. They were kept under quarantine at a military facility in Diyatalawa. In the quarantine facilities, the intervention of the military and national career Sri Lankan airline to provide facilities within a short period was praised and highlighted. This incident boosted the heroic nationalistic and patriotic feelings among Sri Lankans (Sri Lankan Airlines, 2020; Daily FT, 2020c). This was the first popular experience the military intervened in controlling Coronavirus in Sri Lanka.

The Sri Lankan authorities were very cautious of the arrival of the European variant of Coronavirus while dealing with the Chinese variant. Sri Lankan officials made it mandatory for passengers arriving from European, the Middle East, and other Asian countries to be quarantined for 14 days. By 10 March 2020, there were 186 people placed under quarantine including 164 Sri Lankan nationals, 20 Italian nationals, and two South Korean nationals (Kohona, 2020). On 10th March, it was reported that the virus was first contracted by a 52-year-old Sri Lankan tour guide, guiding a group of Italians who were infected with the virus. Since then, the numbers of patients have increased, identified in various clusters related to mosques, fish markets, navy, and military camps and never named such clusters connected to high class or elites. Initially, the deaths were connected to those with long-term chronic diseases such as diabetes, high blood pressure, heart issues, and age factor. Eventually the Corona cases increased out of control, especially today in the starting of fourth wave of spreading.

The national data released by the Epidemiology Unit of the Ministry of Health Sri Lanka on the 10th of September 2021 lists 480,478 of the total number confirmed cases while the total number recovered cases were 409,628 while 10,995 deaths reported. The total number of confirmed and hospitalised or home-based cases was 59,855. Moreover, the number of citizens who took first dose of the vaccination were 13,264,806 while 10,211,537 received the second dose (Epidemiology Unit, 2021). When compared with the pre- and the post-Sinhala-Tamil New Year celebration between 13 and 17 in April, there has been a rapid increase after the festival, which has marked the beginning of the third wave of the Coronavirus infection spread in the country. This was considered as an outcome of the militarised approach of the political leadership, which crippled the independent health and other professional approach to deal with a pandemic, which can be considered as a barrier for modernising the society (see Höglund and Piyarathne, 2009).

Following the first reported case of Coronavirus, shortage of face masks followed by face masks being sold at over ten to 20 times the original price was noted. People also created their own face masks made of clean cloth initially, in the absence of various masks recommended by the health authorities.

Local Political Context of the COVID-19 Pandemic

In general, in South Asia, party politics and party-led regimes play a key role in shaping everyday social lives of the people. Citizens always expect politicians to play a key role in assuring the welfare and well-being of the people, which is connected to politics of patronage in general and state-based political patronage in particular (see Höglund and Piyarathne, 2009). This was very significant in the crisis period of Tsunami and presently in Corona. By the time Coronavirus started creating a fear psychosis in the minds of the people shattering their everyday lives, Sri Lanka was being governed by President Gotabaya Rajapaksa who won the 8th Presidential Election conducted on 16 November 2019. Gotabaya Rajapaksa had served as defence secretary in his brother Mahinda Rajapaksa's government. He came to power during the post-Easter period due to the disappointment that people had towards the "yahapalana" government (S: good governance), which had promised to protect the people (Chandrapema, 2020). There was a lot of appreciation from the locals for the successful control of the virus spread in the country. He used state officials, the military, and the police to implement health regulations. The parliamentary election was conducted on 5 August 2020 to elect members for the 16th Parliament in Sri Lanka, amidst viewpoints expressed in favour of and against the election. This election further assured people's support for the Sri Lanka People's Freedom Alliance (SLPFA), that is a left-wing nationalist political alliance formed in 2019 by the Sri Lanka Podujana Peramuna (SLPP), which contested under the lotus flower bud as the symbol. The election results have decided whether Sri Lanka is aligned towards the western democratic nations including India or China which gave over one billion dollar pandemic relief (Baumgart, 2020).

Disappointing the people's expectation of having a stronger intervention to control the spread of coronavirus in Sri Lanka, the government made changes in the key positions of the health ministry. Dr. Anil Jasinghe, who played a major role in the suppression of Coronavirus in Sri Lanka as the Director General of Health Services, was appointed as the Secretary to the Ministry of Environment. Dr. Jasinghe also held the position of vice chair of the Executive Board of the World Health Organization (WHO) for several months since 6 February 2020. There was a lot of discussion and arguments about this transfer. People tend to believe that state intervention under the president prior to the parliamentary election was better than the post-Parliamentary election period (Mendis, 2020).

Parallel to the transfer of Dr. Jasinghe, the Director of the Medical Research Institute (MRI) Dr. Jayaruwan Bandara was also transferred creating controversy in the country (Mendis, 2020). The debate on these transfers in the political arena seems to benefit both the ruling and the opposition parties, to continuously engage in party politics. For example, during the election, the opposition party members questioned the authenticity of the number of victims given by Jasinghe to influence the election results, while later they questioned the void created by his removal (Mendis, 2020). Moreover, another rumour is that his media portrayal as the "man of the match" saving lives from Coronavirus did not go down well among some interested parties (Perera, 2020). Anyway, the politicians show a trend of not tolerating popularity of the persons not connected to leading political families fearing that they would be a threat for the kith and kin of current political leaders who consider politics as a "way of life" (Piyarathne, 2008: 103).

Intervention of the State in Controlling Coronavirus

The new government (appointed in August 2020) took measures as the second and third wave of Coronavirus infections occurred after the election of the new parliament with increased suffering of the people and complex vaccine diplomacy. The Sri Lankan government adopted basically four lines of operations. They are: (1) military, police, and intelligence operations; (2) medical and health care; (3) psychological aspects; and (4) economic and community well-being (Amaratunga et al., 2020).

The state health authorities from the beginning followed strategies such as "social distancing", making it compulsory to wear masks and washing hands before entering public buildings, case detecting, contact tracing, spraying disinfectants intended to kill the virus, travel restrictions within and between districts, introduction of laws connected to passenger transport services, establishing roadblocks with military and police checkpoints to monitor people's travel, adherence to health policies and issuing health guidelines to various sectors, quarantining, lockdowns, identifying local curfew zones, travel restrictions, and isolation of villages. PCR and antigen tests were done in randomly selected places according to the requirements of the health officials and politicians. Conducting similar tests established inter-district and inter-province border crossing areas. Home quarantining under the supervision of Public Health Inspectors (PHIs) came to be implemented at a very late stage of the Coronavirus spread. Sri Lanka relied heavily on controlling human mobility as a main method of preventing the spread of Coronavirus in the country (Erandi et al., 2020: 1).

The government's approach always gave much prominence to the military officials rather than the civil health authorities under the Gotabaya

Rajapaksa's rule. There were lots of criticism against the militarisation of civil space hiding behind the Coronavirus through "contact tracing", "lock down", "monitoring of people wearing face masks and other guidelines", "imposing laws", and "intelligence reports" (also see Satkunanathan, 2021).

Furthermore, this shows a trend of "Sri Lanka's defence establishment emerging as the most powerful political actor" in the country according to Jayadeva Uyangoda, an internationally recognised local Political Scientist (quoted from Sheikh, 2021). The chief of the military and the police media spokesperson were the ones who always gave instructions to the public about the medical guidelines on having social lives, that is "social distance" maintenance, travelling, working and mask wearing. The National Operation Centre for Prevention of COVID-19 Outbreak [NOCPCO] is led by the Chief of Defence Staff and Commander of the Army. The police spokesperson always referred to various legal frameworks and acts, which would enable to punish people. Thus, some people followed health guidelines out of fear than from an enlightened mind-set.

While professional bodies such as the Government Medical Officers Association (GMOA) came forward from time to time pointing out weaknesses of the government's approach, that is need of taking right decisions on time and zonal lockdown (News1st, 2020b), serious commitment towards treating patients at home or at intermediary centres. This organisation in general and its current president Dr. Anuruddha Padeniya in particular was heavily involved in bringing the existing government into power by actively participating in election rallies as well as movements such as "Viyathmaga" (Professionals for a Better Future), a network of Sri Lankan scholars, academics, and professionals with an intrinsic passion for the country (Daily News, 2018; LNW, 2019).

Similarly, many associations such as the Federations of University Teachers Association (FUTA) did not actively involve themselves in using the knowledge they had to educate and guide people and the policy-makers to take a professional approach to address Coronavirus scientifically. However, The Public Health Inspectors Union has been very critical of the government's approach and they withdrew from offering their services several times regionally as a way of showing their displeasure towards certain measures taken by the government, that is, the health minister stating via a media briefing that the power of implementing health guidelines related to COVID-19 for election in 2020 will not be given to PHIs in order to avoid inconvenience to the public (Ranasinghe, 2020). Limitations in physical, human, and information sources, lack of consistency in government's decision-making, establishment of haphazard structures, and short-term orientation prioritising emergency relief were some shortcomings. Concerns raised regarding militarisation and human rights violations hint at the lack of preparedness for pandemics and the absence of a national framework to guide such preparedness in Sri Lanka' (Amaratunga et al., 2020).

Indigenous Solution: Promoting Superstitious and Mythological Practices Over Science

Local people used various traditional herbs and tactics to get support from supernatural forces such as goddess Kāli (West and Dodan Godage, 2021). The three Sri Lankan ministers of Health, Energy and Tourism were seen dropping gallons of holy water on the Lankan land (Manu, 2020) collected from the three holy rivers of the land. In almost every house, people used various boiled herbs, gargled with salt water, and drank hot water daily. Miraculously most of the people, who always visited private dispensaries (for fever, cough, and cold) run by medical officers as after-office private practice reduced their visits to the doctors as they did not have serious issues with drastic cut down in medical expenditure.

Two types of syrup "Dhammika paniya" (Dhammika syrup associated with Goddess Kāli) and Ritigala Devendra's Ravana Paniya (syrup associated with the ancient King Ravana) became popular with the former getting support of the ruling politicians of the government that came into power by arousing patriotic feelings and highlighting threats for the nation and the country (Policy Statement of Gotabaya Rajapaksa, 2020; France 24, 2019).

The national newspapers and other media covered how Dhammika syrup concoction was tried out by the Minister of Health, Pavithra Wanniarachchi, The speaker Mahinda Yapa Abeywardena, and the State Minister for Promotion of Indigenous Medicine, Sisira Jayakody by consuming spoons of honey at the Parliament premises (BBC, 2021; Daily News, 2021). Mr. Dhammika (a mason who apparently got this mysterious medical formula from Goddess Kāli) offered this syrup to the Temple of the Tooth Relic in Kandy and to the Jaya Sri Maha Bodhiya, which is a sapling of the Bōdhi Tree (tree of awakening), which shaded prince Siddhartha to attain enlightenment or to realise the way of ending rebirth or suffering.

Dhammika, who went into a trance at Anuradhapura, shouted at the chief incumbent, the most venerable Pallegama Siriniwasa Thero saying "I am Kāli. I am your mother . . . ", which can be interpreted as a way of showing his authority over the chief monk. Thousands of people gathered and queued along the road, which led to his house in Hettimulla, Kegalle, violating all the health guidelines and travel restrictions (The Guardian, 2021). The government deployed police officials and in one of the media footages, military soldiers were also seen standing in the queue to get the Dhammika syrup. This syrup was advertised even in eBay at the price of US$250 introducing it as a locally developed Corona vaccination. His popularity came down when the Minister of Health tested positive for Coronavirus and survived after undergoing a lot of treatment in the ICU at the IDH hospital. Not only she but a few other ministers who consumed the Dhammika paniya also got infected (The Guardian, 2021; BBC, 2021). Also introduction of foreign-developed vaccines made the syrup not politically marketable anymore.

The third local syrup called "Sudarshana Paniya" was introduced by Sri Jayewardenepura University (USJ) and the University Business Linkage Cell (UBL), as an Ayurvedic medicine to improve the health and well-being of Sri Lankans (Daily FT, 2020b). The university recommended it for all types of fevers and cold. Prof. Channa Jayasumana, the State Minister for Production, Supply and Regulation of Pharmaceuticals, addressing the event organised to launch the product said that a similar drug has been approved for treating COVID-19 patients in Thailand (Daily FT, 2021).

Groups Affected: Vulnerable Communities Sandwiched by Unethical Socio-economic Forces

Initially, restaurants, bars, wine stores, night clubs, spas, casinos, and salons were closed until further notice. People in manufacturing, agriculture, and service sectors were affected with infection spreading from various special entities such as garment factories, fish markets, and navy camps with majority of the workers in the garment factories coming from low-income backgrounds. There are more than one million workers out of which 8.6 million of economically active population in Sri Lanka are serving in nearly 350 apparel manufacturing establishments which were seriously affected by the pandemic (Kodippili et al., 2020; Hewamanna, 2021; The New Indian Express, 2020).

The second wave of Coronavirus emerged mainly in garment factories in Minuwangoda, in the western province in Sri Lanka with the factories losing income sources by cancellation of export orders and workers forced to resign or work with reduced salaries (Kodippili et al., 2020).

A narrative shared with the author by Nalin,[2] whose wife working in the garment factory in Kalutara tested positive for the virus and was quarantined emphasises the struggle of families during the pandemic. Nalin had been responsible for looking after his aged in-laws. When Nalin's wife went into quarantine, the father-in-law was in a very bad health condition caused by a heart ailment and was continuously confined to his bed. When the PCR tests conducted on Nalin and his children became positive, he requested his wife's brother to come home and look after his father until Nalin or his wife returned home (Nalin's entire family was at a quarantine facility provided by the factory). However, disinterest from the family members compelled Nalin to send his father-in-law to a hospital according to the instructions given by the PHI where he died. Nalin believes that attention by hospital staff could not have equalised with the care they gave at home. The dead body was kept in a parlour, which was an unusual way of conducting final rites to a person in a village context, assuming that there would not be anyone even to carry the coffin to the village burial ground located just 200 metres away from his home.

Those engaged in self-help employment and the employees in sectors other than the government sector, that is local lunch packet sellers, wholesale and retail trade, tourism, transportation of goods and services, were heavily affected by the pandemic. According to the Sri Lanka Labour Force Survey 2019, 4,698,187 (57.4%) of working people were engaged in the informal sector (Department of Census and Statistics, 2019). Out of the total workers, 2,854,997 (46.7%) were non-agricultural, low skilled workers engaged in elementary occupations such as craft and related trade work, and plant and machine operations and as assemblers (also see Arunatillake, 2020). There are over 1.2 million registered three wheelers out of which 800,000 three wheelers are engaged in the profession and around three million family members live on that income (Economynext, 2020a). According to de Silva and Arunatillake (2019), the three-wheel taxi drivers who usually earned an average of 2,000–3,000 Sri Lankan Rupees per day were not able to earn at all due to the curfews imposed with the number of passengers travelling in them being very low in non-curfew times too.

During the lockdown period, the government gave a six-month moratorium on leasing loan instalments for all three-wheel owners on 23 March 2020 (Ada Derana, 2020; ColomboPage, 2020a). However, the three-wheel taxi owners lamented that they did not get this facility. It was during this period that news bulletins showed the fatal assault of Sunil Jayawardena, the Chairman of the Self-Employed Professionals' Three-Wheeler Association who was murdered after a heated argument he had with one of the staff members of the leasing company when he visited a leasing company (Economynext, 2020b; News1st, 2020a).

The government relaxed the regulations applicable to people such as farmers who are engaged in paddy, chena (slash and burn cultivation), or any form of agriculture-related work including the Indian origin plantation Tamil tea-plucking community who serve in estates in the hill country and the rubber tappers in the lowlands. This move was supported by the plantation Tamil community in Sri Lanka who earn about US$3–6[3] per day (Hapuarachchi, 2021).

Effects on the Muslims: Ethno-religious Nationalism in Global Pandemic

Even when Coronavirus was very active, the continuous maintenance of ethno-national divisions was witnessed, which always worked, as voting machines to win elections for political parties in Sri Lanka (Piyarathne, 2018: 65). The discussion with reference to Muslims was observed in key areas such as (1) contribution of the spread of the virus deliberately by not maintaining or following health guidelines, (2) not collaborating with the health officials and medical staff, and (3) not following the commonly accepted cremation as shown in the media (Farzan, 2020b; Tennakoon, 2020; Shehadi, 2020; Silva, 2020). In March 2020, the government authorities imposed regulations making cremation of all the Coronavirus-infected dead bodies to be compulsory. This was challenged by the Muslims of the country who demanded that the government lift this regulation as it was against the Islamic faith. Since then, the debate of burying dead bodies, which may cause contamination of the ground water, and other reasons have continued (Jabbar, 2020). Prime Minister Mahinda Rajapaksa announced that the government would take steps to lift this barrier allowing burial just before the Pakistan Prime Minister Imran Khan visited the country with the latter's tweets welcoming the Sri Lankan government's decision (Aljazeera, 2020).

However, when Organisation of Islamic Cooperation (OIC) raised the forced cremation policy at the Human Rights Council in Geneva in February 2021, Michelle Bachelet, the Chairperson of the Office of the High Commissioner for Human Rights (OHCHR), said in her statement, "The policy of forced cremation of COVID-19 victims has caused pain and distress to the minority Muslim and Christian communities" (Aljazeera, 2020). The government regulation was seen as an anti-Muslim cremation order with people protesting on the streets, filing cases in courts, and multiple religious and world leaders issuing various statements. When a 20-day-old baby was forcefully cremated by the health authorities, protests spread around the country. People who protested against this act tied strips of white cloth on the fence of the crematorium in Borella (Human Rights Watch, 2021).

At one point, the Sri Lankan government also explored the possibility of burying dead bodies of the Muslims in the neighbouring country of Maldives and several internal locations which were far away from the victim's hometown. Commenting on this step, Ahmed Shaheed, the UN special rapporteur on freedom of religion or belief, stated that the plan "could end up enabling the further marginalisation of Muslim communities in Sri Lanka" (Human Rights Watch, 2021). Summarising the sentiments of all the Muslims in the country Ali Zahir Moulana, a former parliamentarian of the Muslim community had told, "we want to be buried on our own soil" (Human Rights Watch, 2021). Analysis of media reporting of some of the popular Sinhala medium television channels proved the attempts of inciting ethnonational feelings against the Muslim community in Sri Lanka (Silva, 2020; Tennakoon, 2020). This attempt worked to some extent as people are still worried about the well-coordinated three suicide bomb attacks launched by members of extremists' groups on 21 April in 2019 which killed over 260 Sinhala and Tamil Christians who were taking part on Easter services in three churches (Imitiyaz, 2020).

Cash to the Needy: Politics of a Welfare State

In March 2020, the Sri Lankan government announced a package of welfare payment, 5,000 Sri Lanka rupees, as a single payment for low-income families. All senior citizens (559,109), disabled persons (119,300), farmers (160,675) registered under the Farmers Insurance Scheme, kidney patients (39,170), and Samurdhi recipients (2,398,994) benefitted (ColomboPage, 2020b). The government made this payment for at least two months in

2020 and in the month of April in 2021 with cabinet approval being sought for the payment in the month of May 2021 (News.Lk, 2021).

Though this was only a small payment, it helped to prevent people suffering from extreme hunger. However, there are allegations of corruption, various malpractices, and political manipulations (Transparency International, 2020) within the context of state administration shaped by the patronage-based political culture, which functions through political parties (Höglund and Piyarathne, 2009: 288).

In the year 2020, the National Election Commission (an independent body) wanted to remove the local politicians from the allowance distribution programme (Farzan, 2020a). The government in 2020 adjourned the Rs. 5,000 allowance for the month of June that year giving consideration to a letter sent by the Election Commission (EC) regarding its impact on voters due to the forthcoming Parliamentary elections (Daily FT, 2020a).

Surviving Democracy Amidst the Pandemic

There were lot of discussions insinuating the role of the above-mentioned welfare package on the election results (elections were held on 5 August 2020) contributing to the victory of the ruling Sri Lanka People's Freedom Alliance (SLPFA). This was a novel experience for the people and the election officials who worked under the leadership of an independent election commission in Sri Lanka, which developed health guidelines, trained officials and voters, planned a counting mechanism, and ran mock election centres. The voters were requested to bring their own ballpoint pens, wear face masks, use hand sanitisers, wash hands when entering and leaving polling stations, and keep adequate physical distance. However, by the time this chapter is finalised, the ruling government is accused of using coronavirus as an opportunity to favour the business community associated with the ruling party via importations of medical supplies and quarantining business and suppressing democratic rights of the people, that is using quarantine laws to suppress freedom to dissent and protests, arresting teachers and other trade union activists protested for their rights, adopting laws of emergency regulations to give police powers to the military posing serious threat for the normal function of the civil society (Economynext, 2021).

Vaccination: International Power Battles at Play

In the recent past, Sri Lanka has become a battle ground for the political economies of China, India, and the United States. While India is allowed to operate commercial flights in Mattala airport, the Hambantota harbour located in close proximity of the Mattala Airport, built using a loan given by China, is given to China to manage on a 99-year lease. For the people, it appeared that India was imposing certain conditions to issue doses of Oxford AstraZeneca vaccine produced by Serum Institute India. Initially

India gifted 500,000 doses of Oxford AstraZeneca vaccines to Sri Lanka (The Hindu, 2021a), which kicked off its vaccination programme in late January 2021. Sri Lanka also was to buy six million more Sputnik V (The Hindu, 2021b). However, post-March, people who received their first dose were nervous as the time to get injected with the second dose was almost past as Serum Institute officially notified the Sri Lankan authorities on its inability to provide additionally ordered doses of the vaccination due to the high demand for vaccinations in India.

One of my colleagues from Jaffna said that people in Wellawatta, Colombo, rushed to get the AstraZeneca vaccine showing higher interest in it before the government made it compulsory for people to take the Chinese Sinopharm vaccine. This sentiment is uniform across communities. The recently received 600,000 doses of China's Sinopharm vaccine, which was used initially for the vaccination of Chinese workers living in the island nation (The Hindu, 2021c), is now being given to locals as well.

The complexities involved in vaccination highlight the need for WHO's monitoring especially when SAARC's role is diminishing. In the meantime, there are discussions that Sri Lanka is going to get six million Russian produced Sputnik V vaccines, raising the total it plans to purchase from Russia to 13 million doses (The Hindu, 2021a).

The third wave (May 2021) witnessed acute politicisation of the vaccination process with competition among the elites and professional groups for vaccines. Sri Lanka's move towards Russian SputniK V and Chinese Sinopharm vaccines and the idea of setting up a factory to produce Chinese Sinovac vaccine became a much discussed issue. From receiving the first batch of COVID-19 vaccines from the COVAX facility to the World Bank promising to give Sri Lanka 80.5 million US dollars to buy vaccines in a programme that has already provided 298 million US dollars to the country to fight the Coronavirus pandemic created hope. India sending oxygen while China supplying the highest number of COVID-9 vaccinations to Sri Lanka can be considered as symbolically balancing Asian powers in pandemic led global political economy.

Conclusion

It seems that Sri Lanka has increased its understanding of Coronavirus. They think of the possibility of shaping their everyday lives amidst the spread of the virus in the country. One has to also negotiate ethnonationalist political forces and international geopolitics. While the welfare state operates with the government trying to protect people, it seems to have divided and maintained the ethnoreligious divisions for use in elections. The geopolitical and economic competition among powerful nations such as India, China, and the United States on Sri Lankan grounds also has put citizens of the country in a more vulnerable position. Vaccine diplomacy and vaccines are being used to create corridors of geopolitical influence with limited options available for a developing country like Sri Lanka. The concerted efforts of citizens in a multi-religious and multi-ethnic society like Sri Lanka has the capacity to construct a social space in which existential needs can be met which I call constructing "commongrounds".

Notes

1 Name changed.
2 Name changed
3 According to the Indicative US Dollar SPOT Exchange Rate issued by the Central Bank of Sri Lanka for 10–12 May 2021, selling price of US$1 is Sri Lankan rupee 202.2820.

References

Ada Derana (2020), "President announces several relief measures due to Covid-19 outbreak", *Ada Derana.lk*, 23 March, www.adaderana.lk/news_intensedebate.php?nid=61738, accessed 15 May 2021.
Aljazeera (2020), "Sri Lanka finally lifts ban on burial of COVID victims", 26 February. www.aljazeera.com/news/2021/2/26/sri-lanka-finally-lifts-ban-on-burial-of-covid-victims, accessed 15 May 2021.
Amaratunga, D., Fernando, N., Haigh, R. and Jayasinghe, N. (2020), "The COVID-19 outbreak in Sri Lanka: A synoptic analysis focusing on trends, impacts, risks and science-policy interaction processes", *Progress in Disaster Science*, 8, https://doi.org/10.1016/j.pdisas.2020.100133, accessed 10 May 2021, 14 May 2021.
Arunatillake, N. (2020), "Easter attacks in 2019 vs. COVID-19 outbreak of 2020: What lies ahead for Sri Lanka?" *Talking Economics*, the blog of the Institute of Policy Studies of Sri Lanka (IPS), Sri Lanka's apex socio-economic policy think tank, 3 April, www.ips.lk/talkingeconomics/2020/04/03/easter-attacks-in-2019-vs-covid-19-outbreak-of- 2020-what-lies-ahead-for-sri-lanka/, accessed 14 May 2021.
Baumgart, P. (2020), "Sri Lanka's parliamentary elections will shape its political future – likely for the worse", *Atlantic Council*, 30 July.
BBC (2021), "Sri Lanka minister who promoted 'covid syrup' tests positive", 23 January, www.bbc.com/news/world-asia-55780425, accessed 15 May 2021.
Bourdieu, P. (1990), *The Logic of Practice*, Cambridge: Polity.
Chandrapema, C. A. (2020), "Why the Yahapalana project failed", *Island, Online*, 16 August.
ColmboPage (2020a), "President announces several relief measures due to Covid-19 outbreak effective from today", 24 March, www.colombopage.com/archive_20A/Mar24_1584988408CH.php, accessed 14 April 2021.
ColmboPage (2020b), "Sri Lanka government grants more concessions to public affected by COVID-19 pandemic", 31 March, www.colombopage.com/archive_20A/Mar31_1585667258CH.php, accessed 20 April 2021.
Daily FT (2020a), "Govt. Suspends Rs. 5,000 allowance payment for June", 22 May, www.ft.lk/front-page/Govt-suspends-Rs-5-000-allowance-payment-for-June/44-700570, accessed 25 April 2021.

Daily FT (2021), " 'Sudarshana Paniya' released to market as treatment for all types of fevers, common cold", 2 April, www.ft.lk/news/Sudarshana-Paniya-released-to-market-as-treatment-for-all-types-of-fevers-common-cold/56–715742, accessed 14 May 2021.
Daily FT (2020c), "Chartered from Wuhan and quarantined at Diyatalawa: A Sri Lankan story on coronavirus", 18 February, www.ft.lk/news/Chartered-from-Wuhan-and-quarantined-at-Diyatalawa-A-Sri-Lankan-story-on-coronavirus/56–695847, accessed 14 May 2021.
Daily News (2018), "Hidden political agendas behind crippling medical and transport strikes", 20 August, www.dailynews.lk/2018/08/20/local/160170/hidden-political-agendas-behind-crippling-medical-and-transport-strikes, accessed 13 May 2021.
Daily News (2020), "Speaker, MPs try herbal syrup concoction", 11 December, www.dailynews.lk/2020/12/11/local/235803/speaker-mps-try-herbal-syrup-concoction, accessed 15 May 2021.
De Silva, T. and Arunatillake, N. (2019), "Allowing youth to tuk-tuk or not tuk-tuk: Should access to three wheeler market in Sri Lanka be regulated?" The blog of the Institute of Policy Studies of Sri Lanka (IPS), Sri Lanka's apex socio-economic policy think tank, 30 January, www.ips.lk/talkingeconomics/2019/01/30/allowing-youth-to-tuk-tuk-or-not-tuk-tuk-should-access-to-three-wheeler-market-in-sri-lanka-be-regulated/, accessed 15 May 2021.
Department of Census and Statistics (2019), "Sri Lanka labour force survey-annual report – 2019", www.statistics.gov.lk/LabourForce/StaticalInformation/AnnualReports/2019, accessed 20 April 2021.
Economynext (2020a), "Truck drivers demand regulatory body, accuse minister of buying time", 17 January, https://economynext.com/tuk-drivers-demand-regulatory-body-accuse-minister-of-buying-time-45013/, accessed 20 April 2021.
Economynext (2020b), "Leasing mafia blamed for alleged beating to death of three-wheeler trade union leader Jayawardena", 11 June, https://economynext.com/leasing-mafia-blamed-for-alleged-beating-to-death-of-three-wheeler-trade-union-leader-jayawardena-70975/, accessed 14 May 2021.
Economynext (2020c), "Sri Lanka locks down navy camp, villages after sailor coronavirus cluster balloons amid testing gap", 24 April, https://economynext.com/sri-lanka-locks-down-navy-camp-villages-after-sailor-coronavirus-cluster-balloons-amid-testing-gap-68002/, accessed 14 May 2021.
Economynext (2021), "Sri Lanka parliament passes emergency regulations to seize food stocks", *Warehouses*, 6 September, https://economynext.com/sri-lanka-parliament-passes-emergency-regulations-to-seize-food-stocks-warehouses-85840/, accessed 11 September 2021.
Epidemiology Unit (2020), *Coronavirus disease 2019 (COVID-19) – Situation Report – 19.02.2020–10.00am*, Colombo: Ministry of Health & Indigenous Medical Services. www.epid.gov.lk/web/images/pdf/corona_virus_report/sitrep-sl-en-19-02_10.pdf, accessed 13 May 2021.
Epidemiology Unit (2021), *Coronavirus Disease 2019 (COVID-19) – Situation Report – 15.06.2021–10.00am*, Colombo: Ministry of Health & Indigenous Medical Services, www.epid.gov.lk/web/images/pdf/corona_virus_report/sitrep-sl-en-15-06_10_21.pdf, accessed 16 June 2021.
Erandi, K. K. W. H. A. C., Mahasinghe, S. S. N. and Perera, S. Jayasinghe (2020), "Effectiveness of the strategies implemented in Sri Lanka for controlling the

COVID-19 outbreak", *Journal of Applied Mathematics*, 1–10. https://doi.org/10.1155/2020/2954519, accessed 20 April 2021.

Farzan, Z. (2020a), "National elections commission wants local politicos removed from allowance program", *News First*, 20 May, www.newsfirst.lk/2020/05/20/national-elections-commission-wants-local-politicos-removed-from-allowance-program/, accessed 23 April 2021.

Farzan, Z. (2020b), "COVID-19 patient who spat on PHI's face, arrested and remanded", *News First*, 4 December, www.newsfirst.lk/2020/12/04/covid-19-pa tient-who-spat-on-phis-face-arrested-and-remanded/, accessed 6 June 2021.

France 24 (2019), "Sri Lanka's Gotabaya Rajapaksa sworn in as new president", 18 November. www.france24.com/en/20191118-sri-lanka-s-gotabaya-rajapaksa-sworn-in-as-new-president, accessed 15 May 2021.

Hapuarachchi, C. (2021), "Plantation workers demand hike in daily wage", *News 1st*, 31 January, www.newsfirst.lk/2021/01/31/plantation-workers-demand-hike-in-daily-wage/, accessed 15 May 2021.

Hewamanna, S. (2021), "Pandemic, lockdown and modern slavery among Sri Lanka's global assembly line workers", *Journal of International Women's Studies*, 22(1), 54–69. https://vc.bridgew.edu/jiws/vol22/iss1/3/, accessed 15 May 2021.

The Hindu (2021a), "Sri Lanka receives 500,000 doses of COVID-19 vaccines from India", 25 February, www.thehindu.com/news/international/sri-lanka-receives-500000-doses-of-covid-19-vaccines-from-india/article33933291.ece, accessed 15 May 2021.

The Hindu (2021b), "Sri Lanka to buy 6 million more Sputnik V vaccines", 6 April, www.thehindu.com/news/international/sri-lanka-to-buy-6-million-more-sputnik-v-vaccines/article34253931.ece, accessed 1 May 2021.

The Hindu (2021c), "Sri Lanka receives 600,000 doses of China's Sinopharm vaccine: Official", 31 March, www.thehindu.com/news/international/sri-lanka-receives-600000-doses-of-chinas-sinopharm-vaccine-official/article34207607.ece, accessed 15 May 2021.

Höglund, K. and Piyarathne, A. (2009), "Paying the price for patronage: Electoral violence in Sri Lanka", *Commonwealth & Comparative Politics*, 47(3), 287–307.

Human Rights Watch (2021), "Sri Lanka: Covid-19 forced cremation of Muslims discriminatory", 18 January, www.hrw.org/news/2021/01/18/sri-lanka-covid-19-forced-cremation-muslims-discriminatory, accessed 15 May 2021.

Imitiyaz, A. R. M. (2020), "The Easter Sunday bombings and the crisis facing Sri Lanka's Muslims", *Journal of Asian and African Studies*, 55(1), 3–16. https://journals.sagepub.com/doi/pdf/10.1177/0021909619868244, accessed 15 May 2021.

Jackson, Michael (1998), *Minima Ethnographica: Intersubjectivity and the Anthropological Project*, Chicago: University of Chicago Press.

Jowsi Abdul Jabbar, J. A. (2020), "Groundwater contamination due to burial of Covid-19 dead bodies", *Colombo Telegraph*, 11 April. www.colombotelegraph.com/index.php/groundwater-contamination-due-to-burial-of-covid-19-dead-bodies/, accessed 15 May 2021.

Kodippili, A. P. S., Premaratne, S. P. and Maurice, D. (2020), "Impact of COVID 19 on garment sector workers in Sri Lanka", Paper presented at the Annual Research Symposium on COVID-19 Pandemic: Development Challenges and Opportunities 2020, Faculty of Graduate Studies, University of Colombo, December 15.

Kohona, P. (2020), "Sri Lanka has been successful in countering COVID-19", *IDN-InDepthNews*, Online, 6 May, www.indepthnews.net/index.php/

opinion/3518-sri-lanka-has-been-successful-in-countering-covid-19, accessed 6 June 2021.

LNW: Lanka News Web.Net (2019), "GMOA Padeniya seen on Gota's stage breaking election laws?" 26 October, www.lankanewsweb.net/67-general-news/50586-GMOA-Padeniya-seen-on-Gota%E2%80%99s-Stage-breaking-Election-Laws, accessed 15 May 2021.

Manu, D. (2020), "Has govt's strategy to dam COVID spread gone to pot?" *The Sunday Times*, Online, 8 November, www.sundaytimes.lk/201108/columns/has-govts-strategy-to-dam-covid-spread-gone-to-pot-421850.html, accessed 15 May 2021.

Mendis, I. P. C. (2020), "The recall of Dr. Anil Jasinghe", *The Island*, Online, 24 November, https://island.lk/the-recall-of-dr-anil-jasinghe/, accessed 6 June 2021.

News.lk (2021), "7.4 million to receive Rs. 5000 Allowance in April – Min", *Bandula Gunawardena*, 20 April, www.news.lk/news/political-current-affairs/item/30133-7-4-million-to-receive-rs-5000-allowance-in-april-min-bandula-gunawardhena, accessed 20 April 2021.

News1st (2020a), "Trade union leader beaten to death", 11 June, www.newsfirst.lk/2020/06/11/trade-union-leader-beaten-to-death/, accessed 14 May 2021.

News1st (2020b), "GMOA says Colombo at risk due to COVID-19", 19 March, www.newsfirst.lk/2020/03/19/gmoa-says-colombo-at-risk-due-to-covid-19/, accessed 15 May 2021.

Perera, S. (2020), "Jasinghe's sudden exit as DGHS raises eyebrows: No word on successor yet", *Island*, Online, 23 August, https://island.lk/jasinghes-sudden-exit-as-dghs-raises-eyebrows-no-word-on-successor-yet/, accessed 13 May 2021.

Piyarathne, Anton (2008), "Have politicians succeeded in earning respect among the youth in Sri Lanka? Problems and dynamics", *Vistas: Journal of Humanities and Social Sciences, 2008*, 87–107.

Piyarathne, Anton (2018), *Constructing Commongrounds: Everyday Lifeworlds Beyond Politicized Ethnicities in Sri Lanka*, Nugegoda: Sarasavi Publishers.

Policy Statement of Gotabaya Rajapaksa (2020), "The policy statement made by his excellency Gotabaya Rajapaksa, president of the democratic socialist republic of Sri Lanka at the inauguration of the fourth session of the 8th parliament of Sri Lanka", 6 January, www.parliament.lk/news-en/view/1820, accessed 15 May 2021.

Ranasinghe, M. (2020), "Sri Lanka's public health inspectors withdraw from pandemic work", *Economynext*, 17 July, https://economynext.com/sri-lankas-public-health-inspectors-withdraw-from-pandemic-work-72097/, accessed 20 April 2021.

Satkunanathan, A. (2021), "Securitisation and militarisation in Sri Lanka: A continuum", *Daily FT*, Online, 20 January, www.ft.lk/columns/Securitisation-and-militarisation-in-Sri-Lanka-A-continuum/4-711827, accessed 13 May 2021.

Shehadi, L. (2020), "Coronavirus: Muslims in Sri Lanka forced to cremate dead, stigmatized under lockdown", *Al Arabiya English*, 20 April, https://english.alarabiya.net/coronavirus/2020/04/20/Coronavirus-Muslims-in-Sri-Lanka-forced-to-cremate-dead-stigmatized-under-lockdown, accessed 15 May 2021.

Sheikh, S. R. (2021), "Rajapaksas marching Sri Lanka towards military rule", *Asia Times*, 21 January, https://asiatimes.com/2021/01/rajapaksas-marching-sri-lanka-towards-military-rule/, accessed 14 May 2021.

Silva, K. T. (2020), *Identity, Infection and Fear: A Preliminary Analysis of Covid-19 Drivers and Responses in Sri Lanka*, Colombo: International Centre for Ethnic Studies.

Tennakoon, T. (2020), "Implications of COVID-19 on ethno-religious tensions in Sri Lanka. Official blog of the Berkeley Centre for religion, peace and world affairs", 26 May, https://berkleycenter.georgetown.edu/posts/implications-of-covid-19-on-ethno-religious-tensions-in-sri-lanka, accessed 15 May 2021.

The Gazette of the Democratic Socialist Republic of Sri Lanka (2020), No. 2160/28, Wednesday, January 29, 2020. https://nmra.gov.lk/images/PDF/gazzet/MRP-for-medical-devicesFace-masksEN.pdf, accessed 20 April 2021.

The Guardian (2021), "Sri Lankan holy man's 'miracle' potion for Covid turns sour", 19 January, www.theguardian.com/world/2021/jan/19/sri-lankan-holy-mans-miracle-potion-for-covid-turns-sour, accessed 20 April 2021.

The New Indian Express (2020), "Over 300 garment factory workers contract COVID-19 in Sri Lanka, Total Cases Cross 3,700", 6 October 2020, www.newindianexpress.com/world/2020/oct/06/over-300-garment-factory-workers-contract-covid-19-in-sri-lanka-total-cases-cross-3700–2206556.html, accessed 6 June 2021.

Transparency International (2020), "Ensuring Covid-19 relief reaches Sri Lanka's people", 10 December, www.transparency.org/en/blog/ensuring-covid-19-relief-reaches-sri-lankas-people, accessed 6 June 2021.

West, C. and Dodan Godage, K. (2021), "Miracle cure for COVID-19 in Sri Lanka: Kali and the politics behind 'Dhammika Paniya'. The official blog of the Asia Research Institute, National University of Singapore (NUS)", 3 March, https://ari.nus.edu.sg/20331-77/, accessed 6 June 2021.

Glossary

Homovivah Same-Sex Marriage
Pardah Veil
Sadharan Chutti General Holiday
Taqdeer Predestination/Destiny

Index

For Product Safety Concerns and Information please contact our EU representative GPSR@taylorandfrancis.com
Taylor & Francis Verlag GmbH, Kaufingerstraße 24, 80331 München, Germany

www.ingramcontent.com/pod-product-compliance
Ingram Content Group UK Ltd.
Pitfield, Milton Keynes, MK11 3LW, UK
UKHW021308260926
475702UK00048B/915
* 9 7 8 1 0 3 2 2 0 6 6 4 6 *